MANAGEMENT OF COMPLICATIONS IN GYNECOLOGIC ONCOLOGY

MANAGEMENT OF COMPLICATIONS IN GYNECOLOGIC ONCOLOGY

Edited by

Gregorio Delgado, M.D.
Associate Professor
Department of Obstetrics and Gynecology
Georgetown University
Chief, Division of Gynecologic Oncology
Lombardi Cancer Center
Washington, D.C.

Julian P. Smith, M.D.
Professor of Gynecology and Obstetrics
Wayne State University School of Medicine
Director, Division of Gynecologic Oncology
Hutzel Hospital
Detroit, Michigan

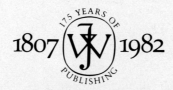

175 YEARS OF PUBLISHING

1807 · 1982

A WILEY MEDICAL PUBLICATION
John Wiley & Sons
New York · Chichester · Brisbane · Toronto · Singapore

Library of Congress Cataloging in Publication Data

Main entry under title:
Management of complications in gynecologic
    oncology.

   (A Wiley medical publication)
   Includes index.

   1. Generative organs, Female—Cancer—Complica-
tions and sequelae—Treatment.   2. Generative organs,
Female—Cancer—Surgery—Complications and sequelae
—Treatment.   I. Delgado, Gregorio, 1941-
II. Smith, Julian P.   III. Series. [DNLM:
1. Genital neoplasms, Female—Complications.
2. Genital neoplasms, Female—Therapy, WP 145
M266]

RC280.G5M36   616.99′46506   81-16135
ISBN 0-471-05993-5   AACR2

Printed in the United States of America

10 9 8 7 6 5 4 3 2 1

To our wives, Mary and Eleanor

Contributors

Neil Angerman, Ph.D., M.D.
Resident in Gynecologic Surgery
Mayo Graduate School of Medicine
Rochester, Minnesota

Richard C. Boronow, M.D.
Clinical Professor
Department of Gynecologic Oncology
University of Mississippi Medical
    Center
Jackson, Mississippi

Gregorio Delgado, M.D.
Associate Professor
Department of Obstetrics and
    Gynecology
Georgetown University
Chief, Division of Gynecologic
    Oncology
Lombardi Cancer Center
Washington, D.C.

Joseph Giordano, M.D.
Associate Professor
Department of Surgery
Director of Vascular Laboratory
George Washington University
    School of Medicine
Washington, D.C.

Mario N. Gomes, M.D.
Associate Professor
Department of Surgery
Georgetown University School of
    Medicine
Washington, D.C.

Jeane P. Hester, M.D.
Associate Professor of Medicine
Associate Internist
Chief, Supportive Therapy
M. D. Anderson Hospital and
    Tumor Institute
Texas Medical Center
Houston, Texas

Richard W. Holt, M.D.
Department of Surgery
Division of Surgical Oncology
Georgetown University School of
    Medicine
Washington, D.C.

Herbert L. Kotz, M.D.
Clinical Professor
Departments of Obstetrics and
    Gynecology and Gynecologic
    Oncology
George Washington University
    School of Medicine
Georgetown University School of
    Medicine
Washington, D.C.

Shashikant B. Lele, M.D.
Senior Cancer Research Surgeon
Roswell Park Memorial Institute
Buffalo, New York

William Maxted, M.D.
Director, Division of Urology
Georgetown University School of
    Medicine
Washington, D.C.

M. Steven Piver, M.D.
Clinical Professor
Associate Chief, Gynecology
Roswell Park Memorial Institute
New York State Department of
    Health
Buffalo, New York

Karl C. Podratz, Ph.D., M.D.
Assistant Professor
Department of Obstetrics and
    Gynecology
Mayo Medical School
Rochester, Minnesota

Peter E. Schwartz, M.D.
Associate Professor
Department of Obstetrics and
    Gynecology
Yale University School of Medicine
New Haven, Connecticut

Julian P. Smith, M.D.
Professor
Department of Gynecology and Obstetrics
Director, Division of Gynecologic
    Oncology
Hutzel Hospital
Detroit, Michigan

C. Robert Stanhope, M.D.
Associate Professor
Department of Obstetrics and
    Gynecology
Wayne State University School
    of Medicine
Assistant Director, Gynecologic
    Oncology
Hutzel Hospital
Detroit, Michigan

Richard E. Symmonds, M.D.
Professor
Department of Obstetrics and
    Gynecology
Mayo Medical School
Chairman, Division of Gynecologic
    Surgery
Mayo Clinic and Mayo Foundation
Rochester, Minnesota

Maurice J. Webb, M.D.
Associate Professor
Department of Obstetrics
    and Gynecology
Division of Gynecologic Surgery
Mayo Clinic and Mayo Foundation
Rochester, Minnesota

Preface

Management of Complications in Gynecologic Oncology will satisfy a definite need in the field of gynecologic oncology. There are several textbooks on the management of complications in surgery, urology, and plastic surgery, but no text deals explicitly with complications related to the management of gynecologic malignancies. This lack became evident when time arrived for the authors to prepare for their specialty boards. Several different books had to be consulted: texts in urology, surgery, plastic surgery, radiotherapy, chemotherapy, and several other fields. The gynecologic approach was not available in a comprehensive publication.

This book does not pretend to be an atlas of surgery but, rather, a rational approach to preventing and managing complications. The emphasis is on management of complications that arise from multidisciplinary therapy for female cancer: surgery, radiation therapy, and chemotherapy. Part 1 of this text explains proper techniques in exploratory laparotomy. Part 2 discusses surgical complications and Part 3, medical complications. The content on surgical complications has been subdivided into separate chapters on radiated and nonradiated tissues because radiation therapy requires a unique approach to each surgical procedure. Part 3 on medical complications covers the most frequent complications in gynecologic oncology: those related to chemotherapy and to hyperalimentation, thromboembolic disease, and infections.

There are several books on standard gynecologic operations such as radical vulvectomies, radical hysterectomies, and pelvic exenteration, but they do not include the prevention and management of complications when radiation has been part of the treatment.

Gynecologic oncologists are pelvic surgeons who must deal with diseases and disorders of the female organs, the gastrointestinal system, and the urological tract in addition to problems caused by previous surgery, radiation therapy, and/or chemotherapy. Since no one person can be thoroughly familiar with all aspects of our growing specialty and, in particular, the prevention and management of complications, authorities on various aspects of gynecologic cancer have combined their knowledge and skills to produce this book. The authors have worked with expert medical illustrators to provide a good understanding of the problems encountered by the gynecologic pelvic surgeon.

It is hoped that this book will be used not only by obstetrics and gynecology residents and fellows but also by experienced gynecologic oncologists in pelvic surgery, radiation therapy, and chemotherapy for the treatment of pelvic malignancies. Every gynecologic oncologist is called upon to treat the types of complications described in this book and so must be competent in assessing the modalities of their management. Finally, it is the purpose of this book to provide a foundation for innovations in the care of female cancer patients.

Gregorio Delgado
Julian P. Smith

Acknowledgments

The editors of this book acknowledge with profound gratitude the cooperation and collaboration of the original corps of authors who made this book possible. We would also like to thank the contributing artists for the consistently high quality of their work. The administrative problem of handling several manuscripts by several authors was efficiently managed by the editors' administrators, Ellen King, R.N., and Jane M. Wittersheim. The skill, cooperation, and dedication of the staff of our publisher should also be acknowledged in the publication of this book.

We wish to pay a special acknowledgment to our teacher Felix Rutledge, M.D., Chief of Gynecology at the M. D. Anderson Hospital, Houston, Texas. His expert training of a great number of gynecologic oncologists was an important factor in the creation of the gynecologic oncology specialty.

Gregorio Delgado
Julian P. Smith

Contents

PART 3   MEDICAL
COMPLICATIONS

Part 1

INTRODUCTION

1
Exploration
of the Abdomen

Richard W. Holt

At the completion of an exploratory laparotomy, the surgeon should be confident that no significant pathologic condition has been overlooked. It is particularly important to accurately stage patients with gynecologic malignancies. However, even after surgery, some patients thought to have disease confined to the pelvis actually have disease that has spread to the major viscera, the para-aortic lymph nodes, the diaphragm, or the greater omentum. Properly performed, the techniques of abdominal exploration presented here will minimize errors of both omission and commission.

A high priority of the surgical team must be to prevent iatrogenic injury. Fabri et al. (1) concluded that an inadvertent injury to the spleen, for example, could significantly affect operative morbidity and mortality. Tissues are handled gently and careful hemostasis is observed. Adequate general anesthesia with relaxation and endotracheal intubation is mandatory, as is adequate lighting. A Foley catheter is inserted to decompress the urinary bladder. The abdomen is carefully prepared with an iodine-containing solution and draped for a midline incision. Towels are held in place by clips.

A vertical midline incision extending from the pubis to the upper abdomen is employed. The umbilicus is skirted to the right or left side. This incision may be made and closed quickly. Exposure of the pelvic organs is excellent, and the upper abdominal viscera can be safely examined. A colostomy and/or other stoma can be placed with ease. While making the incision and conducting the exploration, the surgeon should take every precaution to avoid potential contamination of the wound and peritoneal cavity. Before entering the peritoneal cavity, he takes care to remove the starch powder from his gloves. Aarons and Fitzgerald (2) attributed a foreign-body granulomatous reaction of the peritoneum to this powder.

Exploration is both visual and palpatory. The wound is elevated by hand to determine if the peritoneum is free in the midline. Retractors are placed within the abdominal cavity by the surgeon, and the assistants move these only on instructions from the surgeon. Kocher clamps are placed on the peritoneum and posterior rectus sheath, to facilitate exposure. Usually there is a relatively avascular zone where adhesions are attached to the peritoneum, bowel, or other structures. After being placed under gentle tension, this avascular area may usually be incised sharply without significant bleeding. Once the peritoneal cavity is entered, the presence and character of any fluid should be noted. An aliquot should be sent to the surgical pathologist for immediate examination. The parietal peritoneum is now palpated for evidence of peritoneal seeding. While the sequence of exploration may be influenced by the type and extent of the pathology, usually the major pathology is evaluated last. In this way, attention is not diverted from the goals of a complete and safe abdominal exploration. Thus, in patients with gynecologic malignancies, the pelvic organs are examined last.

Some surgeons explore the abdomen by means of systems (e.g., gastrointestinal, biliary). Others separate the abdomen into compartments (e.g., supramesocolic and inframesocolic). Thorek (3) has presented a somewhat clockwise plan, and the method suggested here is modeled after Thorek's. The sequence of examination is as follows: esophageal hiatus, left lobe of the liver and gastric cardia; spleen and splenic flexure of the colon; stomach; pylorus and duodenum; pancreas; biliary tract; right lobe of the liver; omentum and transverse colon; small intestine; appendix and cecum; ascending colon and right kidney; descending colon; sigmoid colon and left kidney; rectosigmoid; retroperitoneum; and, finally, the pelvic viscera. Several of the organs and areas deserve special comment.

STOMACH

As the first part of the exploration, both leaves of the diaphragm should be palpated, particularly in cases of ovarian carcinoma. Bagley et al. (4) reported that the diaphragm may be the only site of metastatic ovarian carcinoma above the umbilicus and that there is no correlation between the side of primary ovarian carcinoma and the side of diaphragmatic involvement. A search should be made for a diaphragmatic hernia. The esophageal hiatus should admit two fingertips. Care should be taken not to force the examining fingers along the side of the esophagus. The cardia of the stomach can be more easily palpated after the left liver lobe is mobilized by division of the left triangular ligament (Fig. 1). Although this ligament is relatively avascular, it may be necessary to apply metal clips on the liver side to prevent bleeding. If the stomach is distended, a nasogastric tube is inserted. Decompression of the stomach not only will permit proper examination of the stomach but will provide access to the left lobe of the liver, spleen, and splenic flexure of the colon. If necessary, the midline incision may be extended to the left of the xiphoid process. The cardia of the stomach is palpated for tumors and induration. Gentle rubbing with a gauze pad may produce petechiae if the area is overlying an ulcer. Also at this time the left lobe of the liver is examined for nodularity suggestive of metastases. The anterior surface of the body of the stomach is now palpated down to the pylorus. The pylorus is identified by a circular muscular constriction and by the prepyloric vein of Mayo descending over its anterior surface. The pylorus will usually admit a fingertip. The lesser and greater gastric curvatures and the omenta with their lymph nodes are inspected and palpated (Fig. 2).

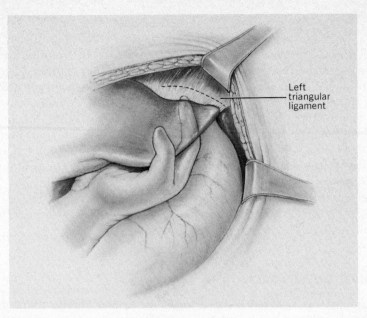

Figure 1. Division of the left triangular ligament of the liver aids exposure of the esophagogastric junction.

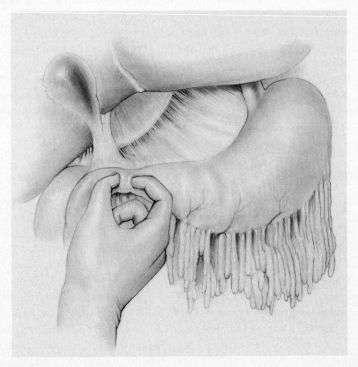

Figure 2. The patency of the pylorus is determined by compression between the thumb and index finger.

LESSER SAC

The lesser sac is an irregular space that lies mostly behind the stomach and the lesser omentum. The posterior surface of the stomach is explored through an incision made in the relatively avascular gastrohepatic omentum.

By blunt digital dissection, the posterior wall of the stomach is separated from the often adherent transverse mesocolon. Then the index finger is advanced through an opening in an avascular area of the gastrocolic ligament. The stomach may then be surrounded by a rubber drain for traction. Madden (5) prefers this method of entry into the lesser sac to the alternative approach through the gastrocolic ligament because the possibility of compromise of the arterial supply of the transverse colon by injury to the middle colic artery is lessened (Figs. 3a and 3b). With the gastrocolic ligament divided, the neck, body, and tail of the pancreas are exposed. The posterior wall of the stomach may now be carefully palpated.

INTERIOR OF THE STOMACH

Mobilization of the stomach as previously described should allow adequate assessment of its interior. However, if difficulty remains, the stomach may be opened for direct inspection and palpation. The stomach is walled off with tapes. A stab wound is made into the gastric wall at the site of the proposed gastrotomy. One fork of a GIA auto suture stapler is inserted into the lumen of the stomach, and the second fork is placed on the serosal surface. Firing of this instrument creates a 5-cm opening. The incision may be lengthened by additional applications of the instrument. The interior of the stomach may now be explored and tumors or ulcerations more precisely evaluated. With the right index finger inserted through the pylorus, the ampulla of Vater may be identified by palpation along the posteromedial surface of the second portion of the duodenum. After the interior of the stomach is explored, the gastrotomy incision is closed with a TA 90 stapling instrument.

SMALL INTESTINE

The small intestine extends from the ligament of Treitz to the cecum. The ligament of Treitz, a band of fibromuscular tissue, extends from the duodenojejunal angle to the right pillar of the diaphragm (Fig. 4). It is identified by elevating the transverse colon, stretching the transverse mesocolon, and putting traction on the first loop of jejunum. The entire small bowel may then be eviscerated and examined along with its mesentery, loop by loop from the ligament of Treitz to the ileocecal valve. The upper portion of the small intestine is thicker, and its diameter becomes diminished from above downward. If the serosa of the bowel is torn while adhesions are being freed, the defect need not be repaired; however, if the muscle layer is torn as well, closure should not be delayed. Failure to recognize full-thickness injuries carries serious consequences. Mesenteric fat growing over an engorged serosal surface of a thickened bowel with a thick mesentery containing enlarged lymph nodes is suggestive of regional enteritis. Donaldson (6) states that if there is appendiceal and/or cecal involve-

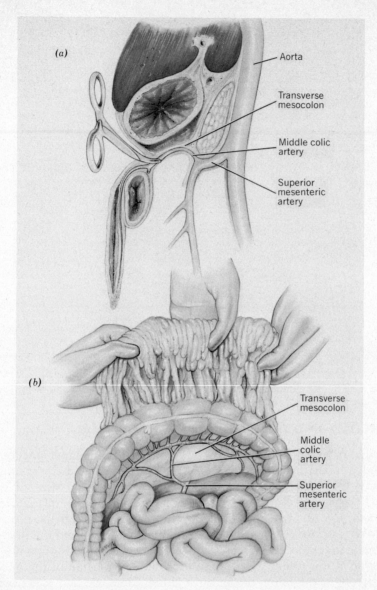

Figure 3. (*a*) Cutaway view of the region of the gastrocolic ligament showing inadvertent clamping of the middle colic artery. The middle colic vessels may be injured during division of the gastrocolic ligament. (*b*) The greater omentum reflected superiorly, exposing the middle colic artery and transverse mesocolon.

ment, incidental appendectomy should not be performed for fear of a leak at the appendiceal stump. Otherwise incidental appendectomy may be performed. In the distal ileum of approximately 2% of the population, a Meckel's diverticulum will be found arising from the antimesenteric border. This outpouching usually occurs within the terminal 2 feet of ileum and is usually 2 inches long—hence the Rule of Two's. Buchsbaum and Lifshitz (7) report that incidental diverticulectomy is recommended by most surgeons.

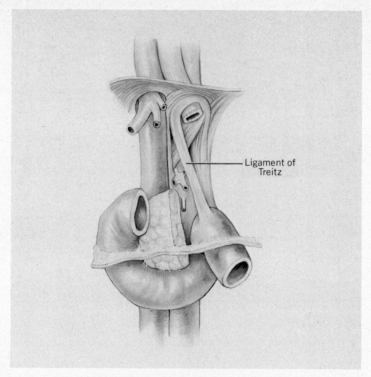

Figure 4. The duodenojejunal junction is suspended by the ligament of Treitz.

FIRST, SECOND, AND THIRD PORTIONS OF THE DUODENUM

The duodenum extends from the pylorus to the duodenojejunal junction, which is suspended by the ligament of Treitz. It makes a C-shaped curve, and within the concavity of that curve is the head of the pancreas. Most of the first (superior) portion of the duodenum consists of the slightly dilated duodenal bulb. Thompson (8) states that approximately 95% of duodenal ulcers occur here. There is a close relationship between the gallbladder and the first portion of the duodenum, and the chronically inflamed gallbladder is often adhesed to the intestine at this point. The second (descending) portion of the duodenum passes in front of the hilum of the right kidney. The bile and pancreatic ducts enter this part of the duodenum posteromedially. Kocher's maneuver of mobilizing the first and second portions may be necessary to fully assess this part of the intestine (Fig. 5). The third (horizontal) portion of the duodenum passes to the left. It crosses the right ureter, inferior vena cava, and abdominal aorta. Anteriorly it is crossed by the superior mesenteric vessels. Finally, there is a very short, fourth (ascending) duodenal portion that turns upward along the left side of the aorta to join with the jejunum at a point marked by the ligament of Treitz. The fourth portion of the duodenum may be mobilized beneath the mesenteric vessels by incising the ligament of Treitz.

COLON

The cecum is the widest and thinnest portion of the large bowel. The internal diameter of the colon diminishes distally. The taeniae coli of the cecum, the

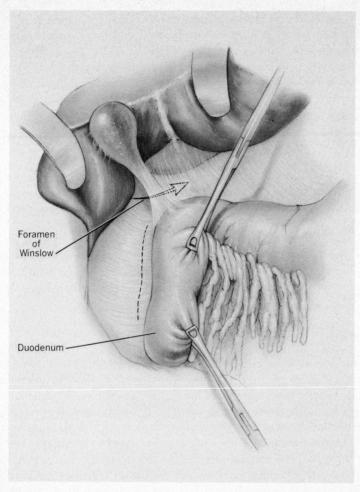

Foramen
of
Winslow

Duodenum

Figure 5. The Kocher maneuver is performed by incising along the lateral peritoneal reflection of the duodenum, allowing medial displacement of the duodenum.

three bands of outer longitudinal muscle, converge on the base of the appendix, sometimes aiding in its identification. The entire colon is palpated for the presence of polyps or tumors. Adequate preoperative mechanical cleansing of the large bowel aids immeasurably in the identification of smaller intraluminal lesions. The colon has small fatty tags—appendices epiploicae—extending from the serosa. In the cecum they contain little fat but are often prominent in the descending and sigmoid colon. In obese patients they may complicate examination of the large bowel. Tumors of the cecum and ascending colon tend to be bulky, fungating lesions, whereas tumors of the left colon tend to be annular. Mobilization of the right and left colon along the lateral peritoneal reflections will aid in exposure of the adrenal glands, kidneys, ureters, and blood vessels to the respective ovary. These reflections are usually relatively avascular except at the flexures. The transverse colon from hepatic to splenic flexure and the greater omentum are examined together. The mobility of this portion of the colon is limited only by the length of its mesentery and the attachments at the flexures. The transverse colon is lifted upward into the wound to expose the transverse mesocolon and its blood vessels. The root of the mesentery is visually and manually examined. It must be emphasized that the spleen is easily injured if traction on the splenic flexure is too vigorous. The descending colon and sigmoid colon are inspected for diverticula and inflammatory masses. The sigmoid colon is usually the most mobile portion of the large intestine because of its long mesentery. Finally, the rectosigmoid and rectum are examined down to the pelvic diaphragm.

LIVER

The liver is explored by placing a hand over the exposed surface of the right lobe up to the dome of the liver. This procedure allows air between the diaphragm and liver, aiding in displacing the organ downward. Ordinarily the left lobe has already been examined during exploration of the stomach. The convex diaphragmatic surface of the liver is smooth and shaped so that it fits the diaphragm. Small hemangiomas and cysts of the liver are not uncommon and are not of consequence. The presence of hard, umbilicated white nodules is highly suggestive of metastatic disease, and representative biopsy specimens should be taken if such nodules are found.

GALLBLADDER

The gallbladder is a thin-walled, hollow, pear-shaped, sea-green organ attached to the inferior surface of the right lobe of the liver. The gallbladder capacity is 30−60 cc. The cystic duct is 2−4 cm long and joins the gallbladder to the right lateral aspect of the common hepatic duct to form the common bile duct. The common bile duct is between 8 and 15 cm in length and 5 and 10 mm in diameter. It enters the descending duodenum about 10 cm distal to the pylorus. Injuries to the bile ducts during elective cholecystectomy result from failure to recognize the many anatomic variations in the biliary tree and its blood supply.

Orloff (9) states that gallstones occur in 10% of adults in the United States (4:1 female:male ratio) and are one of the most common incidental findings during laparotomy. Suggestive of chronic cholecystitis along with gallstones are adhesions between a gray-green gallbladder and the duodenum,transverse colon, and/or greater omentum. A gallbladder distended with bile may obscure calculi. With gentle compression, the gallbladder can be partially emptied through the cystic duct. Stones could be forced into the common bile duct if palpation is too forceful. The common bile duct is palpated by placing the index finger on the free right edge of the lesser omentum until the foramen of Winslow is located. The inserted finger now enters the lesser omental sac. The thumb is then placed on the anterior surface of the duct. Between the thumb and the finger are the common bile duct, the portal vein, and the hepatic artery. Behind the finger is the inferior vena cava (Fig. 6). The common bile duct is then palpated for stones or tumors.

KIDNEYS

The kidneys are retroperitoneal organs, and they lie close to the spinal column, just below the diaphragm. Anterolaterally the kidneys are covered by the surfaces of the respective adrenal gland. The adjacent organs vary on the right

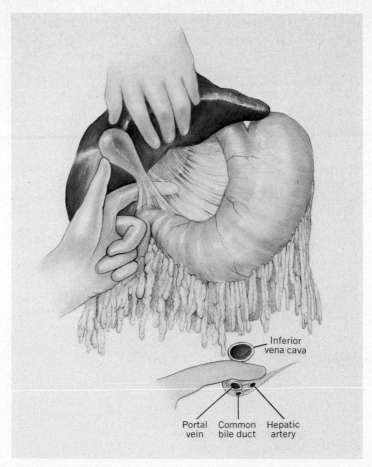

Figure 6. Anterior to a finger placed in the foramen of Winslow are the common bile duct, portal vein, and hepatic artery; posterior to the finger is the inferior vena cava.

and left sides. The right renal pedicle is closely related to the descending duodenum. The lower renal poles are crossed by the hepatic and splenic flexures. The tail of the pancreas crosses the upper pole of the left kidney. The kidneys are palpated for tumors or cysts. This examination is usually performed after examination of the right or left colon (Figs. 7 and 8).

RETROPERITONEAL SPACE

The retroperitoneal space is bounded anteriorly by the peritoneum, posteriorly by the spine and psoas and quadratus lumborum muscles, superiorly by the twelfth ribs and attachments of the diaphragm, and inferiorly by the brim of the pelvis. The retroperitoneal space contains the kidneys, ureters, adrenal glands, elements of the autonomic and peripheral nervous systems, pancreas, lymphatics, blood vessels (including the abdominal aorta, inferior vena cava, and ovarian vessels), fatty and connective tissue, and retroperitoneal portions of the intestinal tract, notably the duodenum. Thus the retroperitoneum has the potential to give rise to a multitude of pathologic entities. Of particular interest is the status of the

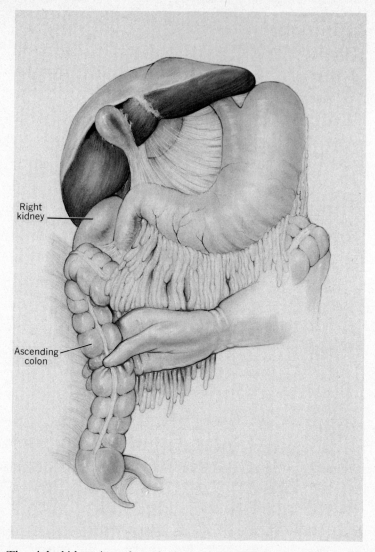

Figure 7. The right kidney is evaluated after palpation of the ascending colon.

paraaortic lymph nodes. As described by Delgado et al. (10), the peritoneum is opened at the level of the aortic bifurcation, and the incision is extended cephalad for approximately 5 cm. The mesentery of the small bowel is retracted and the abdominal aorta and inferior vena cava visualized. The ureters and ovarian vessels are identified. Lymph nodes on either side of the aorta are exposed (Fig. 9). Metal clips should be placed at biopsy sites.

SPLEEN

The care with which the spleen must be examined cannot be overemphasized. Morgenstern (11) states that operative injury to the spleen accounts for 20–40% of splenectomies in this country. Danforth and Thorbjarnarson (12) state that

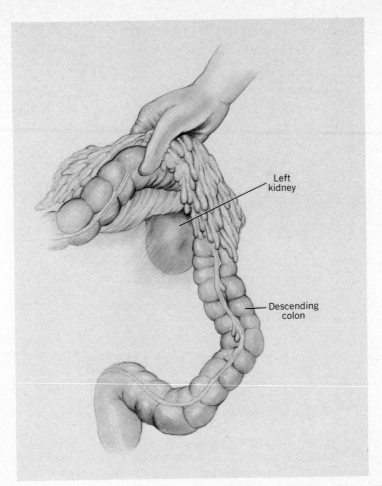

Left
kidney

Descending
colon

Figure 8. The left kidney is evaluated after palpation of the descending colon.

incidental splenectomy occurs most frequently during gastric or left colon resections. However, Prian (13) reported splenic injury as a complication of laparoscopy and pelvic laparotomy. Access to the left upper quadrant and visualization of the spleen through a midline vertical incision are limited, and it is safer to confine exploration and palpation of this highly vascular organ to its lower and anterior border. This is usually adequate to determine splenic size and configuration. The major ligamentous attachments of the spleen converge on the hilar and perihilar fat rather than the spleen itself and are generally not responsible for capsule avulsion injuries, the most common cause of accidental splenectomy. As Morgenstern (11) has emphasized, a variable number of thin peritoneal folds attach the capsule of the spleen to the greater omentum, the gastrosplenic omentum, and the diaphragm. Of particular importance are the folds that attach to the lower pole of the medial surface of the spleen. Traction on these inferomedial folds is the most common cause of capsular avulsion injuries.

   Before the definitive steps of any surgical procedure in the left upper abdominal quadrant are begun, the splenoperitoneal folds should be visualized

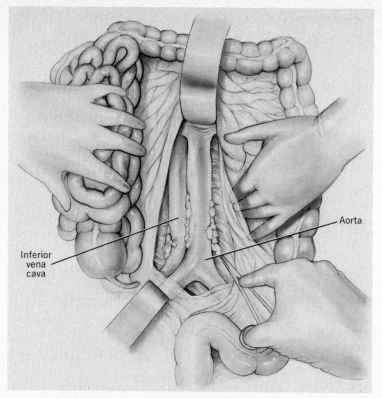

Figure 9. Exploration of the periaortic lymph nodes.

and divided. Gentle traction on the omentum and stomach exposes these folds. If avascular, they are simply divided sharply. If they contain fat or obvious vessels, they may be divided between metal clips.

The splenic capsule lacks muscular tissue. If a capsular tear occurs after even slight traction on the stomach or omentum and if it takes a portion of splenic parenchyma with it, the spleen cannot contract and parenchymal bleeding continues. Standard surgical teaching is to remove the spleen in that circumstance. New hemostatic agents such as microfibrillar collagen hemostat (Avitene) may control bleeding, making splenectomy unnecessary. Generally, such agents will not be effective if there is a hilar injury.

PANCREAS

The neck, body, and tail of the pancreas have been exposed by entry into the lesser omental sac. The duodenum must be mobilized medially (Kocher maneuver) to allow complete bimanual examination of the head of the pancreas. Elevation of the previously mobilized stomach will allow definition of the upper border of the gland (Fig. 10). An enlarged gland suggests a recent episode of acute pancreatitis. In chronic pancreatitis, the gland will be firm, secondary to the fibrous replacement of pancreatic parenchyma. There may be calcifications

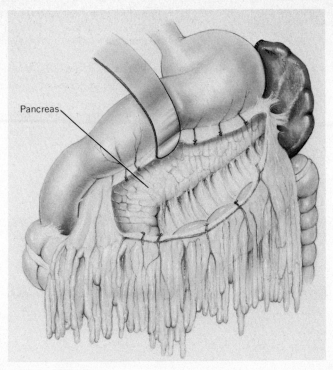

Pancreas

Figure 10. Upward traction on the stomach exposes the neck, body, and tail of the pancreas.

palpable within the pancreatic duct system. Pancreatic tumors or cysts may be palpated.

The preliminary portion of the exploratory laparotomy has now been completed. The surgeon may now direct his full attention to the pelvic viscera, confident that no significant pathologic condition has been overlooked.

REFERENCES

1. Fabri PI, Metz EN, Nick WV, et al: A quarter century with splenectomy: Changing concepts. *Arch Surg* 108:569, 1974.

2. Aarons J, Fitzgerald N: The persisting hazards of surgical glove powder. *Surg Gynecol Obstet* 138:385, 1974.

3. Thorek P: *Atlas of Surgical Techniques.* Philadelphia, JB Lippincott CO, 1970, p 10.

4. Bagley CM Jr, Young RC, Schein PS, et al: Ovarian carcinoma metastatic to the diaphragm— frequently undiagnosed at laparotomy: A preliminary report. *Am J Obstet Gynecol* 116:397, 1973.

5. Madden JL: *Atlas of Techniques in Surgery,* ed. 2. New York, Appleton-Century-Crofts, 1964, p. 263.

6. Donaldson LB: Crohn's disease: Its gynecological aspect. *Am J Gynecol* 131:196, 1978.

7. Buchsbaum HJ, Lifshitz SG: Bowel complications in gynecologic surgery, in Wynn RM (ed): *Obstetrics and Gynecology Annual.* New York, Appleton-Century-Crofts, 1976, p 226.

8. Thompson JC: The stomach and duodenum, in Sabiston DC (ed): *Textbook of Surgery,* ed. 11. Philadelphia, WB Saunders CO, 1977, p 912.

9. Orloff, MJ: The biliary system, in Sabiston DC (ed): *Textbook of Surgery,* ed. 11. Philadelphia, WB Saunders CO, 1977, p 1249.

10. Delgado G, Chun B, Cagler H, et al: Paraaortic lymphadenectomy in gynecologic malignancies confined to the pelvis. *Obstet Gynecol* 50:418, 1977.

11. Morgenstern L: The avoidable complications of splenectomy. *Surg Gynecol Obstet* 145:525, 1977.

12. Danforth DN, Thorbjarnarson B: Incidental splenectomy: A review of the literature and the New York Hospital experience. *Ann Surg* 183:124, 1976.

13. Prian DV: Ruptured spleen as a complication of laparoscopy and pelvic laparotomy. *Am J Obstet Gynecol* 120:983, 1974.

Part 2

SURGICAL COMPLICATIONS

2
Vascular Complications in Gynecologic Surgery

Mario N. Gomes

A century has passed since Freund performed in 1878 the first successful abdominal hysterectomy for carcinoma of the uterus. Continuous progress in gynecologic oncology has been made since then. Wertheim, who, early in this century, performed a radical operation for cancer of the cervix, and Brunschwig (1), who, in 1951, performed exenterative pelvic surgery for advanced or recurrent cervical cancer, are two of the many contributors to the development of pelvic surgery.

More extensive and aggressive surgical procedures in the treatment of vulvar, vaginal, uterine, and ovarian carcinomas are now performed with increasing frequency. Metastatic spread of the primary lesions to the regional lymphatics often requires retroperitoneal node dissection that may include the hypogastric, iliac, and aortic systems. Serious damage to the adjacent vascular structures can occur during the removal of the regional lymph nodes, particularly in older patients in whom significant atherosclerotic changes are present. Venous and arterial vessels can be acutely injured by external compression or by disruption of the vessel wall. The advent and popularity of laparoscopy as a diagnostic and therapeutic procedure has also added a number of arterial and venous injuries to the list of gynecologic operative complications. Penetration of the terminal aorta (2, 3), vena cava (2), mesenteric vessels (4), and iliac arteries and veins (2, 3) has been reported. The few reports in the literature confirm the rarity of the cases, but the high morbidity warrants their description. Early recognition and effective surgical management by vascular reconstruction will generally produce the most satisfactory results.

Advances in the treatment of vascular injuries have been made by employing principles acquired from military experience. A ligature to control bleeding in war wounds was first used by Ambrose Paré during the sixteenth century and remained the main method of treatment of arterial injuries throughout World Wars I and II despite very high amputation rates. In spite of successful animal experiments on arterial reconstruction, which had been reported by Carrel (5) during the early 1900s, arterial repair was used only in selected instances during World War II.

   The Korean War established the routine use of sutures to repair acute arterial injuries and, with their use, the incidence of limb amputation was markedly reduced. Autogenous vein grafts were used regularly only at this time although good results with this technique had been previously obtained by German surgeons during World War I in patients with traumatic aneurysms and arteriovenous fistulas. More recently, during the war in Vietnam, vascular surgeons, who were readily available, clearly demonstrated improved results by performing early vascular reconstruction. The value of concomitant venous repair in some of these injuries was also recognized at this time.

ARTERIAL INJURIES

Etiopathogenesis

Blunt and penetrating trauma are the two basic mechanisms of arterial injuries. Compression of an artery seldom causes permanent damage unless the compression is excessive or prolonged enough to reduce or stop blood flow and, eventually, cause thrombosis. Arteriosclerotic vessels are much more likely to be injured by blunt trauma producing intimal disruption or a subintimal hematoma. Intimal damage will lead to deposition of platelets, fibrin, and red cells at the site of injury and to gradual thrombus formation (Fig. 1). In some instances the torn intima may be lifted by the flow of blood, creating a false channel; in this manner, the arterial lumen can be occluded by the intimal flap. A less common mechanism of obstruction is intramural hemorrhage. The internal and external vessel layers remain intact, but the blood accumulating within the wall itself may create variable degrees of luminal narrowing.

   Arterial contusions may appear to be innocent if external findings are minimal. Without bleeding or disruption of the vascular wall, a serious injury may often be underestimated or initially go undetected. Signs of distal ischemia

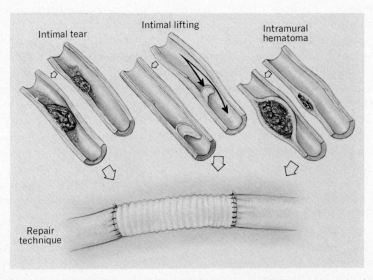

Figure 1. Causes of arterial obstruction in blunt trauma and the usual method of repair.

and the loss of distal pulses will develop subsequently, hours or even days later, when thrombosis occurs.

Occasionally, vessel spasm alone is the cause of the physical findings of ischemia in traumatized arteries. Generally, an underlying anatomic abnormality is present and should always be ruled out. Underestimating the severity of the problem and attributing the arterial insufficiency to the associated spasm is a common error.

Punctures, lacerations, and transections are the manifestations of penetrating vascular wounds (Fig. 2). Hypovolemia, local hematoma, and distal ischemia are the immediate common complications; false aneurysms and arteriovenous fistulas may also occur but in general do not become clinically apparent until later. The ends of a completely severed normal artery will generally constrict and retract, cessation of bleeding occurring spontaneously. The clot forming at the two ends tends to extend proximally and distally, maintaining the hemostasis after relatively little initial bleeding. The common iliac arteries are exceptions to this rule, possibly because the adjacent tissues provide inadequate compression of the divided arterial ends. Vasoconstriction of a significant degree may also not occur in arteriosclerotic vessels; in this case, severe bleeding and arterial transection can be present. Disappearance of distal pulses is the basis for the diagnosis of arterial division and may be the only sign. Its presence does not rule out a significant injury. Pulses may be palpable when the arterial flow is already decreased if the injured vessel is not yet thrombosed; transmission of pressure waves through a soft thrombus or a large collateral branch is also a possible mechanism. Evidence of distal ischemia may not be immediately apparent and will depend on the site of injury and degree of collateral development.

Arterial lacerations usually result in more serious blood loss. Their pathogenesis depends on two basic factors: incomplete vessel constriction because of the intact segment of the arterial wall, and retraction of the divided portion that further separates the edges of the arterial wound. A major hemorrhage can take place immediately if the vessel is exposed; otherwise, the

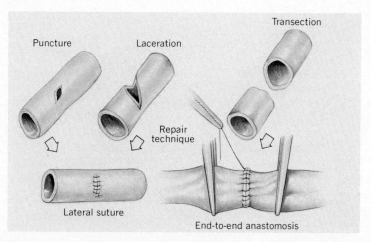

Figure 2. Common vascular wounds in penetrating trauma and the standard operative reconstruction.

adjacent tissues may contain the hematoma temporarily. The size of the arterial laceration will determine the immediate outcome. If the penetrating wound is small, it may become sealed by a hematoma, which ultimately results in formation of a false aneurysm (Fig. 3). In spite of the organization of the hematoma and its replacement by fibrous tissue, progressive expansion will take place. A rapid increase in the size of the pulsating hematoma, creating the potential for sudden, massive bleeding, is seen with larger lacerations. In either case, distal pulsations are generally present without evidence of distal ischemia. Transmission of the pulse wave with a systolic thrill is done by the intact vessel wall, and major arterial flow remains if the hematoma is contained.

Simultaneous injury to the adjacent veins can also take place. An arteriovenous fistula may be formed if the arterial flow from the disrupted artery enters the lacerated vein (Fig. 3). A minimal hematoma can be seen at the site of injury. Given the differential pressures between the systems, blood flow will enter the vein during systole and diastole, generating the typical continuous murmur and palpatory thrill. Most patients will have palpable pulses distal to the injury.

Management

The diagnosis and type of injury encountered during the original surgical procedure are, in general, easily determined. In some cases of delayed thrombosis, the assessment of false aneurysm and arteriovenous fistula secondary to small penetrating lesions may require more than physical examination. Doppler ultrasonic flow studies and angiography are valuable additional diagnostic techniques in the delineation of arterial patency, site, and extent of the injury.

As a rule, acute arterial injuries should be repaired promptly. Delay will increase the damage due to distal ischemia and will reduce the likelihood of a favorable outcome.

Major vessel injury during laparoscopy, although relatively unusual, must be recognized. Significant blood loss may take place, retroperitoneally or intraperitoneally, and serious morbidity or even death may occur. The withdrawal

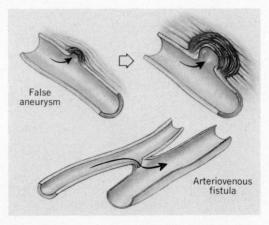

Figure 3. Associated complications of a partially divided artery, with and without disruption of an adjacent vein.

of blood after needle insertion carries a high index of suspicion. On the other hand, a large retroperitoneal hematoma can accumulate with a drop in blood pressure but an initially negative peritoneal aspiration. Preparations for laparotomy should be made while the patient is kept under close observation. Prompt exploration should follow if the patient's vital signs change or the abdomen seems to be enlarging.

Temporary control by direct pressure over the site of the unexpected arterial bleeding is practical and adequate. This measure will allow for placement of large-bore venous cannulas and a monitoring central venous pressure catheter for restoration of blood volume. Typing and cross-matching for more bank blood, if the injury does not seem easily repairable, can take place during the time required to stabilize the patient with the necessary fluid replacement. Autotransfusion should be considered if significant blood loss has occurred or seems likely to occur, during the impending vascular reconstructive procedure. If the use of venous autografts seems indicated, a lower extremity should be prepared and draped at this time, for ready access to the saphenous vein.

Proximal and distal control should be obtained before any attempt at reconstruction is made. The incision should be extended along the pathway of the involved vessel and the bleeding controlled by digital pressure. The artery above and below the injury can be encircled with umbilical tapes and atraumatic vascular clamps applied 2–3 cm from the site of injury. Temporary intraluminal occlusion with a Fogarty catheter, or even a Foley catheter for a much larger vessel such as the aorta, can also be used for initial control of difficult bleeding (6).

Once the involved arterial segment is isolated and adequately exposed, evaluation of the damage can take place and careful examination of the surrounding structures.

Maintenance of the distal arterial circulation is fundamental to the patency of the repair. Systemic anticoagulation with heparin (5,000–10,000 units, I.V.) can be employed at this time, particularly if the aorta needs to be clamped. Because of the original operative procedure, regional heparinization with 30–40 cc of a saline solution containing a 1:100 dilution of heparin (100 units/ml) can be used, instead, to irrigate the distal arterial system, in order to retard or prevent intravascular thrombosis.

The presence of a distal thrombus should always be ruled out. Back-bleeding is an unreliable sign, and a thrombectomy with the Fogarty catheter should probably be performed routinely to ensure complete removal of thrombi (7). The catheter should be advanced as far as possible distally and the balloon inflated with saline, to the volume required, and then withdrawn. Gentleness and some experience are required for proper use of the catheter. Distal arterial perforations from excessive roughness on insertion have been reported. Over-distension of the balloon can also produce severe spasm or even arterial rupture. A proximal thrombus can be removed by flushing or by using the Fogarty catheter, just before completion of the arterial reconstruction.

A concomitant venous injury should be repaired first, in order to enhance the patency of the arterial repair by providing a better outflow (8).

The type and extent of damage will determine the appropriate reconstruction (Figs. 1, 2). Synthetic sutures (Dacron/Teflon) or monofilament polypropylene sutures size 5-0 or 6-0 are the commonly used and favored sutures. A size 4-0 suture may be required for aortic repair or grafting.

The basic purpose of arterial reconstruction is to reestablish blood flow without any significant luminal narrowing. The need for graft interposition is determined by the length of the damaged vessel since excessive tension should not be present at the anastomosis. The common techniques used are lateral repair, lateral repair with patch angioplasty, primary end-to-end anastomosis, and graft replacement. Appropriate but conservative debridement may be necessary before the vascular repair. Excess adventitia, that is, adventitia protruding into the lumen, should be removed, but the surgeon should keep in mind that the arterial tensile strength derives mainly from this layer. Detached or injured intima should be excised; the integrity of the distal intima should be ascertained in order to prevent thrombosis.

Lateral arteriorraphy is all that is generally necessary in the repair of puncture wounds or minor arterial lacerations. Interrupted or continuous sutures placed approximately 2 mm apart and everting the wound edges can be used. This technique is safe for larger arteries but should not be used for lacerations comprising more than 30% of the vessel circumference (9) because of the luminal constriction that will result.

In smaller vessels or longer lacerations, stenosis at the suture line can be prevented by using a widening patch. In potentially contaminated wounds, an autogenous vein graft should be used, tailored in size and width, to restore the normal arterial lumen. On a clean surgical field, particularly if the aorta or common iliac arteries are the vessels involved, a Dacron patch can be used. Narrowing may occur at the proximal and distal angles of the patch if a large amount of the arterial wall is incorporated in the suture line.

A transected artery can usually be repaired without tension by direct anastomosis of the divided ends. Restoration of normal vessel diameter and intimal coaptation, without excessive anastomotic tension, are fundamental for the patency of the repair. If necessary, proximal and distal dissection of the divided arterial segments will provide extra length, thus decreasing the tension of the repair. An end-to-end anastomosis with a continuous suture is the standard method of repair. In one technique (Fig. 4) two double-needle sutures are placed directly posteriorly and anteriorly, approximating the divided arterial ends. An everting over-and-over stitch, starting posteriorly, will bring the suture line toward the anterior fixation point. With the posterior quadrants completed, the same maneuver will be carried alternately from the anterior needles around the remaining circumference of the artery. Of various techniques, this four-quadrant method is a simple and practical one.

If a loss of 2 cm or more of the arterial wall has taken place, a graft replacement may be necessary, especially if significant intimal damage to a contused artery (Fig. 1) will require excision of the involved arterial segment. Excessive pressure by a retractor is not an uncommon cause of intimal fracture or lifting. When an arterial vessel is transected, the normal retraction of the artery magnifies the length of the gap between the divided ends. In these cases, the decision regarding direct anastomosis versus grafting should be made only after placing vascular clamps on the arterial ends and, then, judging the degree of tension necessary to their approximation. In larger arteries, such as the aorta

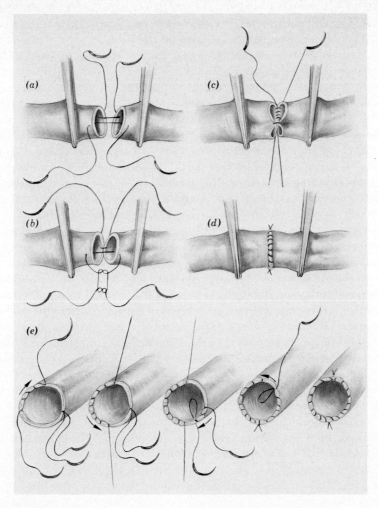

Figure 4. Arterial repair by an end-to-end anastomosis using a four-quadrant technique.

or common iliacs, prosthetic grafts are required for replacement; in other vessels they should be avoided, whenever possible, since prostheses increase the risk of infection in the presence of a contaminated field. The reversed saphenous vein is the recommended prosthesis in smaller vessels. As a rule, the graft should be slightly larger than the vessel that it is replacing.

Before the completion of the anastomosis, the vascular clamps are momentarily released, first the distal and then the proximal, in order to remove any residual air or thrombi. Gentle pressure over the suture line, for a brief period, will control the usual oozing of blood from the needle holes.

Upon release of the clamps, a strong pulsation should be felt, beyond the anastomosis, over the distal vessels. A significant pressure gradient across the suture line may indicate mechanical narrowing, or thrombus, and revision will be necessary. If the reason for the poor quality of the distal arterial pulses is not obvious, an intraoperative arteriogram should be performed. The anastomotic site, as well as the distal arterial circulation, can be adequately investigated in this manner. The presence of spasm can also be ruled out.

A high degree of success should be expected in the repair of arterial injuries if meticulous surgical technique is applied.

The reconstructed artery should be covered by soft tissue, namely peritoneum, for the aorta and iliac vessels. Neutralization of the heparin at the end of the operation is usually not necessary since its effect will have practically disappeared during the several hours of the surgical procedure.

Ligation of an injured artery is generally not indicated unless the vessel is small or not contributing significantly to the major blood flow. An exception will be the rare circumstance when the patient's life is being compromised by prolonged attempts to repair the involved artery. The viability of the area supplied will depend on the adequacy of the collateral circulation; an extraanatomic bypass may be considered later if ischemic changes are manifest.

The inferior mesenteric artery is a very important vessel to be aware of during the para-aortic lymphadenectomy. It has been reported (10) that about 0.5 – 1% of the gynecologic patients who undergo para-aortic node dissections will have some degree of left colon ischemia, because of the surgical trauma to that artery. If the inferior mesenteric artery is transected or ligated distal to the origin of the left colic artery, its first branch, the viability of the descending and rectosigmoid colon may be seriously impaired. The anastomoses from the superior to the inferior mesenteric systems are established between the middle and left colic arteries via the marginal artery of Drummond. Ligation of the inferior mesenteric artery proximal to the takeoff of the left colic will preserve these anastomoses. The presence of good pulsation in the divided distal stump will provide further reassurance of the adequacy of the blood supply. In questionable circumstances, or if this vessel seems unusually large, reimplantation into the aorta should be done. An increase in vessel size, particularly in older people, often indicates obstruction of the superior mesenteric artery. A button of aortic wall should be excised, over a partial occlusion clamp, and the inferior mesenteric artery anastomosed, in a continuous manner, with a 5-0 vascular suture.

An acute occlusion of the common or external iliac arteries, either by ligation or thrombosis, is followed by a high rate, about 50%, of gangrenous changes in the involved extremity (11). The hypogastric artery may be ligated without harm (12, 13). A secure arterial ligation can be obtained with a double ligature, the distal one being a transfixing suture. A sufficient cuff is necessary to prevent the distal ligature from slipping, which may compromise a collateral branch in that area. A continuous running suture of a larger artery can be used instead and, being equally secure, will also preserve any collateral vessels.

Postoperative Care

Anticoagulation is rarely used postoperatively because of the danger of bleeding in the operative area. Its use will not keep an artery patent if the anastomosis is technically inadequate or thrombi are present in the distal arterial vessels. Adequate blood flow and perfusing pressures should be maintained after the operation, to preserve patency of the reconstructed vessel.

The arterial pulses distal to the area of repair should be checked at hourly intervals, in the immediate postoperative period, by direct palpation or by use of the Doppler ultrasound technique. Serial measurement of ankle pressures by means of the Doppler flow probe is a useful indicator of the degree of perfusion, particularly if the distal pulses cannot be felt. The absence or disappearance of arterial pulses after arterial reconstruction is an indication for angiography or reexploration. Vasospasm is seldom, if ever, the reason for absent pulses. Intravenous papaverine can be tried, to rule out the presence of arterial spasm.

The viability of a limb can usually be estimated by the signs of ischemia and, particularly, by its neurologic function. The loss of sensation and motion generally indicates impending gangrene unless the arterial circulation can be promptly restored.

Infection with secondary bleeding due to suture line disruption can be fatal in some areas of the body. A large retroperitoneal hematoma can be present without any external signs until significant hypotension is apparent. Immediate reintervention is necessary.

The use of prophylactic antibiotics is generally accepted in arterial surgery, particularly if a prosthetic graft is inserted. Unless there is secondary contamination, such as from bowel contents, antibiotic coverage is directed to the most common organism in wound infections, the staphylococcus.

VENOUS INJURIES

Etiopathogenesis

Isolated major venous trauma, particularly to the inferior vena cava and common iliac veins, is not an infrequent occurrence during their dissection from the accompanying arteries. Iatrogenic lacerations of these vessels, in the course of other major operative procedures, have been described and the incidence is probably much higher than reported. Partial tears of the inferior vena cava during nephrectomy for malignant disease are the most frequent injuries (14). Damage to the vena cava or iliac veins can also be caused during surgery of the distal aorta or urinary tract, or even during lumbar sympathectomy. Cases have been reported in which these vessels have been injured in the course of an abdominoperineal resection (15) or, more frequently, in the resection of a prolapsed intervertebral disk (16).

The common iliac vessels are in very close proximity, the veins being partially behind the arteries and, sometimes, fairly adherent to them. Unintentional trauma to these major veins, during lymph node dissections, is not uncommon, given the surgical anatomy of these structures. Seldom when radical surgery is indicated is resection in continuity of the vena cava and pelvic vessels required. Distant metastases or other local organ involvement is also frequently present when there is tumor invasion of the pelvic vessels, which narrows down considerably the number of instances in which extensive vessel resection is indicated in the field of surgical oncology. This procedure should be considered only in cases of invading carcinoma of the female genital organs, bladder, or sigmoid colon in which there is no evidence of distant metastases. Even in these cases the prognosis is poor. In a series of 840 cases of pelvic exenterations, resection and reconstruction of the iliac vessels was done in only 55 of these patients. The survival rate after 5 years was 20%. When malignant involvement of the pelvic veins was present, the survival rate after 5 years was only 11% (17).

Perforations of the inferior vena cava (2) and iliac veins (2, 3) during laparoscopy have also been reported.

Iliac vein stenosis can be seen after radiotherapy to the pelvic area. Often there is also damage to the pelvic lymphatic system and, frequently, this is responsible for the leg edema. The true cause of the stenosis should be clearly identified before venous reconstruction is attempted.

Management

Suture repair of venous injuries and reconstruction have been described and recommended since the nineteenth century. Murphy (1897), Schede (1882), and Kummel (1899) (18), among others, successfully performed venous repairs. In spite of these reports, ligation of major veins, concomitant with acute ligation of traumatized limb arteries, was widely advised. This concept of limb protection was not refuted until after World War II (19).

Even after the Second World War, ligation of major injured veins continued to be a frequent method of repair. Interest in venous repair arose again after the Korean War, when a relatively large number of arteriovenous fistulas were successfully reconstructed. During the Vietnam conflict the number of venous repairs significantly increased. Approximately one-third of the venous injuries (20) were thus treated, mostly by lateral suture (21).

Many veins of small dimensions can be ligated with minimal or no disability. Sometimes, because of technical difficulties or the need to reduce operating time, a major vein is ligated and minimal or no immediate disability occurs. In these cases, early supportive measures, such as elevation and the use of Dextran and anticoagulants, should be instituted to prevent extension of venous thrombosis.

As a rule, major veins should be preserved. Their ligation impairs venous return although chronic venous insufficiency may not be apparent until months or years later (21). In some circumstances, such as when severe injuries to the infrarenal vena cava have caused extensive loss of the venous wall, ligation may be required. Whenever possible, the site of ligation should be immediately below a major tributary or the renal or lumbar veins, to prevent formation of a cul-de-sac, where stagnant blood will thrombose or even embolize (2%−6% of the cases) (14).

Ligation of the inferior vena cava, in its renal or suprarenal segment, is poorly tolerated and carries a very high mortality rate (80%−90%) although some survivors have been reported (22, 23). Every effort should be made to repair the cava at this level. An occluding balloon catheter or an internal shunt may be necessary for temporary control of bleeding in these very challenging situations (24).

Two potential complications of venous injury, thrombophlebitis and pulmonary embolism, are sometimes attributed to venous repairs. However, this supposition has not been substantiated. Data obtained from the Vietnam Vascular Registry seem to refute this belief (20). Other investigators, also, have reported the absence of pulmonary embolism after venous reconstruction (25).

The iliac veins are the main vessels through which venous return occurs in the lower half of the body. Any interruption of the venous system between the femoral veins and the inferior vena cava markedly impairs venous return, particularly in the standing position. In order for chronic venous insufficiency to be prevented, reconstruction should be done routinely for any injured large vein proximal to the profunda femoris.

Although the trend in venous injuries is to repair, instead of ligate, the injured vein, certain anatomic and physiologic factors make venous repair a more difficult technique than arterial repair, and the incidence of thrombosis is higher. The thinness and fragility of the venous wall, the low intravenous pressure, and the relatively slow venous flow are some of these factors.

Bleeding from vena caval or iliac vein injuries is best controlled by direct digital compression (Fig. 5). An attempt to suture the lacerated veins, when distended, is usually followed by further extension of the injury. In some instances, a partial occlusion clamp, such as a Satinsky, can be applied to the vein, without further dissection, and lateral suture of the laceration can then be performed. Direct control of the venous tear can sometimes be done, simply and effectively, by sequential application of Allis clamps (26). While bleeding is being controlled by digital pressure, the first Allis clamp is placed immediately above the upper part of the laceration. A second clamp is applied just below it while the first one is gently lifted. Further clamps are placed until the venous edges are approximated. The laceration is then repaired with a continuous running stitch using a 5-0 or 6-0 monofilament suture.

This method of lateral suture repair is a common one, but care must be taken to avoid unduly narrowing the vein. In both methods the repair is done without interrupting the venous return.

When these techniques are not possible, decompression of the vein and control of the hemorrhage can be accomplished by direct compression, above and below the laceration, using a folded 4 × 4-inch sponge held in a ring forceps clamp. This is done by the first assistant while the surgeon initially controls the bleeding by digital compression. Atraumatic vascular clamps can then be used more effectively, replacing the external compression, after further mobilization of the injured vein.

Direct suture repair is possible in most instances and, generally, it is the method of choice. In order for excessive constriction of the venous lumen to be avoided, an autogenous venous patch, usually from the saphenous vein, may be necessary. Local or systemic heparinization is generally not indicated unless the venous occlusion is needed for a long time.

End-to-end reconstruction can sometimes be done after further mobilization of the divided venous segments. Given the greater incidence of thrombosis in venous than in arterial repairs, meticulous technique is imperative. Any thrombus in the afferent or efferent ends should always be cleared before the repair.

The long-term results of venous reconstruction are definitely better when direct repair is used instead of vascular grafts. The autogenous veins, particularly the saphenous or internal jugular, are satisfactory for venous grafts. Prosthetic grafts have generally been disappointing because of a high incidence of thrombosis. Technical precision, avoiding any compromise of the lumen or tension at the anastomosis, is again emphasized. Constriction or turbulence of

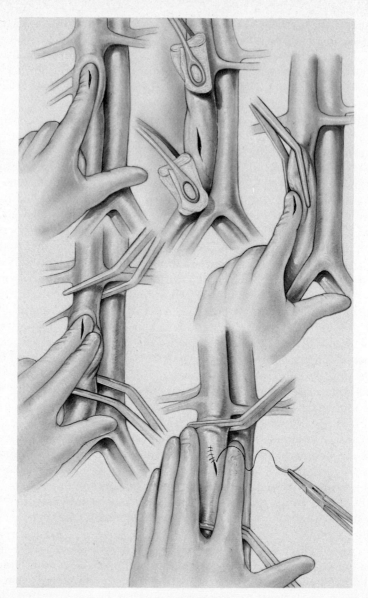

Figure 5. Common techniques of bleeding control and repair in lacerations of the inferior vena cava.

the venous flow in this low-pressure system is conducive to thrombosis. Some of the technical details that enhance the patency of graft interposition in venous repairs, particularly in smaller veins, are the use of slightly longer venous grafts, but with the same approximate diameter; obliquity of the anastomotic ends of the vein and prosthesis; and the avoidance of tension in the continuous suture line (27).

Most investigators (8, 9, 28) believe that even short-term patency, such as from 24 to 72 hours, is beneficial because it allows for additional collateral venous flow and prevents chronic venous insufficiency. Recanalization of the thrombosed vein is usually established 4−6 weeks later, providing further venous return. Systemic heparinization and low-molecular dextran have been advocated as adjuncts in venous reconstruction. There is experimental evidence (29) to suggest an improvement in venous patency after venous repair with the use of low-molecular dextran. Some authors (30) have also reported an improvement with heparinization, but this has not been proven experimentally (29).

Until recent years the failure rate of venous reconstruction by grafting the iliac veins and inferior vena cava has been as high as 50%−80% (14). Improved surgical techniques have made reconstructive venous surgery more successful, particularly by adding a temporary arteriovenous fistula. Since the first clinical use of an arteriovenous fistula, by Johnson and Eiseman in 1969 (31), a revival in venous reconstruction of large veins has taken place. The incidence of venous thrombosis has, thus, been markedly reduced after grafting in which an autogenous vein or even a Dacron prosthesis has been used. The hemodynamics created by the temporary distal arteriovenous fistula account for the patency of a synthetic graft interposed in the inferior vena cava or iliac veins. A significant increase in the venous flow rate and velocity, and a small rise in the venous pressure take place, changes that are favorable to the patency of the proximal venous repair (32).

These new techniques can be applied not only to traumatic lesions but also to extensive radical tumor surgery in which resection of the iliac veins or inferior vena cava is indicated. Selection criteria should be strict because of the frequent association with metastatic spread. In cases in which there is a reasonable chance of complete surgical resection of the tumor, a Dacron prosthesis, with the protection of a temporary distal arteriovenous fistula, can be considered.

When the patient has sustained concomitant injuries to arteries and accompanying veins, the venous repair should ordinarily be performed first. This step will not only prevent the inconvenience of venous bleeding after the arterial repair but also contribute to the success of the arterial reconstruction by the better outflow (20).

Postoperative Care

Assessment of venous patency is not so easy to establish as arterial patency. Clinical accuracy is poor, and the diagnosis can be made only by venography or by the use of the Doppler ultrasound unit. The accuracy of the Doppler examination for venous obstruction is high, particularly in the lower extremities. Depression and rapid elevation with the Valsalva maneuver indicate adequate venous flow. For more central veins, venography, particularly intraoperative, may be indicated to demonstrate the adequacy of the repair. Narrowing of the anastomosis or the presence of a thrombus will necessitate revision given the inevitability, in those circumstances, of graft thrombosis.

After venous reconstruction, early and intensive supportive care of the affected extremity should be given, to minimize edema of the involved extremity. Elevation and appropriate elastic support ought to be instituted immediately after the operation, particularly if a major vein, such as the inferior vena cava, was ligated. Adequate early measures will result in less disability from chronic venous insufficiency at a later time.

Critical judgment should be exercised regarding the feasibility of an adequate repair, given the disastrous consequences of reconstructive failures in some cases.

Some of the basic principles of diagnosis and management of vascular injuries have been delineated in this chapter.

These general guidelines are intended to be of help in an emergency, but they are not a replacement for the direct advice or participation of an experienced and skilled vascular surgeon.

REFERENCES

1. Brunschwig A: Operative treatment of carcinoma of cervix: Radical panhysterectomy with pelvic lymph node excision. *Am J Obstet Gynecol* 61:1193, 1951.

2. McDonald PT, Rich NM, Collins GJ, et al: Vascular trauma secondary to diagnostic and therapeutic procedures: Laparoscopy. *Am J Surg* 135:651, 1978.

3. Katz M, Beck P, Tanler ML: Major vessel injury during laparoscopy: Anatomy of two cases. *Am J Obstet Gynecol* 135:544, 1979.

4. Esposito J: Hematoma of the sigmoid colon as a complication of laparoscopy. *Am J Obstet Gynecol* 177:581, 1973.

5. Carrel A: The surgery of blood vessels. *Bull Johns Hopkins Hosp* 190:18, 1906.

6. Smiley K, Perry MO: Balloon catheter tamponade of major vascular wounds. *Am J Surg* 121:326, 1971.

7. Hardy JD, Raju S, Neely WA, et al: Aortic and other arterial injuries. *Ann Surg* 181:640, 1975.

8. Hewitt RL, Drapanas T: Vascular injuries, in Haimovici H (ed): *Vascular Surgery: Principles and Technics.* New York, McGraw-Hill Book Co, 1976, p 560.

9. Rich NM, Spencer FC: Management of acute arterial injuries, in *Vascular Trauma.* Philadelphia, WB Saunders Co, 1978, p 75.

10. Belinson JL, Goldbert MI, Averette HE: Paraaortic lymphadenectomy in gynecologic cancer. *Gynecol Oncol* 7:188, 1979.

11. Rich NM, Spencer FC: Iliac artery injuries, in *Vascular Trauma.* Philadelphia, WB Saunders Co, 1978, p 475.

12. Cranley JJ, Meese EH: Vascular trauma, in Cranley JJ (ed): *Vascular Surgery.* Hagerstown, Md., Harper & Row Publishers Inc., 1972, p 187.

13. Thal ER, Perry MO: Peripheral and abdominal vascular injuries, in Rutherford R (ed): *Vascular Surgery.* Philadelphia, WB Saunders Co, 1977, p 433.

14. Vollmar J: Reconstruction of the iliac veins and inferior vena cava, in Hobbs JT (ed): *The Treatment of Venous Disorders.* Philadelphia, JB Lippincott Co, 1977, p 320.

15. Gaspar MR, Treiman RI: The management of injuries to major veins. *Am J Surg* 100:171, 1960.

16. Moore CA, Cohen A: Combined arterial, venous and ureteral injury complicating lumbar disk surgery. *Am J Surg* 115:574, 1968.

17. Barber HRK, Brunschwig A: Excision of major blood vessels at the periphery of the pelvis in patients receiving pelvic exenteration: Common and/or iliac arteries and veins, 1947 to 1964. *Surgery* 62:426, 1967.

18. Hobson RW, Rich NM, Wright CB: Concepts in venous trauma and reconstruction, in Hobbs JT (ed): *The Treatment of Venous Disorders.* Philadelphia, JB Lippincott Co, 1977, p 355.

19. DeBakey ME, Simeone EA: Battle injuries of the arteries in World War II. *Ann Surg* 123:534, 1946.

20. Rich NM, Hughes CW, Baugh JH: Management of venous injuries. *Ann Surg* 171:724, 1970.

21. Rich NM, Spencer FC: Venous injuries, in *Vascular Trauma.* Philadelphia, WB Saunders Co, 1978, p 156.

22. Cassebaum WH, Bukanz SL, Baum V, et al: Ligation of the inferior vena cava above the renal vein of a sole kidney with recovery. *Am J Surg* 113:667, 1967.

23. Ramnath R, Walden EC, Caguin F: Ligation of the suprarenal vena cava and right nephrectomy with complete recovery. *Am J Surg* 112:88, 1966.

24. Bricker DL, Morton JR, Okies JE, et al: Surgical management of injuries to the vena cava: Changing patterns of injury and newer techniques of repair. *J Trauma* 11:725, 1971.

25. Drapanas T, Hewitt RL, Weichert RE, et al: Civilian vascular injuries: A critical appraisal of three decades of management. *Ann Surg* 172:351, 1970.

26. Lim LT: Management of aorto-vena caval injury, in Bergan JJ, Yao JST (eds): *Surgery of the Aorta and Its Body Branches.* New York, Grune & Stratton Inc, 1979, p. 307.

27. Rich NM, Hobson RW, Wright CB, et al: Techniques of venous repair, in Swan KG, et al (eds): *Venous Surgery in the Lower Extremity.* St Louis, Warren H Green Inc, 1975, p. 243.

28. Freeark RJ: Arterial injuries, in Davis-Christopher L (ed): *Textbook of Surgery.* Philadelphia, WB Saunders Co, 1977, p 1954.

29. Hobson RW, Croom RD, Rich NM: Influence of heparin and low molecular weight dextran on the patency of autogenous vein grafts in the venous system. *Ann Surg* 178:173, 1973.

30. Baird RJ, Lipton IH, Mivagishima RT, et al: Replacement of the deep veins of the leg. *Arch Surg* 89:797, 1964.

31. Johnson V, Eiseman B: Evaluation of arteriovenous shunt to maintain patency of venous autograft. *Am J Surg* 118:915, 1969.

32. Hobson RW, Wright CB: Peripheral side to side arteriovenous fistula: Hemodynamics and application to venous reconstruction. *Am J Surg* 126:411, 1973.

3
Arterial Hemorrhage in Gynecologic Malignancies

Peter E. Schwartz

Massive arterial hemorrhage is an uncommon complication in the management of patients with gynecologic malignances. It most often occurs in debilitated women who have previously been treated with extensive radiation therapy, surgery, and/or chemotherapy. Frequently these patients are in shock, unable to tolerate immediate surgical procedures to control the hemorrhage; at times their bone marrow may be suppressed as a result of previous chemotherapy.

The surgical management advocated for massive pelvic hemorrhage has been bilateral hypogastric artery ligation (1). Often this is an impractical solution because of the patient's debilitated state. In addition, hypogastric artery ligation may be technically difficult to accomplish because of prior radiation resulting in marked fibrosis, making a rapid surgical approach technically impossible. Bleeding from gastrointestinal sources may also be difficult to control surgically because of the patient's medical condition and the difficulty in determining the bleeding site.

Recent advances in selective arteriography for identifying the sites of abnormal bleeding in both the gastrointestinal tract and pelvis have led to the development of arterial catheter techniques to control the bleeding (2). These techniques include infusion of vasoactive material to produce vasoconstriction, particularly for gastrointestinal tract bleeding (3); transcatheter embolization of autologous and synthetic materials (4, 5); and balloon catheter insertions to control bleeding from major blood vessels (6). Also, clinical investigators are evaluating transcatheter occlusive therapy with liquid tissue adhesives and stainless steel coils (7, 8).

ARTERIOGRAPHIC TECHNIQUES FOR ESTABLISHING BLEEDING SITES

Arteriography is readily accomplished using the technique described by Seldinger. A needle is inserted into the femoral artery and a guide wire is then inserted through the lumen of the needle and advanced under fluoroscopy through the lumen of the femoral, external iliac, and common iliac arteries into the aorta. The needle is then removed over the guide wire, and a polyethylene catheter is directed over the guide wire into the artery. The catheters employed are flexible and can be preformed so that they may be readily advanced into the takeoffs of the branches of the aorta and iliac arteries. As the catheter tip is advanced beyond the guide wire, the preformed curve will appear at the catheter tip. The exact catheter tip curvature is determined by preforming the curve before the catheter is advanced over the guide wire. The catheter may then be inserted in sequence into the celiac, superior mesenteric, and inferior mesenteric arteries and an arteriographic survey of these vessels and their branches performed to determine bleeding sites from the gastrointestinal tract. Similarly, bleeding from the pelvis can be evaluated by directing the guide wire around the bifurcation of the aorta and into the common iliac, external iliac, or hypogastric artery. The catheter is then advanced over the guide wire into these vessels and arteriographic surveys performed to evaluate the pelvic structures. Finally, the catheter may be withdrawn to evaluate the ipsilateral iliac vessels.

It should be noted that successful identification of the active bleeding site depends upon the presence of active bleeding at the time of the arteriography (2). In addition, it is most important to survey for dual blood supplies for the site of the arterial bleeding. Obviously, the uterus has dual blood supplies, but when dealing with gastrointestinal bleeding, one must consider the fact that the stomach, duodenum, and transverse colon also have dual blood supplies; thus it is most important to eliminate the possibility of a second source of arterial hemorrhage before attempting catheter techniques to control the arterial hemorrhage.

SELECTION OF CATHETER OCCLUSION TECHNIQUE

Vasopressin Infusion

Vasopressin infusion has been successfully employed in managing gastrointestinal bleeding from esophageal varices and subsequently demonstrated to be effective in managing bleeding secondary to ulcers (3). Patients with gynecologic cancer infrequently have gastrointestinal bleeding requiring catheter techniques. These techniques, however, have been employed in managing entercolonic anastomosis leaks secondary to managing complications of intense radiation therapy for the treatment of gynecologic malignancies and benign ulcer disease associated with advanced gynecologic cancers (2).

Selective arteriography should be employed to identify the exact source of the gastrointestinal bleeding. Vasopressin may then be infused through the same arterial catheter at an initial dosage of 0.2 units/minute. Within 20 minutes the effects of the vasopressin should be quite obvious and injection of radiographic dye through the arterial catheter should demonstrate control of the hemorrhage. If it appears that the hemorrhage has not been controlled, the dose should be increaseed by 0.1 units/minute until control is established. The infusion should continue for 6–12 hours after hemostasis. The vasopressin infusion may then be stopped, but the catheter should be left in place for at least another 12–24 hours with saline infused through it. This is important because bleeding may recur, and having the catheter in place will allow rapid retreatment of the bleeding. Vasopressin infusion may not completely control bleeding, but it may provide time to stabilize a patient in shock and get her in proper medical condition for definitive surgical hemostasis. An additional advantage of the catheter is that it may be used to control recurrent bleeding after vasopressin infusion failure by embolizing material through it.

An example of the role of intra-arterial vasopressin infusion to control massive hemorrhage is seen in Figures 1a and b. Massive arterial bleeding from the gastrointestinal tract of this patient occurred 1 day after an ileoascending colostomy for small bowel obstruction secondary to recurrent cancer and severe radiation enteritis. The patient's prior therapy included a selective lymphadenectomy, intense radiation to the pelvis and lower para-aortics, and intracavitary radiation therapy for management of a Stage IIIA squamous cell carcinoma of the cervix. Arteriography demonstrated the bleeding site to be at the region of the enterocolostomy (Fig. 1a). Vasopressin infusion was initiated at 0.2 units/minute, and a repeat arteriogram 1 hour later (Fig. 1b) showed a

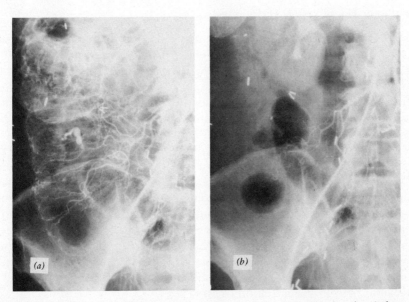

Figure 1. (a) Postoperative hemorrhage from an ileocolic anastomosis. A late-phase superior mesenteric arteriogram reveals contrast media in the ascending colon. (From Schwartz PE, et al: Control of arterial hemorrhage using percutaneous arterial catheter techniques in patients with gynecologic malignancies. *Gynecol Oncol* 3:276–288, 1975. Reprinted with permission.) (b) Control of bleeding demonstrated 1 hour after initiation of vasopressin infusion into the superior mesenteric artery.

dramatic reduction in the amount of bleeding present. Three hours after vasopressin infusion was begun, the patient became dyspneic and a chest x-ray film indicated pulmonary edema, which promptly cleared when the infusion was stopped. The bleeding subsequently resumed and on laparotomy an anastomotic leak was revealed on the colonic side of the ileocolic anastomosis. This leak was oversewn and the patient did well postoperatively.

Complications using vasopressin infusion are associated with fluid and electrolyte balance, which must be closely monitored. Vasopressin is virtually pure posterior pituitary extract, and infrequently acute water retention may occur (9–11). This water retention does not usually become clinically significant unless the patient has been exposed to a prolonged infusion. It is most likely that the patient presented here did not have acute water retention but rather had excessive fluid replacement during the course of treatment for massive hemorrhage. There are occasional reports of prolonged vasopressin infusion causing bradycardia and, at times, hypertension (12). In general, the low dose of vasopressin infused infrequently results in systemic pharmacologic effects. Ischemic damage to the bowel is extremely infrequent. The prolonged duration of insertion of the arterial catheter may lead to sepsis, which can be treated by removing the catheter and administering appropriate antibiotic therapy. Other infrequent complications include migration of the catheter tip, catheter occlusion, and bleeding from the catheter insertion site and thrombosis of the femoral artery (3).

Transcatheter Embolization Techniques

Transcatheter embolization techniques are indicated for control of bleeding from large vessels (3, 13), tumor vessels (14, 15), arteriosclerotic vessels (16, 17), and lesions with dual blood yupply (3, 12, 16) because such vessels do not usually respond to vasopressin infusion. The choice of embolization material is diverse and includes autologous blood and autologous tissue as well as synthetic material such as surgical-type gelatin sponge (Gelfoam) (5, 15), polyvinyl alcohol (Ivalon) (3), and oxidized cellulose (Oxycel) (4). Autologous blood clot is the tissue of choice to control bleeding from benign disease because the clot will lyse 12–36 hours after embolization and will be present for a sufficient period of time of control hemostasis (18). Unfortunately, the blood of patients with massive arterial hemorrhage secondary to gynecologic malignancies does not clot rapidly unless thrombin and platelets or epsilon-aminocaproic acid is added to maintain the clot (4). Autologous tissue requires an incision to be made and offers no particular advantage over gelatin sponge. Experience employing gelatin sponge has been most gratifying because it can be embolized through arterial catheters, provokes very little tissue reaction, and persists for 20–50 days after the embolization before recanalization occurs (19).

The gelatin sponge embolization technique requires that standard gelatin sponge pads routinely used in the operating room be diced into small particles 2–3 mm in maximum diameter. The particles are then placed in a syringe containing 2–3 ml of saline. The syringe is shaken and attached to the arterial catheter, and the particles are rapidly infused through the catheter. This technique can be employed routinely for hypogastric artery occlusion but requires multiple embolizations of gelatin sponge particles to accomplish occlusion of the vessel. With the catheter left in place, one can evaluate the effect of the embolization radiographically. When control of bleeding is documented, the catheter may then be removed. Transcatheter gelatin sponge embolization has an advantage over surgical ligation of the hypogastric artery in that the embolization technique occludes peripheral branches of the artery, thereby reducing the component of bleeding from collateral circulation. Hypogastric artery ligation, on the other hand, is confined to the main vascular trunk and does not interrupt collateral circulation (20).

Complications following the transcatheter embolization technique have been infrequently reported. Long-term complications from an indwelling catheter are not a problem. However, occasional instances of an asymptomatic embolus to the lower extremities have been reported (5). Such an embolus is more likely to occur as a result of embolization of the renal artery than the hypogastric artery (20). An occasional episode of an ischemic injury to the bowel has been reported; however, the ischemic injuries resolved spontaneously (4).

An example of the gelatin sponge embolization technique may be seen in Figures 2a and 2b. This 20-year-old patient presented with massive uterine hemorrhage after treatment for high-risk gestational trophoblast disease that became unresponsive to standard therapy. At the time of presentation the patient was febrile to 103°, was found on chest x-ray to have widespread metastases and intrapulmonic hemorrhage, and was unsuited to any form of anesthesia. She was in hemorrhagic shock at the time the procedure was

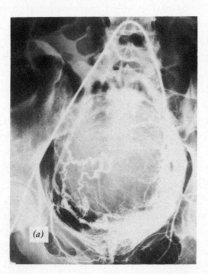 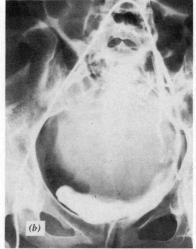

Figure 2. (a) A left hypogastric arteriogram reveals marked hypervascularity of the uterus in a patient with choriocarcinoma. (From Schwartz PE, et al: Control of arterial hemorrhage using percutaneous arterial catheter techniques in patients with gynecologic malignancies. *Gynecol Oncol* 3:276–288, 1975. Reprinted with permission.) (b) Left hypogastric artery occlusion demonstrated following embolization of gelatin sponge particles.

initiated. Bilateral hypogastric arteriograms revealed the bleeding site to be branches of the uterine vessels, and arteriovenous communications compatible with choriocarcinoma were present (Fig. 2a). Bilateral gelatin sponge embolization was performed and the bleeding immediately stopped (Fig. 2b). The patient later received experimental chemotherapy, which was unsuccessful in treating massive recurrent choriocarcinoma.

Balloon Catheter Techniques

Arterial balloon catheter techniques are indicated for control of bleeding from major blood vessels. This technique employs multilumen catheters with inflatable balloons that may be controlled from the distal end of the catheter (6). The balloon should be left inflated for 12–24 hours and subsequently must be removed. The catheter is inserted percutaneously and advanced to the site immediately proximal to the site of arterial injury. The catheter will produce instant control of the bleeding when the balloon is inflated, which can be documented arteriographically. Balloon catheters have an advantage over gelatin sponge embolization in that their position may be readily changed. However, a balloon catheter must be left in place for a prolonged period of time and eventually removed, and it does not occlude peripheral branches of the artery. It will allow the patient to become hemodynamically stable so that she can then undergo a major surgical precedure under more suitable conditions. Catheters with detachable balloons are currently being clinically investigated (21).

An example of control of arterial hemorrhage using a balloon catheter is shown in Figures 3a and 3b. This 59-year-old patient experienced massive hematuria and shock 2 years after treatment for a Stage IIIA squamous cell carcinoma of the cervix. She had undergone a pretreatment selective lymphadenectomy, and bilateral lymphocysts developed postoperatively. The patient then received intense intracavitary and external beam radiation therapy. One year after this treatment the patient underwent an ilioascending colostomy and descending loop colostomy for management of radiation enteritis and proctitis and a ureteroileoneocystotomy for treatment of bilateral hydroureter secondary to the lymphocysts. On admission the patient was in shock. Arteriographic evaluation revealed that the patient had what appeared to be an infected lymphocyst secondary to necrosis of the bladder and was hemorrhaging from a site in the external iliac artery into which the infected lymphocyst had eroded (Fig. 3a). Under these circumstances neither vasopressin infusion nor gelatin sponge embolization would have been appropriate. A Wholey-Edwards balloon catheter was inserted into the right femoral artery and advanced to the site immediately proximal to the injury in the external iliac artery (6). Following inflation of the balloon, hemostasis was observed (Fig. 3b). The patient had excellent collateral circulation that extended to the femoral artery, so ischemic injury to the leg did not occur. The balloon catheter was left inflated for 48 hours. Twenty-four hours later the patient underwent surgical ligation of the external iliac artery. Several hours were required intraoperatively to identify the vessel because the patient had intense scarring in the pelvis due to the initial operation, lymphocyst formation, radiation, and reoperation. The

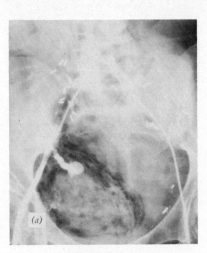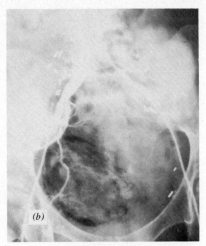

Figure 3. (*a*) A right external iliac arteriogram demonstrating massive hemorrhage into an infected lymphocyst (mottled area) that communicates with the urinary bladder. (From Schwartz PE, et al: Control of arterial hemorrhage using percutaneous arterial catheter techniques in patients with gynecologic malignancies. *Gynecol Oncol* 3:276–288, 1975. Reprinted with permission.) (*b*) A balloon catheter has been inserted via the right femoral artery and advanced to a site immediately proximal to the rent in the right external iliac artery. Complete control of bleeding has been achieved with inflation of the balloon. Collateral circulation to the right femoral artery is demonstrated.

ureteroileoneocystotomy was brought out as an ileal conduit. The patient died 6 weeks postoperatively from sepsis unrelated to the arterial occlusion.

ADDITIONAL INDICATIONS FOR TRANSCATHETER ARTERIAL OCCLUSION

Transcatheter arterial occlusion techniques have been most successfully employed in patients who are actively hemorrhaging from gynecologic malignancies or complications related to the management of gynecologic malignancies (2). However, an occasional patient requires multiple transfusions over prolonged periods of time for minimal but persistent bleeding from tumor sites. These patients often fail to respond to local attempts to control bleeding and may require hospitalization and multiple blood transfusions when symptomatic. A case in point is a patient with vulvar melanoma who, over a 14-year period, had multiple recurrences, including a vaginal recurrence that failed to respond to surgery and radiation treatment. Because this patient required numerous transfusions and hospitalizations to receive the transfusions, it was elected to palliatively occlude the hypogastric arteries. Interestingly enough, the search for the bleeding site revealed that the arterial supply came not only through hypogastric vessels but also from a branch of the femoral artery, as shown in Figure 4*a*. Gelatin sponge transcatheter embolization into the hypogastric artery and the branch of the femoral artery completely stopped the bleeding (Fig. 4*b*) in this unfortunate patient, who eventually died from widespread melanoma.

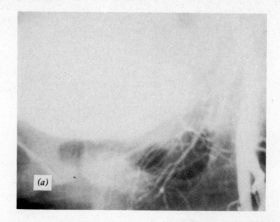

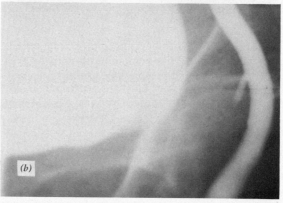

Figure 4. (*a*) Abnormal vascularity to the area of the vagina from the left hypogastric and femoral arteries in a patient with recurrent malignant melanoma. (*b*) Complete occlusion of branch of left femoral artery following selective gelatin sponge embolization of this vessel and left hypogastric artery embolization.

Another use of selective arterial catheterization and transcatheter embolization is in patients who are about to undergo radical cancer surgery and are at high risk for massive bleeding. Such techniques may reduce the risk for these patients and are frequently employed in preoperative management of selected tumors to reduce blood loss (20). An example of this approach to gynecologic malignancies was a patient with recurrent leiomyosarcoma that had originated in the uterus but had metastasized to the buttock. The tumor was causing severe pain, had infiltrated into the bony pelvis, resulting in an unstable pelvis, and had failed to respond to chemotherapy and radiation therapy. Nevertheless, the patient was eager to relieve her symptoms and reduce her functional impairment before receiving experimental therapy. Transcatheter presurgical embolization of the lateral branches of the hypogastric artery dramatically reduced the amount of bleeding from the massive debulking procedure and definitely improved the patient's ability to tolerate the procedure (Figs. 5*a* and 5*b*).

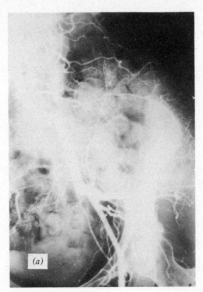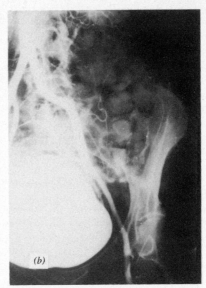

Figure 5. (*a*) An aortogram demonstrating marked vascularity in the area of the left buttock in a patient with a huge metastatic uterine leiomyosarcoma to this site from the left lumbar and hypogastric arteries. (*b*) An aortogram demonstrating a marked decrease in vascularity of the left buttock following gelatin sponge embolization of the left hypogastric and two lumbar arteries.

REFERENCES

1. Benjamin HB, Becker AB, Aquino E: Collateral circulation after massive occlusion of pelvic vessels. *Surg Gynecol Obstet* 117:20–24, 1963.

2. Schwartz PE, Goldstein HM, Wallace S, et al: Control of arterial hemorrhage using percutaneous arterial catheter techniques in patients with gynecologic malignancies. *Gynecol Oncol* 3:276–288, 1975.

3. Waltman AC, Greenfield AJ, Novelline RA, et al: Pyloroduodenal bleeding and intraarterial vasopressin: Clinical results. *Am J Roentgenol* 133:643–646, 1979.

4. Bookstein JJ, Chlosta EM, Foley D, et al: Transcatheter hemostasis of gastrointestinal bleeding using modified autologous clot. *Radiology* 113:277–285, 1974.

5. Tadavarthy SM, Knight L, Ovitt TW, et al: Therapeutic transcatheter arterial embolization. *Radiology* 111:13–16, 1974.

6. Wholey MH, Stockdale R, Hung TK: A percutaneous balloon catheter for the immediate control of hemorrhage. *Radiology* 95:65–71, 1970.

7. Freeney PC, Bush WH, Kidd R: Transcatheter occlusive therapy of genitourinary abnormalities using isobutyl 2-cyanoacrylate (bucrylate). *Am J Roentgenol* 133:647–656, 1979.

8. Anderson JH, Wallace S, Gianturco C, et al: "Mini" Gianturco stainless steel coils for transcatheter vascular occlusion. *Radiology* 132:301–303, 1979.

9. Baum S, Nusbaum M: The control of gastrointestinal hemorrhage by selective mesenteric arterial infusion of vasopressin. *Radiology* 98:497–505, 1971.

10. Marubbio AT: Antidiuretic hormone effect of Pitressin during continuous Pitression infusion. *Gastroenterology* 62:1103, 1972.

11. Baum S, Rosch J, Dotter CT, Ring EJ, et al: Selective mesenteric arterial infusions in the management of massive diverticular hemorrhage. *N Engl J Med* 288:1269–1272, 1973.

12. Conn HO, Ramsby GR, Storer EH: Selective intraarterial vasopressin in the treatment of upper gastrointestinal hemorrhage. *Gastroenterology* 63:643–645, 1972.

13. Nusbaum M, Baum S: Radiographic demonstration of unknown sites of gastrointestinal bleeding. *Surg Forum* 14:374–375, 1963.

14. Bookstein JJ, Goldstein HM: Successful management of postbiopsy arteriovenous fistula with selective arterial embolization. *Radiology* 109:535–536, 1973.

15. Lang EK: Superselective arterial catheterization as a vehicle for delivering radioactive infarct particles to tumor. *Radiology* 98:391–399, 1971.

16. Rosch J, Dotter CT, Antonovic R: Selective vasoconstrictor infusion in the management of arteriocapillary gastrointestinal hemorrhage. *Am J Roentgenol Radium Ther Nucl Med* 116:279–288, 1972.

17. Brant B, Rosch J, Krippaehne WW: Experiences with angiography in diagnosis and treatment of acute gastrointestinal bleeding of various etiologies: Preliminary report. *Ann Surg* 176:419–433, 1972.

18. Goldstein HM, Medellin H, Ben-Menachem Y, Wallace S: Transcatheter arterial embolization in the management of bleeding in the cancer patient. *Radiology* 115:603–608, 1975.

19. Smith DC, Wyatt JF: Embolization of the hypogastric arteries in the control of massive vaginal hemorrhage. *Obstet Gynecol* 49:317–322, 1977.

20. Athanasoulis CA: Therapeutic applications of angiography. *N Engl J Med* 302:1117–1125, 1980.

21. Debrun G, Legre J, Kasbarian M, et al: Endovascular occlusion of vertebral fistulae by detachable balloons with conservation of the vertebral blood flow. *Radiology* 130:141–147, 1979.

4

Complications Related to the Nonradiated Gastrointestinal Tract

Gregorio Delgado

ANASTOMOSIS TECHNIQUES AND THE MANAGEMENT OF COMPLICATIONS

Although different techniques are used in small bowel anastomosis, certain general principles should be observed to achieve success. Good bowel preparation, including the addition of antibiotics, is an important preventive measure. During surgery, the use of intestinal clamps is advised to prevent spillage of intestinal contents, especially with the open technique. An end-to-end anastomosis provides adequate results. A side-to-side anastomosis ensures a good stoma and, usually, a good blood supply. The drawback of the latter type of anastomosis is the possibility of dilation of the distal portion of the afferent loop. Sometimes, a pouch is created, producing a blind loop syndrome. For this reason, an end-to-end anastomosis is advisable in the intact nonradiated bowel (1, 2).

Ovarian cancer patients may have recurrent cancers that have spread through the peritoneal surfaces, encroaching on and obstructing loops of bowel and other viscera. In such patients, resection is difficult and complicated. Instead, a bypass procedure with mucous fistulas of the proximal and distal ends of the obstructed bowel (Fig. 1) is recommended.

Management of Complications of Anastomosis by the Conventional Suture Technique

After bowel resection, continuity of the gastrointestinal tract can be established by end-to-end or side-to-side anastomosis. For many years, the use of suture material in performing anastomosis has been advocated. Recently, however, the use of a stapler has become very popular because it shortens operating time without ill effects (3).

45

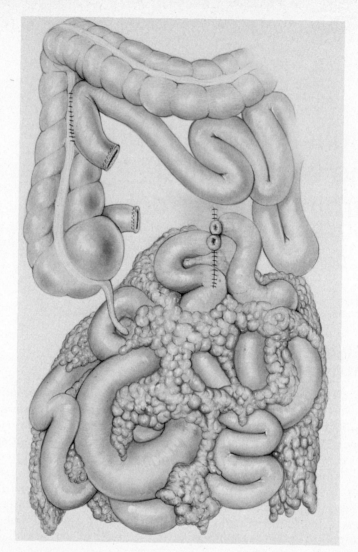

Figure 1. Conventional suture technique. Recurrent cancers spreading through the peritoneal surface encroaching and obstructing several loops of bowel with other viscera. In sick and debilitated patients, a bowel bypass with mucous fistulas is preferable to a total bowel resection.

There has been some reluctance to use staple gun anastomosis in a radiated bowel; nevertheless, there are some reports in the literature of great success using the staple gun after heavy pelvic radiation (4).

Bowel anastomosis techniques can be divided into two classes: those using sutures in either the closed or open method, and those using the staple gun. In the open method of suturing, the full thickness of the bowel, including the mucosa, is closed with an absorbable material, usually 3-0 G.I. catgut. The sutures may be placed in an interrupted or a continuous fashion (Fig. 2a). In the closed method (Fig. 2b), seromuscular sutures are used. A second row of sutures of nonabsorbable material is recommended for both methods.

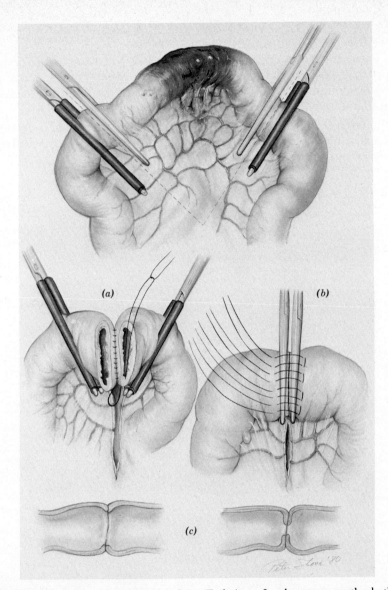

Figure 2. Anastomosis techniques. (*a*) *Open Technique.* In the open method, the full thickness of the bowel, including the mucosa, is closed with an absorbable material, usually 3-0 G.I. catgut. (*b*) *Closed Technique.* In the closed method, seromuscular sutures are used. (*c*) Narrowing of the lumen with the closed technique.

The open method, which assures good closure under direct vision, is preferred because it reduces the chances of narrowing the lumen and facilitates placement of the sutures (2) (Fig. 2*c*). Hamilton (5) has shown that in animals the open method requires fewer sutures for an adequate anastomosis. The advantage of the closed method is that it prevents any abdominal contamination by spillage.

There are several complications in suture anastomosis that should be avoided:

1. Encroachment of the lumen of the bowel with surface tissue should be

avoided because it produces bowel obstruction (Fig. 3a). The open method facilitates prevention of this problem (Fig. 3b).

2. To ensure that the edges of the anastomosis will have a sufficient blood supply, an oblique division of the bowel is advised. This diagonal division gives maximum access to the straight blood vessels that supply the small bowel and that derive from a series of arches (6) (Figs. 4a and 4b).

3. Although a clear surface of the bowel on the mesentery side is needed for a good anastomosis, overdissection of the blood vessels in this area will produce necrosis and leakage (Figs. 5a and 5b).

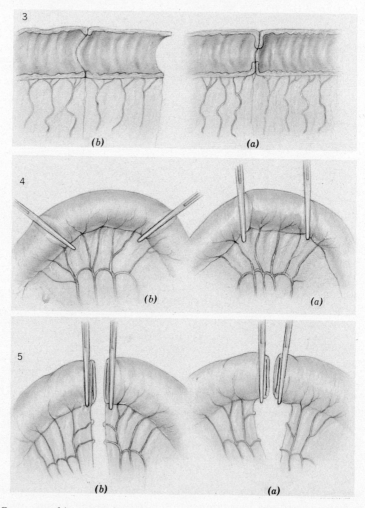

Figure 3. Correct and incorrect bowel anastomoses. (a) Including large amounts of tissue in the bowel can produce bowel obstruction. (b) The open technique prevents encroachment of the bowel lumen.

Figure 4. (a) Clamps indicating incorrect straight incision of the bowel, resulting in a poor blood supply to the anastomosis. (b) Diagonal clamps indicating correct incision of the bowel, ensuring a good blood supply to the anastomosis.

Figure 5. (a) Over dissection of blood vessels, resulting in necrosis and leakage. (b) Proper dissection of blood vessels.

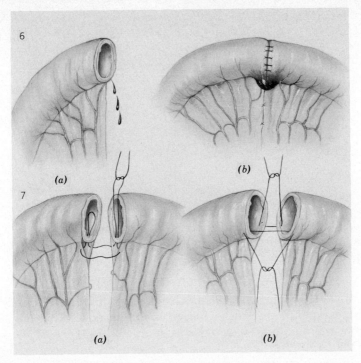

Figure 6. Correct and incorrect bowel anastomoses. (*a*) Careful hemostasis, preventing hematoma. (*b*) A hematoma resulting from lack of hemostasis.
Figure 7. (*a*) Not including the mesentery of the bowel in suturing, resulting in leakage. (*b*) Including the mesentery of the bowel in suturing, preventing leakage.

4. All bleeding vessels on the edges of the bowel should be carefully clamped and ligated, to prevent a hematoma in the mesentery of the bowel (Figs. 6*a* and 6*b*).

5. The mesentery should be included in the suturing of the mesentery angle, to prevent the anastomosis from leaking (Figs. 7*a* and 7*b*).

6. When the second row of nonabsorbable sutures is placed, the mucosa of the bowel should be covered by the serosa and the edges approximated.

7. If there are distended loops of small bowel, they should be decompressed before anastomosis. Decompression is accomplished by first placing a pursestring suture of chromic material in the loop and then inserting a suction catheter.

Management of Complications of Anastomosis by the Automatic Staple Technique

Automatic stapling instruments (Fig. 8) have been viewed with enthusiasm since the publication of several reports of good results in bowel resection and anastomosis. The use of these instruments has become popular in nearly every surgical area associated with the gastrointestinal tract (3, 7–15). They have also been successfully used in cardiovascular surgery (16), bronchial stump closure (17), radiated bowel (4), and pelvic exenteration (20).

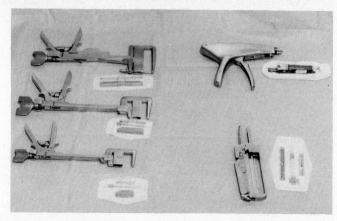

Figure 8. Automatic stapling gun instruments (U.S. Surgical Corporation). The TA instrument in three sizes (left); the LDS instrument (upper right); the GIA instrument (lower right).

Use of automatic stapling instruments is not entirely without complications. Postoperative complications that have been reported include stenosis (21) and bleeding from the anastomosis because of mechanical failure of the stapling instrument (22). Intraluminal extrusion of staples has also been documented (23). Although the formation of stones in ileal conduits closed with staples has been reported (18, 19), this complication may be prevented by using a crushing clamp and suturing with chromic pursestring in front of the metallic clips (20). It is prudent to periodically test the staples to be sure they have not caused complications.

Chassin et al. (3) reviewed 812 operative procedures in the gastrointestinal tract; in 472 of them, staple anastomoses were performed, resulting in a 2.8% complication rate; in 296 suture anastomoses, there was a 3% complication rate. Results were equally good with both techniques. (The remaining 44 procedures combined staples with sutures.) Similar results were found in a study at the Gynecologic Oncology Division of Georgetown University Hospital (20).

The common finding in these reports is that the staple technique has definite advantages over conventional surgical procedures (11, 20). Stapling decreases operating time, results in less contamination of the abdominal cavity, and facilitates a better blood supply because of the B-shaped staples (4). Understandably, there has been some reluctance to use staple anastomosis in the radiated and debilitated patient, but Photopulos et al. (4) performed gastrointestinal resection and anastomosis in 17 patients who had had radiation therapy, and no complications related to the anastomoses occurred.

Several reports have indicated great success using the staple method. Chassin favorably compared use of the staple gun with use of conventional suturing in anastomoses, showing very good results and the shortening of operating time (3). Photopulos et al. (4) reported that 19 patients with radiation therapy had had successful anastomoses performed with staples.

The Gynecology Oncology Division at Georgetown University Medical Center compared the two techniques in 76 patients with major gastrointestinal anastomoses and resections (Table 1). All these patients had had advanced gynecologic malignancies, and the majority had had previous therapy.

Surgical procedures on patients in whom staple anastomosis was performed took less time and caused no serious complications. Results were as good as, if not better than, with the conventional suture technique. Twenty-nine patients underwent 63 stapling procedures compared with 47 patients who underwent conventional suturing procedures. Table 2 lists the different surgical procedures performed in patients with staple and conventional suture anastomoses. Some of these patients had more than one anastomosis procedure. Table 3 shows the different therapies these patients received before bowel surgery. The study included patients with radical pelvic operations—12 with pelvic exenterations and 29 with urinary diversions—as shown in Table 4.

Complications related to the anastomosis procedure itself are shown in Table 5. Fistulas in the bypassed bowel occurred in two staple anastomosis patients, one enterocutaneous fistula and one in the bypassed bowel, 3 and 6 months after

Table 1. Number of Cancer Patients Undergoing Staple and Conventional Anastomoses

Type of Cancer	Staple	Suture	Total
Cervix	14	24	38
Ovary	9	16	25
Uterus	6	5	11
Other	—	2	2
Total	29	47	76

SOURCE: Delgado G: Use of the automatic stapler in urinary conduit diversions and pelvic exenterations. *Gynecol Oncol* 10:1, 1980.

Table 2. Number and Types of Surgical Procedures Received by Cancer Patients Undergoing Staple and Conventional Suture Anastomoses

Type of Surgery	Staple	Suture	Total
Colostomy	13	22	35
Intestinal urinary diversion	16	13	29
Hemicolectomy	1	2	3
Anterior resection of sigmoid colon	4	4	8
Small bowel resection	21	20	41
Bowel bypass	11	13	24
Total	66	74	140

SOURCE: Delgado G: Use of the automatic stapler urinary conduit diversions and pelvic exenterations. *Gynecol Oncol* 10:1, 1980.

Including three ureteroileoneocystotomies.

Including three mucous fistulas.

Table 3. Types of Therapy Received by Cancer Patients Undergoing Staple and Conventional Suture Anastomoses Before Bowel Surgery

Prior Therapy	Staple	Suture	Total
X-ray therapy only	2	5	7
Other single therapy	3	6	9
Surgery and chemotherapy	15	17	32
Surgery, x-ray therapy, and chemotherapy	3	6	9
No prior therapy	—	2	2
Total	23	36	59

SOURCE: Delgado G: Use of the automatic stapler in urinary conduit diversions and pelvic exenterations. *Gynecol Oncol* 10:1, 1980.

Total number of patients undergoing staple anastomoses with prior x-ray therapy: 20.

Total number of patients undergoing suture anastomoses with prior x-ray therapy: 28.

Table 4. Number of Cancer Patients Undergoing Staple and Conventional Suture Anastomoses with Urinary Diversions and Pelvic Exenterations

Type of Surgery	Staple	Suture	Total
Pelvic exenteration	8	4	12
Urinary diversion	16	13	29
Total	24	17	41

SOURCE: Delgado G: Use of the automatic stapler in urinary conduit diversions and pelvic exenterations. *Gynecol Oncol* 10:1, 1980.

Table 5. Number of Patients with Complications After Surgical Staple and Conventional Suture Anastomoses

Complication	Staple	Suture	Total
Enterocutaneous fistula	—	1	1
Enterovaginal bypass bowel fistula	1	1	2
Sepsis	1	1	2
Short bowel syndrome	2	2	4
Small bowel obstruction	—	1	1
Wound infection	6	7	13
Total	10	13	23

SOURCE: Delgado G: Use of the automatic stapler in urinary conduit diversions and pelvic exenterations. *Gynecol Oncol* 10:1, 1980.

Sepsis leading to death.

the operations had been performed. In four patients short bowel syndrome developed.

At the present time, use of the staple gun for intestinal tract anastomoses is preferred, even for low colonic anastomoses and urinary diversions. The staple gun facilitates a clean procedure and minimal spillage of the intestinal contents.

Ligation and Division Stapler

The ligation and division stapler (LDS) permits rapid ligation and division of the mesentery of the bowel. It can also be used to detach the omentum from the transverse colon and the stomach in cases of total omentectomy, or to make an omental lid to cover the pelvic floor after pelvic exenterations (20). Complications (Fig. 9) using the LDS instrument include the following:

1. If too much tissue has been divided, the staples cannot secure the blood vessels and bleeding may occur, necessitating the use of hemostatic clamps and sutures (Fig. 10).
2. If the instrument is not properly assembled, it can lock after it has fired a staple. When locking occurs, the segment of tissue must be divided between two clamps and tied (Fig. 11).
3. A marginal blood vessel may be missed by the staples, a situation leading to bleeding, retraction, and a hematoma. The hematoma should be removed and the blood vessels clamped and ligated.
4. Suddenly moving the stapling instrument may rupture blood vessels and produce bleeding.
5. Bleeding and a hematoma may occur from the two openings created so that the instrument may be easily introduced into the tissue breech. These problems may be corrected with ligation (Fig. 12).

Thoracic-Abdominal Instrument

The thoracic-abdominal instrument (TA) will place a double line of staples, 30 mm, 50 mm, or 90 mm in size. The staples come in 3.5 mm and 4.8 mm sizes, the choice depending on the thickness of the tissue. This stapling instrument can be used to close the cut ends of the bowel with a double row of staples. In side-to-side anastomoses it is also used after the gastrointestinal anastomosis instrument (GIA) to close the remaining open edges of the bowel (Fig. 13c).

Several complications can result from using the TA instruments. One of these is a failure to lift up both edges of the bowel together, so that an opening is left when the staples are fired, which causes the anastomosis to leak (Fig. 14d). This complication is avoided by placing sutures on the edges of the bowel that is to be closed. The edges of the bowel are then lifted by the sutures, to be sure they are at the same level and above the suture line of the staples. If an opening remains after the stapling, it should be closed with suture material (Fig. 14e). Sometimes a few nonabsorbable sutures are also necessary to reinforce the closure.

Gastrointestinal Anastomosis Instrument

The gastrointestinal anastomosis instrument (GIA) places two rows of staples that can be transected in the middle with a knife attached to the instrument. The instrument is used in the following procedures:

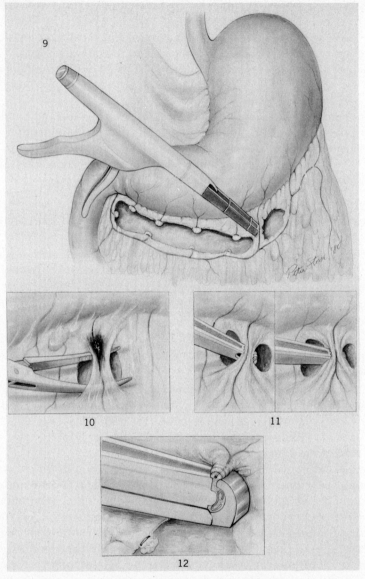

Figure 9. Complications of LDS instruments. The LDS stapler detaching the omentum from the greater curvature of the stomach.

Figure 10. Complications of LDS instruments. Too much tissue to staple adequately, which may result in bleeding.

Figure 11. Complications of LDS instruments. An LDS instrument locking itself after firing.

Figure 12. Complications of LDS instruments. An LDS instrument being introduced into two openings, which may result in bleeding.

54

1. *Side-to-Side and Functional End-to-End Anastomoses* (Fig. 13*b*).
2. *Transection of the Bowel.* Any place in the large or small bowel can be transected because the instrument places rows of staples on each side and the knife can be used to cut between them (Fig. 13*a*).
3. *Pelvic Exenterations.* The GIA instrument may be used to transect the distal and proximal parts of the sigmoid colon, and this segment can be used as a sigmoid conduit. (Figs. 15*a* and 15*b*). The GIA instrument also allows the colostomy end to remain closed until after it has been pulled through the skin (Fig. 15*c*). The mesentery of the bowel and the omentum around the transverse colon and stomach can be easily detached with the use of the LDS (Fig. 9).
4. *Urinary Diversions.* The bowel is transected in two places, and this segment is closed on both ends. If the small bowel is being used as a conduit, the other two ends can be anastomosed using the GIA and the TA instruments.

   There has been some reluctance to use staples in urinary diversions because urine, after coming into contact with a metallic surface, may produce stones (19). After the bowel has been closed clamp with the Kelly. However, 3-0 chromic placed in a continuous fashion in front of the staples will prevent the urine from coming in contact with the metallic surface and thus prevent the formation of calculi (20). (Fig. 15*b* and 15*d*).

Several complications can result from using the GIA instrument:

1. If the mesentery of the bowel is included in the GIA instrument, bleeding occurs because the staples are not hemostatic. The LDS should be used for cutting blood vessels (Fig. 14*a*).
2. After the bowel anastomosis has been performed, the row of staples should be inspected. If bleeding is present, blood vessels should be clamped and ligated with chromic sutures (Fig. 14*b*).
3. Both ends of the bowel should be at the same level in each arm of the GIA instrument. If not, a large opening will remain (Fig. 14*f*), to be closed by the TA instrument.
4. If the arms of the GIA instrument are inserted in the submucosa instead of the lumen, a faulty anastomosis will result (Fig. 14*g*).
5. A hematoma may result if the mesentery of the bowel is stapled and transected by the GIA instrument. The blood vessels must be clamped and ligated and the hematoma removed (Fig. 14*c*).

Enteroenteroanastomosis Instrument
When a resection of the sigmoid colon is very low, anastomosis with the rectal stump can be difficult. If the rectal stump is sufficiently long, the GIA instrument can be used (13). In most rectosigmoid resections for cancer of the female genital tract, the enteroenteroanastomosis instrument (EEA) is useful (14, 12) (Fig. 16). Fain et al. (15) pioneered the use of the EEA in 20 dogs in 1975. Subsequently Goligher et al. (21) reported using the EEA instrument in 62 patients with high anastomoses, without complications. Of 24 patients with low anastomoses, 2 had clinical evidence of dehiscence, 3 had moderate bleeding that stopped spontaneously, and 2 had strictures. Fewer complications were reported

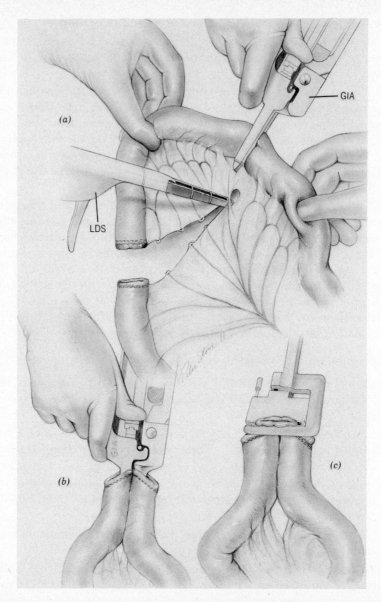

Figure 13. Bowel anastomosis with the automatic stapler. (*a*) The GIA instrument transecting small bowel segments, two rows of staples and a knife cutting between. The LDS instrument is shown cutting the mesentery of the small bowel. (*b*) Using the GIA instrument for end-to-end anastomosis. (*c*) The TA instrument being used to close the remaining open ends of the bowel after the GIA instrument has been used.

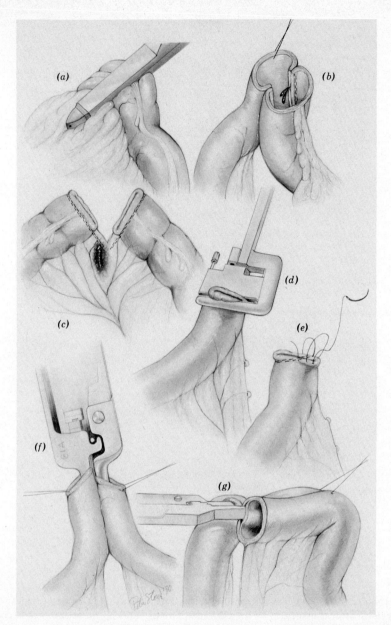

Figure 14. Complications with the automatic stapler. (*a*) Including the mesentery of the small bowel in the GIA instrument, resulting in bleeding. (*b*) Inspection for bleeding after an anastomosis. (*c*) An ovoid hematoma in the mesentery of the bowel after being stapled and transected by the GIA instrument. (*d*) The edges of the bowel not included in the TA instrument, leaving an opening. (*e*) Closing the bowel edges with suture material after incomplete TA instrument stapling. (*f*) The bowel edges at different levels of each arm of the GIA instrument, resulting in a large opening that must be closed. (*g*) An arm of the GIA instrument improperly inserted in the bowel submucosa.

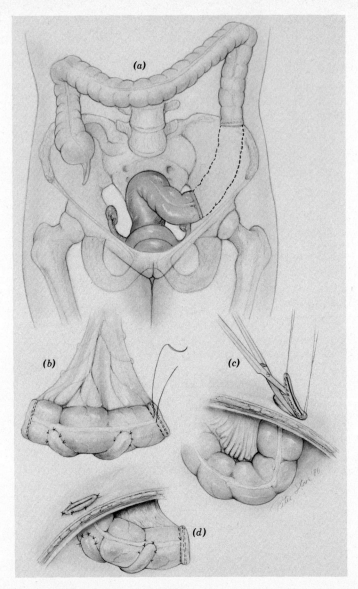

Figure 15. Automatic stapler in pelvic exenteration. (*a* and *b*) The proximal and distal sigmoid colon after transection by the GIA instrument. This segment can now become the sigmoid conduit. (*c*) The proximal end of the colon, which becomes the stoma of the colostomy, closed by the GIA instrument until it has been pulled through the skin. (*b* and *d*) Chromic sutures placed proximal to the metallic staples prevent stone formation.

with this technique when these patients were compared with a group of patients who had had their anastomoses performed with suture material (21).

The EEA instrument is specifically designed for low colon rectal anastomoses, especially in anterior resection or in pelvic exenteration in which preservation of the sphincter is attempted. The instrument is introduced via the anus into the abdomen. The proximal and distal segments of the bowel are approximated and

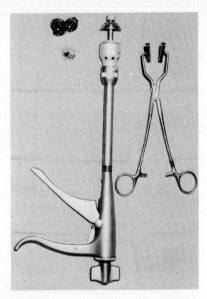

Figure 16. EEA instrument for low colorectal anastomosis. The instrument in the upper right is for putting a pursestring suture around the edges of the sigmoid. The two dougnut-shaped pieces of tissue seen on the left will ensure a good anastomosis.

mechanically anastomosed by a circular double row of staples; a circular knife cuts the excess in between. A secure anastomosis is performed in less time and with a lower rate of complications with the EEA instruments than with suture material (21).

1. If all tissues are not included in the two rows of staples, there may be leakage that can be corrected by hand suturing.
2. Stenosis of the anastomosis may occur. It can be avoided after surgery by giving patients bulky residual types of food that will act as a dilator. Occasional finger dilation may be necessary.
3. Bleeding from the anastomosis site may result. It should stop spontaneously. Occasionally, however, a suture may be necessary.

THE SMALL BOWEL

Management of Complications

Nonviable Bowel
It is essential that the bowel involved in an anastomosis have a good blood supply. If unhealthy bowel is used, major complications will arise. All unhealthy bowel should be resected and anastomosis performed only with the edges of very healthy bowel. Otherwise leakage of the anastomosis will result in generalized peritonitis requiring emergency surgery. If there is any question about the viability of a bowel segment, it should be resected. However, an ischemic and traumatized bowel can resume its normal appearance, regaining its pink color,

after warm packs are placed around it. If pulsation of the small blood vessels and peristalsis can be seen, the bowel can be assumed to be viable.

Inadvertent Laceration of the Bowel Wall

Laceration of the bowel wall is a common complication, especially in gynecologic surgery, because of the multiplicity of surgical procedures, such as successive laparotomies for evaluation of cancer, which may result in multiple adhesions of the abdominal cavity. After radiation therapy, loops of bowel often adhere to the anterior abdominal wall, increasing the risk of injury to the bowel when the abdominal cavity is entered. When possible, previous surgical scars should be avoided when opening the peritoneum by retroperitoneal dissection; the opening should be made laterally away from the previous surgery or the field of radiation.

If a small laceration occurs, the bowel should be freed from adhesions and the edges well identified. The laceration should be closed in two layers with 3-0 chromic catgut interrupted or running sutures, through the full thickness of the bowel. The serosa is then closed with a nonabsorbable material, usually 3-0 silk, using a gastrointestinal needle. Closure should be made perpendicular to the longer axis of the laceration, to avoid decreasing the bowel lumen (Fig. 17).

Obstruction

The most common causes of early postoperative bowel obstruction are adhesions, internal hernias due to a defect in the mesentery of the bowel after anastomosis, excessive narrowing of the stoma after anastomosis, partial volvulus, and acute angulation of the distended loops of the bowel (22, 23).

The first symptom of bowel obstruction is usually abdominal distention, followed by colicky pain, hyperactivity, air and fluid levels that are revealed on a

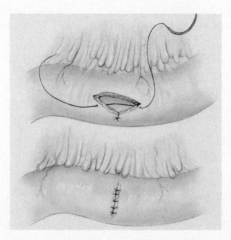

Figure 17. Inadvertent laceration of the bowel wall. Lacerations of the small bowel are repaired with a double layer of sutures perpendicular to the longer axis of the laceration to avoid decreasing the bowel lumen.

flat plate roentgenogram of the abdomen, and the absence of gas in the rectum and colon. Bowel obstruction should be differentiated from an adynamic ileus that also causes abdominal distention but does not cause bowel sounds or colicky pain.

The treatment of bowel obstruction requires adequate fluids and electrolytes and continuous nasogastric suction (24). A long intestinal tube introduced into the small bowel is also of great help if the obstruction results from angulation of the bowel. These measures are often enough to relieve the obstruction. If the patient is improving, the therapy should continue until the tenth or twelfth postoperative day. If the symptoms continue, surgical intervention is required. During this period of observation, the possibility of a compromised blood supply should be kept in mind. If this is a strong possibility, immediate surgical intervention is indicated.

Removal of adhesions is sometimes all that is necessary during surgery. However, a resection with an anastomosis is usually indicated, particularly if several intestinal loops of bowel are involved in the obstruction.

Recurrent Bowel Obstruction

Recurrent bowel obstruction is usually due to adhesions after multiple laparotomies. Sometimes obstruction threatens to create an endless cyclical situation in which removal of adhesions to correct an obstruction is followed by a recurrence of obstruction. Under these circumstances, more conservative management, such as nasogastric suction, is advisable.

When surgery is indicated, the surgical plication procedure described by Noble (25) is appropriate. Important technical points of plication are as follows: (1) The bowel should be sutured along the mesenteric margin starting and ending about 3 cm from turns. (2) All row areas of bowel should be covered with other loops of bowel (26). Others recommend splinting the small bowel with a long intestinal tube up to the ileocecal valve after surgically freeing the intestine from adhesions (27).

Cancer-Related Bowel Obstruction

Bowel obstruction resulting from multiple secondary growths of cancer involving several loops of small bowel is usually associated with ovarian cancer because of the unique conglutinated spread of this type of malignancy. Obstructions of multiple loops of small bowel are also caused by abdominal radiation. Identifying the direction of peristalsis of the bowel is important in evaluating cancer-related obstruction (28). When this type of obstruction is suspected, a long intestinal tube should be introduced; sometimes fluoroscopy helps to pass the long tube through the pylorus. If peristalsis is present, the mercury bagged tube will be carried to the obstructed loop of the bowel. During laparotomy, the long tube can be followed to the tip, to indicate the length of the unobstructed bowel. This unobstructed loop of bowel can then be used for the bypass, especially when large masses of resected tumor or portions of radiated bowel are present. If a bypass procedure is used, the distal and proximal loops of bowel should be exteriorized as a mucous fistula to prevent a blind loop syndrome and to isolate the loops of bypass bowel from the rest of the gastrointestinal tract (Fig. 1).

Before the bypass procedure, a barium enema should be performed to assess the patency of the large bowel (29).

Vascular Compromise of the Bowel

Strangulation of the bowel is a serious complication occurring in protracted mechanical bowel obstruction with overdistention of the intestinal lumen. Failure to diagnose or correct an obstruction causes it to progress to vascular compromise.

Anytime a patient has symptoms of bowel obstruction, the physician should be alert for signs of vascular compromise. If the condition of the patient deteriorates so much that necrosis of the bowel and gangrene occur, death is likely. Barnett and colleagues (23) reported a mortality rate of 39% in 130 patients with gangrenous bowel; 20% of the hernia patients died; 23% of the patients with adhesions died, and, 74% of the patients with mesenteric insufficiency that included arterial and venous thrombosis died (Table 6). The single most important factor in successful outcome in the management of bowel obstruction is early surgical intervention before strangulation and gangrene can occur.

Vascular compromise should be suspected when the following signs and symptoms develop in a patient: continuous and severe abdominal pain, a palpable abdominal mass, generalized rebound tenderness in the abdomen, a pulse rate of 100 (with no other plausible explanation), a leukocyte count of 10,000 or more, and a hypoactive abdomen. Fever and a rigid abdomen are consistent with a strangulated obstruction. Aspiration of the abdominal cavity producing blood or dark abdominal fluid corroborates the presence of strangulation. The differential diagnosis between a simple and a strangulating obstruction is very difficult except in advanced cases (23).

If vascular compromise is suspected, the patient should have surgery for resection of the compromised bowel and possible reanastomosis, if no perforation has taken place. If perforation has taken place and there is massive contamination of the abdominal cavity, resection of the strangulated or necrotic bowel with exteriorization of the proximal and distal loop of the gastrointestinal tract should be performed. The abdominal cavity should be completely lavaged and antibiotic therapy instituted at once. This complication is often fatal, so treatment should be immediate and vigorous, to prevent gangrene (22).

Table 6. Outcome of Patients with Bowel Gangrene

			Mortality Rates	
Etiology	Number of Patients	Total Deaths	Preventable Deaths	Probable Preventable Deaths
Adhesions	43	23%	13%	4%
Hernia	45	20%	23%	9%
Mesenteric insufficiency	42	74%	67%	67%
Total	130			

SOURCE: Adapted from Barnett WO, Pedro AB, Williamson, JW: A current appraisal of problems with gangrenous bowel. *Am Surgery* 183:653, 1975.

Excision of Meckel's Diverticulum

A Meckel's diverticulum in the antimesenteric section of the ileum may be an incidental finding on laparotomy. This problem may lead to complications such as perforation with peritonitis, which closely mimics appendicitis, obstruction, intussusception, hernia, and volvulus of the small intestine.

If the diverticulum is discovered during surgery, it should be removed unless removal increases the operative risk (30). Before removal, the blood vessels coming from the mesentery of the bowel toward the diverticulum should be ligated and transected. The clamp should be placed at about 45 degrees to the transverse axis of the small bowel, to prevent its narrowing. If the base of the diverticulum is wide, it should be excised parallel to the axis of the bowel and sutured transversely. After the diverticulum has been removed, the opening should be closed with an atraumatic needle and 3-0 chromic inverted sutures. Then, the seromuscular layer should be closed in a watertight fashion with a layer of silk (31).

Anastomosis Leakage Leading to an Enterocutaneous Fistula

A watertight anastomosis prevents leakage, a complication that eventually leads to abscess or enterocutaneous fistula formation (Fig. 18). If the leakage is minimal, antibiotic therapy and bowel suction with prevention of bowel distention will probably heal the defect. However, if the leakage is significant, peritonitis and generalized sepsis develop, which may lead to death. If the infection is localized, an abscess may be the only problem. Immediate drainage and antibiotic therapy should be established to prevent deterioration.

If the abscess is not properly diagnosed and corrected, the next step in the progression of the condition is the development of an enterocutaneous fistula (Fig. 19). High intestinal fistulas produce a large output containing pancreatic enzymes that erode the skin, an erosion that is very difficult to control. Low intestinal fistulas have less output and erosion is easier to control. If there is no distal bowel obstruction or tumor, most fistulas, especially low-output fistulas, will close spontaneously (32). High-output fistulas will take longer to close and require therapy. The treatment for this condition is hyperalimentation, continuous nasogastric suction, and continuous suction of the fistula to prevent skin excoriation. Hyperalimentation that facilitates medical management is sufficient for most patients (33). Dudrick (34) reports spontaneous fistula closure in 70.5% of patients treated with hyperalimentation.

If surgery is needed after a fistula develops, there should be a delay of 30−40 days before fistula repair is attempted. The abdomen is then incised in an area of unscarred tissue and the fistula clearly identified and dissected. It is important to identify the afferent limbs of the fistula before repair. A long intestinal tube can be helpful in this identification. If the intestinal tract is free from obstruction and the fistula is small, a diamond-shaped resection of the fistula can be performed and the fistula closed with chromic catgut continuous sutures. A second layer of 3-0 silk is placed in the seromuscular layers with an atraumatic needle; usually, drainage will not be necessary. If the fistula is larger, resection and anastomosis may be required to repair the fistula (35).

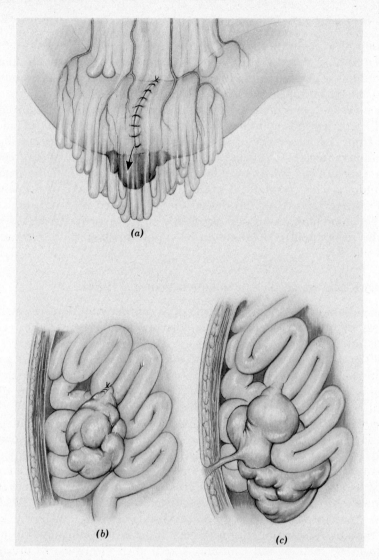

Figure 18. Anastomosis leakage. (*a*) Leakage from an anastomosis. (*b*) Leakage leading to an abscess. (*c*) An abscess developing into an enterocutaneous fistula.

THE LARGE BOWEL, RECTUM, AND ANUS

Complications of Sigmoidoscopy and Colonoscopy Perforation

Perforation of the large bowel can be caused by too much pressure when air is insufflated to obtain complete dilatation. Perforation can also be caused by an explosion of colonic gases when fulguration devices are used. The colon may also be perforated by incorrect application of the sigmoidoscope. Perforation of the colon by the colonoscope occurs rarely, however, with experienced operators. Perforation may also occur with the barium enema procedure. This type of

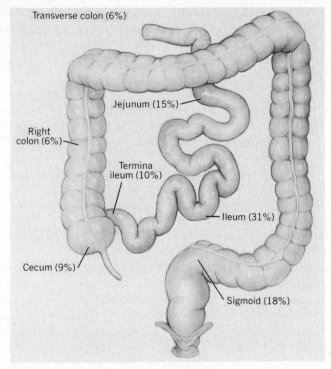

Figure 19. Anatomic locations of enteric and colonic fistulas and percentage of fistula occurrence in each location. (From Edmunds, 1960).

perforation happens when the enema is forced into the colon in the presence of neoplastic growth occluding the colon.

Perforation requires an immediate operation to obtain closure. Sometimes a patient requires a colostomy if contamination of the abdominal cavity has taken place (36).

Cecostomy

Cecostomy is a procedure that may be used very efficiently in a debilitated patient who has an obstruction of the transverse colon. It is a seldom-used procedure because the transverse colostomy tube should be placed appropriately, projecting into the lumen of the cecum. A cecostomy is usually a temporary procedure until the patient is stronger and ready for further treatment. Retention of the cecostomy for too long erodes and perforates the cecum. If a fistulous tract is present after removal of the cecostomy, it will take about 10–12 days to close. In a previously radiated patient, the fistula will not close; it will become permanent (37).

Colostomy

Generally, a colostomy is performed in gynecologic malignancies under two conditions: first, as a replacement of the rectum after radical pelvic surgery in which removal of the rectosigmoid area is required; and second, as a procedure following injury, surgical resection, or anastomosis of the lower rectosigmoid colon. Under the first condition, when resection of the rectum is necessary, the colostomy will be permanent. Under the second condition, a temporary colostomy will suffice.

An end colostomy is the procedure of choice for a permanent colostomy, especially after a rectosigmoid resection. However, a well-placed loop colostomy can meet all the needs of a colostomy. If complete isolation of the gastrointestinal tract is needed, the distal loop can be closed by a pursestring suture (38), with the proximal loop becoming an end colostomy (Fig. 20). If there is a possibility of obstruction in the distal segment of the colon, the distal loop should be left open as a mucous fistula.

There is a tendency to avoid performing protective colostomies after injury, resection, or anastomosis when the tissue is healthy (39). However, for patients who have infection or extensive cancer and are undergoing radiation therapy, a protective colostomy is a good procedure.

A well-planned colostomy includes adequate site selection before surgery. The best site for a colostomy is the junction of the descending colon and the sigmoid colon, so that the distal loop will be fixed to the peritoneal reflexion, thus reducing the possibility of a prolapse (40). With the patient lying supine, a line is traced from the iliac crest to the umbilicus. A point is marked one-third of the distance from the umbilicus as a possible site (41) (Fig. 21a). Next, with the patient in a sitting position, the center of the ring that will be part of the colostomy appliance is placed at the marked point and adjusted so that the stoma will not be in a skin depression or too close to the bone or the incision (Fig. 21b). This area is then carefully marked with a subdermal injection of methylene blue (Fig. 21c).

The main problems related to colostomies result from (1) an abdominal wall opening that is too small or too large; (2) tension building in the colostomy; and (3) colostomy placement in the wrong area on the abdominal wall.

Complications and Their Management

Complications that may occur after a colostomy (42, 43, 40) are shown in Table 7 and in Figure 22.

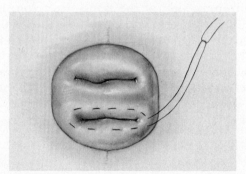

Figure 20. Colostomy. Converting a loop colostomy to an end colostomy.

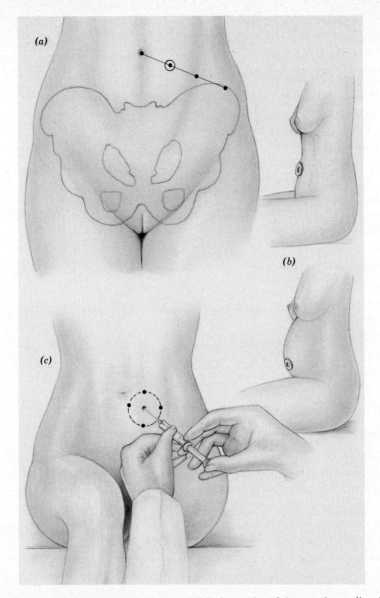

Figure 21. Marking the colostomy site. (*a*) With the patient lying supine, a line is traced from the iliac crest to the umbilicus. A point is marked one-third of the distance from the umbilicus as a possible site. (*b*) Next, with the patient in a sitting position, the center of the ring that will be part of the colostomy appliance is placed at the marked point and adjusted so that the stoma will not be in a skin depression or too close to the bone or the incision. (*c*) This area is then carefully marked with a subdermal injection of methylene blue.

Table 7. Complications After Colostomy
(*N* = 181)

Complication	Number of Patients
Stenosis requiring revision or dilation	11
Prolapse requiring revision	10
Peristomal hernia	6
Redundant mucosa requiring revision	5
Wound infection	3
Recurrent tumor at stoma	3
Severe psychologic problems	3
Severe skin excoriation	2
Evisceration	1
Small bowel obstruction	1
Retraction of colostomy	1
Severe edema of loop	1
Stress ulcer	1
Myocardial infarction	1
Pulmonary embolus	1
Sepsis leading to death	1
Total	51 (28% of patients)

SOURCE: Hines JR, Harris GD: Colostomy and colostomy closure. *Surg Clin N Am* 57:1379, 1977.

Small-Opening Complications

1. Stenosis of the skin can usually be avoided by cutting a circular segment of skin, rather than making a linear incision. If skin stenosis occurs, it can be corrected later under local anesthesia as an office procedure.
2. Stenosis at the fascial level (Fig. 22*c*) with narrowing of the lumen can be corrected by subsequent finger dilation. Occasionally revision of the colostomy with a wider fascial opening may be necessary.
3. Retraction of the stoma (Fig. 22*d*) occurs when tension in the colostomy builds up or when its blood supply is compromised at the edges, causing necrosis of the distal part. In this circumstance, use of the colostomy appliance is very difficult and a revision of the colostomy may be necessary.
4. Swelling of the mucosa resulting from a small opening can usually be treated by applying ice packs around the stoma.

Large-Opening Complications

Complications from large openings are more troublesome than those from small openings.

1. If a bridge put in the loop colostomy is reduced or removed too early, the colostomy can drop into the abdominal cavity and the patient will require an emergency operation to bring the colostomy to the skin level.
2. Evisceration may occur (Fig. 22*a*). If the small bowel prolapses around the

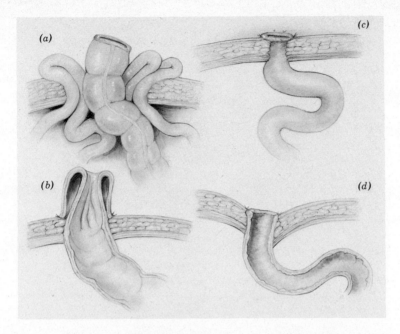

Figure 22. Large opening complications (*a* and *b*). (*a*) The small bowel prolapsing around the stoma. (*b*) A prolapse of the mucosa of the stoma. Small opening complications (*c* and *d*). (*c*) Fascial stenosis with narrowing of the lumen. (*d*) Retraction of the stoma due to tension.

   stoma, surgical correction is required, and sometimes the colostomy site must be removed.

3. Prolapse of the mucosa of the stoma (Fig. 22*b*) occasionally occurs and can be reduced manually by the patient. A prolapsed mucosa may become infected and excoriated. Surgical correction involves removal of the redundant mucosa of the colon and reattachment of the mucosa to the wall of the colon and the abdomen. Recurrence of the prolapse may make resection of the area and construction of a new colostomy necessary (Fig. 23 and 24).

4. Peristomal hernias can usually be corrected by surgery. Some physicians advocate relocation of the original site of the colostomy (44).

Other Complications of Colostomies

1. Careful ligation and hemostasis are mandatory to prevent a hematoma at the mesenteric site during the colostomy procedure.

2. An inadequate blood supply causes a colostomy to become dark and nonviable. Such symptoms should be carefully monitored postoperatively. If the blood supply is reduced only at the edges of the stoma, the colostomy can be observed to determine how much retraction will occur in the stoma. If it appears that retraction will be considerable, the colostomy will have to be revised.

3. Granulation tissue at the colonocutaneous junction develops when the serosa

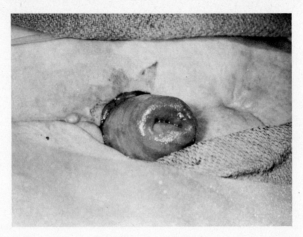

Figure 23. A prolapse of the mucosa of the stoma requiring resection.

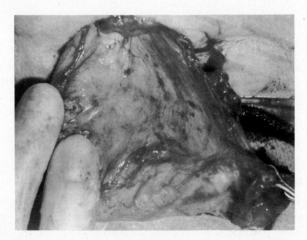

Figure 24. The colostomy has been freed from adhesions. After resection of the colon, the colostomy was placed in a different site.

has been exposed or when inflammation occurs (Fig. 25). Silver nitrate or electrocautery may be used to eliminate this tissue.

4. Excoriation of the skin is treated by cleansing the skin with soap and water and using a protective ingredient such as a mixture of karaya gum, aluminum hydroxide, and zinc oxide. The use of bismuth subgallate, 100 mg taken orally q.i.d., is very helpful to control odor.

Irrigations are sometimes advisable, preferably in patients with left-sided colostomies. One complication of bowel irrigation is colon perforation, especially if a redundant proximal loop is present or if the patient has a stomal hernia. If perforation of the colon occurs from the irrigation catheter, the patient will exhibit signs of peritonitis. In this case, an exploratory laparotomy in which the defect is immediately corrected should be performed.

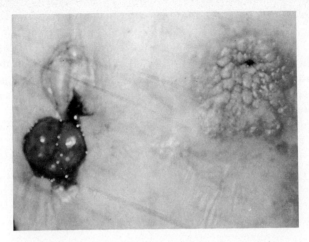

Figure 25. Granulation tissue at the colostomy site.

The stoma therapist is of great help in teaching patients to manage their colostomies and to avoid complications.

Colostomy Closure

Temporary colostomies are usually closed 12–16 weeks after surgery but may be retained longer. Before closure of a colostomy is attempted, proctosigmoidoscopy after a barium enema should be performed. Preparation of the bowel is advisable (45, 46).

Closing a colostomy can cause a significant number of complications (Table 8). Complications resulting from closure have been described by Yakimets (47), Yajko et al. (48), and Finch (49). They can be avoided by a careful and well-planned procedure.

In the colostomy closure procedure (without a laparotomy) a ring of skin and subcutaneous tissue around the stoma are removed (Fig. 26*a*) and all scar tissue

Table 8. Complications After Colostomy Closure
(*N* = 100)

Complication	Number of Patients
Incisional hernia	7
Large bowel obstruction	2
Small bowel obstruction	2
Wound infection	2
Fecal fistula	1
Diarrhea	1
Thrombophlebitis	1
CVA, pneumonia, and fecal fistula	1
Total	17 (17% of patients)

SOURCE: Hines JR, Harris GD: Colostomy and colostomy closure. *Surg Clin N Am.* 57:1379, 1977.

around the colostomy. The colon and abdominal wall are then freed from all adhesions (Fig. 26b). The abdominal cavity must also be free for an adequate anastomosis. The bowel is then closed with a running suture, chromic 3-0, and a second layer including the serosa and muscularis is attached with nonabsorbable material in interrupted sutures. The use of staples can shorten operating time and give a wide anastomosis. Care should be taken that no mesentery is between the loops of the bowel.

When the adhesion cannot be removed easily and the edges of the colon are not free and clean, a laparotomy and closure at the stoma are advised after careful dissection, sometimes with resection of the colostomy and end-to-end anastomosis. This is a very important step, and the patient should be advised of this possibility in advance. Failure to carry out this procedure, particularly when circumstances are difficult, creates unnecessary and troublesome complications, such as an obstruction or a fistula.

1. *Wound Infection.* This common complication of closure is prevented by not closing the wound until 5−7 days after the surgical procedure, when the wound is free from infective microorganisms.
2. *Leakage of the Anastomosis.* A watertight anastomosis with a good blood supply should be ensured to prevent infection and peritonitis.
3. *Obstruction from Stenosis of the Anastomosis.* This complication can often be corrected with nasogastric suction. Sometimes, reoperation is necessary.
4. *Fecal Fistula.* This complication is most likely to occur when scar tissue has not

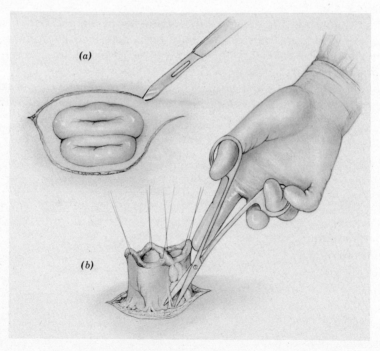

Figure 26. Colostomy closure. (a) Removal of skin and subcutaneous tissue around the stoma. (b) The colon and abdominal wall are then freed from all adhesions.

been completely removed and a good closure has not been obtained. Most fecal fistulas without distal obstruction will close spontaneously in a non-radiated bowel. During the time before closure, the patient should ingest residual bulky-type food and a stool softener, such as Metamucil. The fistula will usually close in 6—8 weeks.

5. *Small Lumen.* If the lumen appears too small, it may be enlarged by an oblique cut in the apex of the bowel. Diarrhea may occur after closure but is usually temporary (50).

ILEOSTOMIES

Ileostomies are seldom used in gynecologic oncology; nevertheless, sometimes they are needed when several loops of bowel are encroached with tumor or when necrosis with perforation has occurred. Ileostomies are very difficult to take care of and are a chronic problem for stoma therapists. The level of intestine used for the ileostomy is directly related to the degree of care that is going to be required. If a proximal segment of ileum is used, the output will be great and high in pancreatic contents that will produce digestion of the tissues around the stoma in the abdominal wall, causing irritation, infection, bleeding, and difficulty in using appliances. A very important way to prevent complications is to create a good stoma in an appropriate place that should be marked in advance (see under "Colostomy" in this chapter). The ileostomy should be mature, and a bud should be created with sutures that will include the skin, the serosa, and the mucosa of the bowel. Problems related to stricture of the stoma can be prevented with finger dilations.

If digestive dermatitis continues to be a major problem and the skin gets so irritated that it is impossible to put on an appliance, a sump pump can be put in the ileostomy and the intestinal contents suctioned while the skin is kept clean with water and antibiotics. The use of karaya gum and local antifungal medicine is helpful. Skin problems will continue to plague some patients for a long time, but in most cases patients will eventually learn to live with an ileostomy. The stoma therapist is a great help in this situation (36).

Large Bowel Obstruction with Blind Loop

Large bowel obstruction resulting from growth of a pelvic tumor or radiation therapy is frequently associated with gynecologic malignancies, especially in the lower rectosigmoid. Surgical correction is eventually required. Occasionally, immediate surgical intervention is necessary, when the ileocecal valve is competent and a blind loop—like obstruction results (Fig. 27). Most patients with this condition have had radiation therapy for cervical cancer or ovarian cancer and then their tumors have recurred, growing and compressing the rectosigmoid until it is completely obstructed (Fig. 28). The status of the ileocecal valve is probably the single most important factor in determining the type of action required to correct this problem.

In a rectosigmoid obstruction, an incompetent ileocecal valve acts as a safety valve so that the gas can be released into the small bowel (51). However, when the ileocecal valve is competent, the whole colon becomes distended. If the dis-

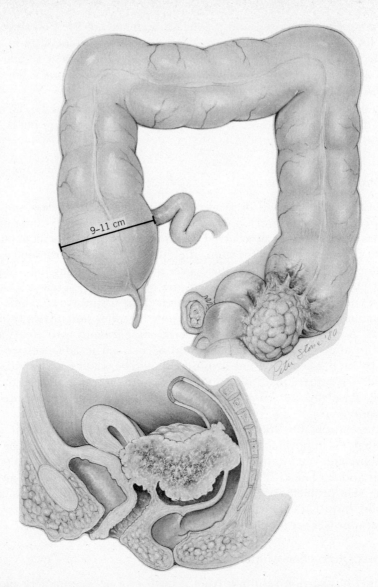

Figure 27. Large bowel obstruction with blind loop. A competent ileocecal valve creating a blind loop obstruction. If the cecum is distended to 9–11 cm, perforation of the cecum is imminent, requiring an emergency decompressive colostomy.

Figure 28. Large bowel obstruction with blind loop. Cervical growth obstructing the rectosigmoid colon.

tention continues and no corrective action is taken, eventually the cecum will perforate, with catastrophic results. (52) The ileocecal valve is believed to be competent in 40%–60% of the patients, but radiation therapy may increase the valve's competence. Gas from the ileum usually stays inside the colon because of the high pressure maintained by a competent valve; the gas cannot move back to the ileum but follows its course through the rectum (53).

Intracolonic pressures have been determined both clinically and experimentally. Wangensteen (54) recorded intraluminal pressures of 12−52 cm of water in patients with large bowel obstruction, with a median pressure of 23 cm. He reported that a patient shown in a flat x-ray of the abdomen to have a cecum distended to 11 cm had an intraluminal pressure of 23 cm. At 20−25 cm of sustained intraluminal pressure, necrosis and perforation of the bowel segment will occur. Because of the impaired blood flow, tissue anoxia and necrosis of the tissue results and there is leakage of intestinal contents into the peritoneal cavity (53).

Anytime a rectosigmoid obstruction is present, the ileocecal valve should be evaluated. If the cecum is seen in an abdominal x-ray film to be distended to 9 cm or more, the risk of impending perforation should be recognized (Fig. 28) and an emergency colostomy performed (55). A transverse loop colostomy will produce decompression of the colon and resolve the emergency.

Rectosigmoid Colon Laceration

Laceration of the sigmoid colon usually occurs during surgery when a large ovarian tumor with multiple adhesions to the sigmoid area is encountered (Fig. 29). The tumor should be removed by sharp dissection. Despite precautions, the colon is sometimes perforated. The dissection should continue until complete resection of the large abdominal tumor is accomplished. One of the following options can then be chosen:

1. The laceration can be repaired with a primary closure, or
2. A protective colostomy can be added.

The surgeon must consider many factors before making this decision. Repair of the laceration without a colostomy should be performed only when the following conditions are present: the laceration is above the retroperitoneal reflexion; the bowel edges are clean and well defined; the bowel was properly prepared before surgery; there is minimal or no spillage of fecal material so that contamination of the abdominal cavity has not occurred; and a good blood supply is assured.

The closure, performed with two layers of 3-0 chromic, should include the entire wall of the colon. Another suture line with permanent material should be placed to include the serosa and muscularis of the wall of the rectosigmoid. Postoperatively, the patient should have I.V. fluids, antibiotics, and continuous gastrointestinal suction until bowel function has been established.

If the laceration is large or irregular; if the edges of the laceration are not well defined; if there are several lacerations of the serosa and muscularis in several other areas around the rectosigmoid; or if there is spillage of fecal material from unprepared colon, a primary closure alone is inadequate and a colostomy is required.

The best approach in the latter situation is to close the laceration with two layers of sutures and then to perform a protective loop colostomy. The colostomy can be closed 6−8 weeks later, if indicated after evaluation of the rectosigmoid with a barium enema and proctosigmoidoscopy.

Lacerations below the retroperitoneal reflexion usually occur during vaginal

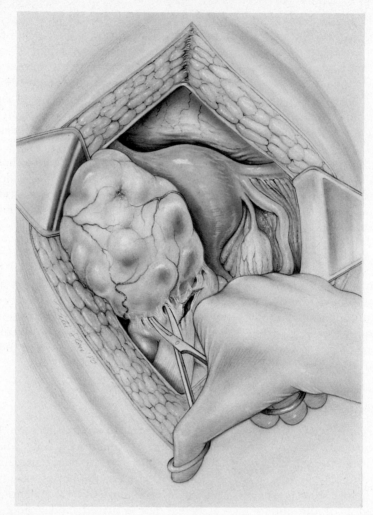

Figure 29. Rectosigmoid laceration. Laceration of the rectosigmoid colon above the peritoneal reflection, an injury usually occurring at the time of dissection of a large ovarian tumor. A diversionary colostomy may be required.

surgeries such as hysterectomies or with the Schauta operation. Such lacerations should be replaced with two layers of sutures, one of chromic 3-0 and the other a nonabsorbable material. The area is then covered with the vaginal mucosa. This procedure is adequate and should not require a colostomy.

VOLVULUS OF THE LARGE BOWEL

The most common site of volvulus of the large bowel is the sigmoid colon (56). The term refers to twisting or torsion of a segment of intestine and its mesentery (Fig. 30). It usually happens in patients with a large colon and a large mesentery that is free and movable. Other factors include closely approximated points of

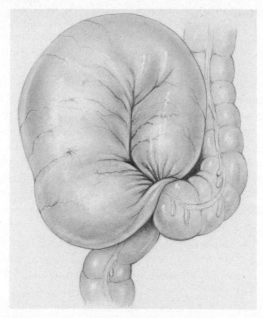

Figure 30. The blind loop. A twisted section of large bowel producing a blind loop that requires resection. If gangrene and perforations are present, resection and exteriorization of the loop of bowel are indicated.

fixation and two loops of bowel close together. Volvulus will eventually produce mechanical obstruction of the lumen and circulatory changes in the wall of the bowel. If the condition remains untreated, necrosis, perforation, and death can occur. The symptoms are similar to those of a blind loop syndrome, and if the blood supply is compromised, strangulation symptoms will be added. Abdominal distention, pain, and marked tenderness in the lower abdomen are characteristic symptoms. In a chronic form, however, the abdominal pain and distention occur over a long period of time and, during the attack, constipation is the rule. When marked abdominal distention is present, a plain x-ray film of the abdomen will show characteristic double-barrel gas. Gerwig (57) classifies volvuluses from Grades I–IV, Grade I being an incidental finding by roentgenologic studies after a barium enema. The importance of a Grade I condition is that it will predispose the patient to the more severe forms of volvulus. In Grade IV volvulus, strangulation and perforation of the bowel have occurred. In Grade III, total obstruction of the loops of the bowel has occurred without perforation. In Gerwig's classification, Grades III and IV are strictly surgical problems. Occasionally in Grade II volvulus, if it is very low in the sigmoid, an enema or passage of a rectal tube will untwist the bowel, but this procedure is associated with the risk of perforation. When surgical resection is indicated, the bowel should be carefully untwisted and, if too distended, decompressed first and then a segment of bowel resected and anastomosis performed. The possibility of a protective colostomy should be considered. However, if the bowel has had vascular compromise with necrosis of the wall, resection and exenteration of the segment should be performed; closure of the bowel should be postponed.

Resection of the Sigmoid Colon

In colonic resection, the anastomosis should not be constructed with tension. If the anastomosis is under tension, leakage, hematomas, and dehiscence can occur.

An anastomosis may fail from an inadequate blood supply. It is therefore very important to understand the blood supply to the colon, lower sigmoid, and rectum. The blood supply to the left colon comes from the inferior mesenteric artery and its branches, the ascending left colic and sigmoid arteries. The superior mesenteric artery and its branches—the ileocolic, right colic, and middle colic arteries—supply the right colon, as shown in Figure 31. The middle colic artery joins the ascending left colic artery, which is a branch of the inferior mesenteric artery. The superior rectal artery joins with the middle and inferior hemorrhoidal branches of the internal and pudendal arteries, supplying blood to the lower sigmoid and the rectum.

When segmental resection of the cecum or ileocecal area is undertaken, the resection should include 7 or 8 cm of terminal ileum, plus the cecum and ascending colon, to ensure a sufficient blood supply (Fig. 32). Otherwise the anastomosis will fail.

If the transverse colon is the area to be resected, the middle colic artery will be ligated and removed. Clean bowel edges and a good blood supply at the end of the bowel, coming from the right colic and the ascending left colic of the inferior mesenteric artery, ensure a good anastomosis (Fig. 33). In resection of the proximal descending colon, the blood supply will come from the middle colic and sigmoid arteries (Fig. 34).

In resection of the distal descending colon and part of the sigmoid, branches of the sigmoid artery 1, 2, and 3 and even the left colic artery can be ligated. The blood supply from the middle colic and superior rectal arteries will still be intact and permit a successful anastomosis (Fig. 35).

When a left hemicolectomy is indicated for the removal of a large growth, the inferior mesenteric artery must also be removed. The rectosigmoid stump should be short enough to ensure a sufficient blood supply from the hemorrhoidal artery (Fig. 35).

Resection of the left colon may result in injury to the spleen when the splenic colon ligament is detached (Fig. 40a). Resection of the right colon carries the risk of injury to the duodenum and the small bowel branches of the superior mesenteric artery.

Anal Fistula

The fistula in ano, usually revealed by drainage in the perianal area, results from infection in the anal crypts. This infection extends through the surrounding subcutaneous tissue and drains into the perineal area. Crohn's disease is a common cause of fistulas (58).

There are different types of fistulas: a complete anal fistula in which there is communication to the anal canal and to the perineal area; an incomplete (internal) fistula in which there is drainage only into the luminal rectum; and an incomplete external fistula in which there is drainage only to the perineal area (Fig. 36). Sometimes fistulas have different tracts and multiple openings because

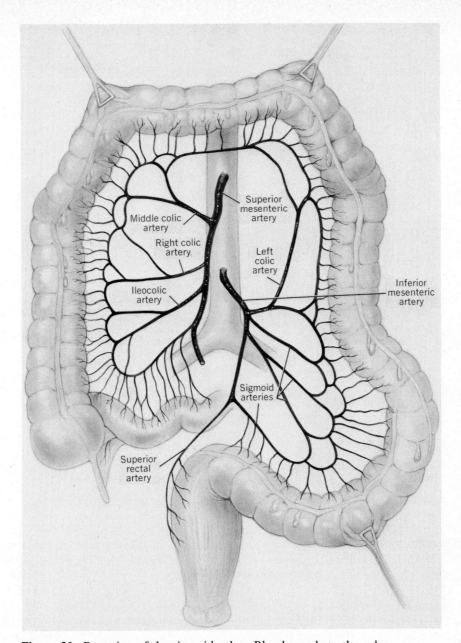

Figure 31. Resection of the sigmoid colon. Blood supply to the colon.

of their special configurations. These fistulas, called horseshoe fistulas, are difficult to manage (59). All acute fistulas should be treated systemically with antibiotics, to prevent sepsis. If an abscess is present, it should be drained immediately.

Surgical management of fistulas requires finding the opening of the fistula and identifying the fistular tract. The Goodsall rule aids in the identification (60)

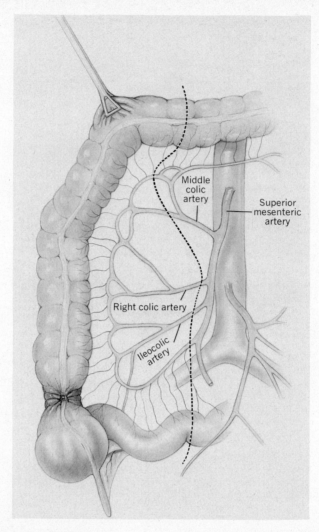

Figure 32. Resection of the sigmoid colon. Resection of the ileocecal area, which should include 6–7 cm of ileum and colon, as shown by the dotted line. The blood supply originates from the ileocolic and right colic arteries.

but is not absolute: (*1*) If the external opening is posterior to the line between the ischial tuberosities, the fistula tends to take a curved course (Fig. 37), terminating in an opening in the midline of the posterior rectal mucosa. (*2*) If the external opening is anterior, the fistula tends to have a radial tract and drain directly into the anal canal (Fig. 37).

There are different surgical techniques for correction of anal fistulas. Identification of the sinus tract is made by inserting a probe and making an incision over the probe from the primary opening to the deep postanal abscess (61). The wound is loosely packed with fine-mesh gauze for 48 hours. Care should be taken not to create a false tract when the probe is introduced. Postoperatively, analgesics, hot Sitz baths, and mineral oil are administered.

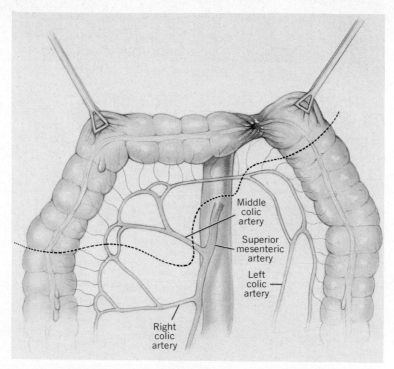

Figure 33. Resection of the sigmoid colon. Resection (following the dotted line) for a lesion located in the transverse colon. The blood supply for the anastomosis will come from the right and left colic artery branches of the inferior mesenteric artery.

PELVIC FLOOR MANAGEMENT

Anterior Resection, Restoring Continuity, and Saving the Sphincter

Anterior resections in gynecology are usually associated with major surgical resections in cancer of the ovary and in advanced cervical cancer that requires pelvic exenteration. Where possible, the surgeon should try to restore continuity and preserve the sphincter. For other conditions such as bowel cancer, a different technique might be selected (62).

The prevention of complications in anterior resection begins with complete bowel preparation. This procedure is performed mechanically with laxatives only or in combination with antibiotics. The insertion of a large intestinal tube is helpful in bowel preparation. The technique chosen for resection and anastomosis should prevent contamination of the abdominal cavity and permit an adequate blood supply at the anastomosis site. This may be accomplished by careful dissection of the retroperitoneal attachments, freeing the bowel without compromising its blood supply. Another important consideration is to avoid tension in the segments of bowel that are to be anastomosed (63).

The technical difficulty and the complications encountered during an anterior resection are related to the location of the anastomosis. When the anastomosis is

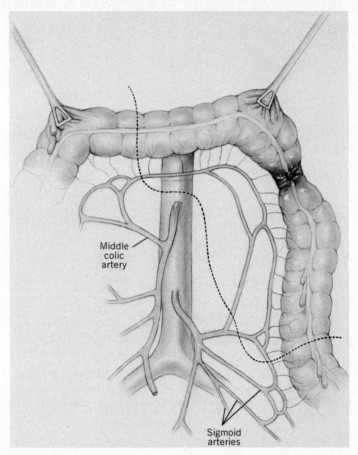

Figure 34. Resection of the sigmoid colon. Resection (following the dotted line) for a lesion located in the proximal portion of the descending colon. The blood supply for the anastomosis will come from the middle colic and sigmoid arteries.

above the peritoneal reflexion, it can be performed under direct vision, which facilitates a watertight closure and a good blood supply. This type of anastomosis can be performed with a double layer of suture material or with a staple gun (64).

When the anastomosis is below the peritoneal reflexion, an anterior resection is more difficult to perform because of the poor exposure and limited mobility of the bowel. In this situation, enteroenteroanastomosis (E.E.A.) can be used in this situation. The E.E.A. instrument is introduced through the rectum; the proximal and distal ends of the bowel are tied to the heads of the instrument and the anastomosis is accomplished by a double row of staples (46) (Fig. 16). This instrument can also be used when the anastomosis is very low, to help preserve the rectal sphincter.

Other sphincter-saving procedures are the pull-through procedure in which the colon stump is pulled through the inverted anal stump and the anastomosis is done outside the body under direct vision, and the D'Allaine's procedure, in

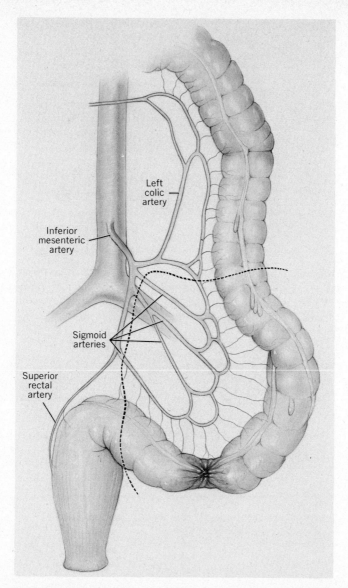

Figure 35. Resection of the sigmoid colon. Resection of a mass located in the descending and sigmoid colon requiring the ligation of the sigmoid arteries and, sometimes, the left colic artery. The blood supply is assured by the superior rectal and middle colic arteries.

which a posterior anastomosis is performed through a paracoccygeal or coccyx resection incision (64, 36).

Management of Complications

1. *Bleeding.* There is usually some bleeding in the perineal area after anterior resection, but the bleeding will usually cease 10–12 hours after surgery. However, if hemostasis is not good and oozing from the dissected area cannot be controlled, suction catheters should be placed for drainage. A small amount of bleeding from the anastomosis will usually subside; however, if

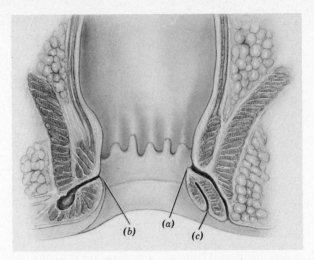

Figure 36. Anal fistulas resulting from an infection of the anal crypts and draining at different levels. (*a*) A complete fistula, draining into the lumen of the rectum and the perineal area. (*b*) An incomplete internal fistula, draining into the rectum only. (*c*) An incomplete external fistula, draining into the perineal area only.

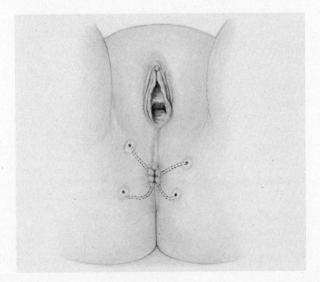

Figure 37. Goodsall rule. Anal fistulas opening posterior to the line between the ischial tuberosities tend to have a curving course. Those fistulas opening anteriorly tend to have a radial course and drain directly into the anal canal.

hemorrhage occurs, a reoperation may be necessary. If the anastomosis is very low, a hemostatic suture through the rectum can be attempted.

2. *Infection.* Infection from leakage, with or without fecal contamination, is caused by separation of the suture line. Partial dehiscence of the anastomosis site often occurs in anterior resection. About 90% of patients will evidence a small amount of leakage (that has no clinical significance) when a barium

enema is performed a week after the operation. In 10% of patients, minor symptoms will be found, and in 5%, enough leakage of the intestinal contents will be present to necessitate vigorous treatment (65). If the separation is small, it will heal spontaneously most of the time. If the separation of the edges of the bowel leads to spillage of fecal material, a colostomy should be performed and the colon irrigated through the colostomy and the anus. If irrigation does not relieve the symptoms, a pelvic abcess is present and must be drained. Any attempt to revise the anastomosis before eliminating the infection will fail.

3. *Stricture.* Most patients with a low anastomosis will have some degree of stricture that will be completely corrected by the fecal motion in about 4–6 months. Few patients require instrument dilation. When required, it is usually performed with Hegar dilators. It should be done very cautiously because the strictures may split, producing an opening directly into the peritoneal cavity (66).

4. *Fecal Incontinence.* Incontinence is directly related to the length of the rectal stump. Usually 7 cm of rectal stump is adequate to ensure spontaneous, although slow, correction of this problem when it occurs. If a colostomy has been performed, before the decision is made to close it, a retention enema should be given to determine whether the patient is continent and the degree of sphincter control.

5. *Urinary Retention.* Although more common in men after anterior resection, urinary retention is also observed in women, especially after a radical pelvic dissection. Urinary incontinence may be troublesome to correct. A patient with this difficulty should have a Foley catheter in place during the post-operative period and an antibiotic to inhibit urinary infection. Stress urinary incontinence may require correction by surgery.

6. *Pelvic Abscess and Peritonitis.* If separation of the anastomosis leads to massive contamination of the pelvis, a pelvic abscess will develop and create a fistula tract unless the abscess is drained immediately and a diverting colostomy performed. Peritonitis and systemic sepsis may also be present. As long as some part of the edges of the bowel are held together, the fistula will eventually close if the infection is controlled, the abscess is drained, and a diverting colostomy has been performed. If the leakage and fistula are entirely extraperitoneal, the presacral cavity will be filled with granulation tissue that will cover the anastomotic site before the colostomy is closed. In order for this condition to be evaluated, sigmoidoscopy and a barium enema of the distal colon should be performed before colostomy closure (63).

Abdominal-Perineal and Pelvic Exenteration

Management of the pelvic floor is very important in order to prevent complications resulting from major surgery in which the pelvic diaphragm is totally or partially removed, as in abdominal, perineal, posterior, or total pelvic exenterations.

When an abdominal-perineal exenteration has been performed and the uterus left intact, the uterus can be sutured posteriorly to the hollow of the sacrum, to occlude this large opening. If the uterus has also been removed, the peritoneum around the pelvic cavity should be carefully preserved, widely dissected, and then closed with suture material. Usually, packing is needed to support the abdominal contents.

In total pelvic exenterations the opening is too large for this procedure; therefore, different procedures may be used to build up a new pelvic floor. These procedures include omental carpeting of the pelvis, grafting myocutaneous muscles to the pelvis, and transplanting muscles from other areas in the abdominal cavity (67, 68).

Management of Complications

1. *Bowel Prolapse.* The major complications of exenterations (68) are due to large defects in the pelvic floor causing prolapse of the small intestine. Prolapse is sometimes fatal because the obstructed (sometimes strangulated) loop of bowel can remain undetected for a long time. When prolapse of the bowel is recognized, it should be corrected immediately by abdominal-route surgery to repair the pelvic floor. If the bowel's vascular supply has been compromised, resection and anastomosis are required. Bowel prolapse results in a large loss of fluid and electrolytes through the raw surface in the pelvic cavity; compensatory fluids and electrolytes must be given.

2. *Bleeding.* Bleeding may take place in the pelvic cavity. The amount of bleeding is related to the amount of dissection and the dimensions of the dead space. Packing may be left in place for 3–4 days if hemostasis is not adequate at the end of the operation. After the packing is removed, the pelvic cavity should be irrigated. If heavy bleeding persists, the patient may require hemostatic sutures.

3. *Infection.* Infection of the open pelvic cavity can be a serious complication, especially if a packing has been left in place for a long time because of hemostatic problems. A large drain should be left in place, and frequent irrigations of the pelvis with Dakin's solution or hydrogen peroxide will help ensure a clean surface. Systemic antibiotics are advisable when this procedure is performed.

Omental Lid

Several techniques have been used to rebuild the pelvic floor after a total pelvic exenteration (68, 69, 70, 71). In one technique the omentum that has been detached from the greater curvature of the stomach and the transverse colon is used (Fig. 38). When the omentum is detached, the left gastroepiploic artery must remain attached, to preserve the blood supply. The omentum is then brought down to the pelvis and attached to the peritoneum (and sometimes, to the periosteum of the pubis) in interrupted sutures with 3-0 chromic material, to make a new pelvic floor for the abdominal viscera (Fig. 39).

Management of Complications

The following complications can arise from the omental lid procedure to rebuild the pelvic floor:

1. Creation of a fistula when the omentum is removed too close to the curvature of the stomach and the stomach wall is included in the transection. This

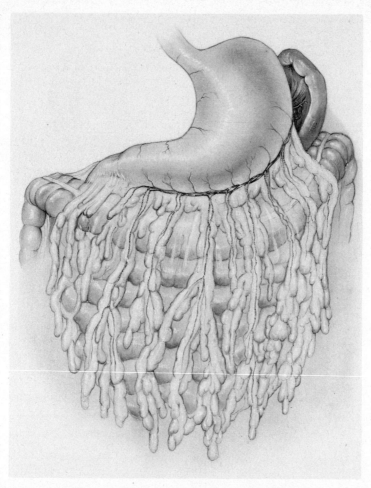

Figure 38. Omental lid. The detached omentum now covering the pelvis. The left gastroepiploic artery supplies blood to the transposed omentum.

complication should be handled as described under "Splenectomy" in this chapter.

2. Failure to preserve the gastroepiploic artery that is closely parallel to the greater curvature of the stomach. When the omentum is detached, this artery must be preserved with the omentum so that an adequate blood supply will be assured after the right gastropiploic artery has been transected.

3. Injury to the capsule of the spleen when heavy traction is used for better exposure. Resolution of this complication will be described under "Splenectomy" in this chapter.

4. Injury to the mesentery of the transverse colon during detachment of the omentum from the greater curvature of the stomach. This complication is prevented by entering the lesser sac before attempting the detachment.

5. Necrosis of the omental lid after it has been placed in the pelvis. This complication occurs if stitches have been placed so that they interfere with the

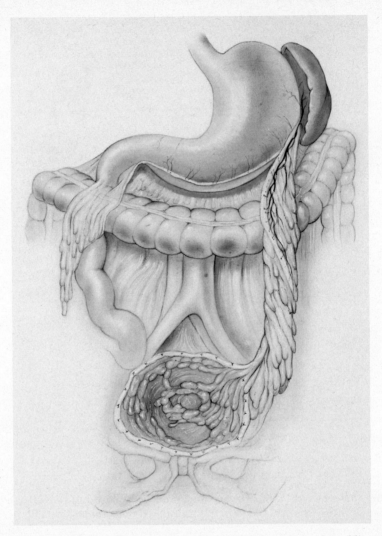

Figure 39. Omental lid. Detachment of the omentum (following the dotted line) from the greater curvature of the stomach and transverse colon. The gastroepiploic artery should be preserved.

marginal blood vessels of the omentum. Correction of this problem may require resection of part of the omentum.

6. Gastric retention because of dissection of the omentum from the stomach. This problem should be corrected as described in this chapter under "Acute Gastric Dilatation."

Splenectomy

Splenectomies in gynecologic oncology are usually associated with ovarian cancer surgery or intraoperative trauma. Laceration of the spleen may occur during surgery if the splenocolic ligament is stretched before it is cut (Fig. 40a).

Lacerations may also occur during total omentectomy if adhesions have attached the omentum to the spleen.

After laceration of the spleen, bleeding can seldom be stopped by hemostatic agents; nevertheless, if the bleeding is not profuse, application of a hemostatic agent should be the first measure taken. Usually, when heavy splenic bleeding occurs in the course of surgery, the only way to control it is by splenectomy.

The major blood supply for the spleen derives from the splenic artery and vein. The splenic artery feeds the left gastroepiploic artery and the short vessels that go to the stomach. Following laceration of a normal-size spleen, the vascular pedicle can usually be identified, clamped, tied, and cut, and the spleen removed (72).

Management of Complications

1. *Intraoperative Hemorrhage.* If a massive hemorrhage occurs, immediate control of the bleeding is required before the spleen is removed. The first step is to quickly open the lesser sac and compress the blood vessels at the tail of the pancreas (Figs. 40*b* and 40*c*). This procedure will usually stop the hemorrhage until adequate exposure is obtained and preparations for the splenectomy are complete. When the blood vessels at the tail of the pancreas have been compressed, they may then be ligated with sutures instead of being individually clamped and tied.

2. *Postoperative Hemorrhage.* Hemorrhage is a complication that can also occur after splenectomy. Hemorrhage from the vascular pedicle requires immediate surgical ligation.

3. *Gastric Fistula.* A gastric fistula can be produced during splenectomy if part of the wall of the stomach is included when the short blood vessels are clamped (Fig. 41*a*). For this reason, the blood vessels should be clamped as close as possible to the spleen. If a gastric fistula occurs and a drain has been left in place, the gastric contents will drain and healing will usually occur spontaneously. However, if peritonitis results, a reoperation may be necessary in which the fistulous tract is resected and the stomach closed in two layers. Following the diagnosis of peritonitis, the patient should be given I.V. fluids, nasogastric suction, and antibiotics as indicated.

4. *Pancreatic Fistula.* If the tail of the pancreas is included when the vascular pedicle is clamped, a pancreatic fistula can develop (73) (Fig. 41*b*). This complication frequently leads to peritonitis.

5. *Thromboses.* Martin et al. (74) found an incidence of 3.7% of portal and peripheral thromboses in 777 patients with splenectomies (74). The pathophysiology is not well understood, but an elevated platelet count in the range of 500,000–700,000 is not uncommon and a hypercoagulability state also may be present. Heparin does not appear to prevent splenectomy-associated thrombosis, which occurs usually in the second or third week after splenectomy.

Appendectomy

Major gynecologic surgery frequently includes an appendectomy. Sometimes specific complications result from the appendectomy.

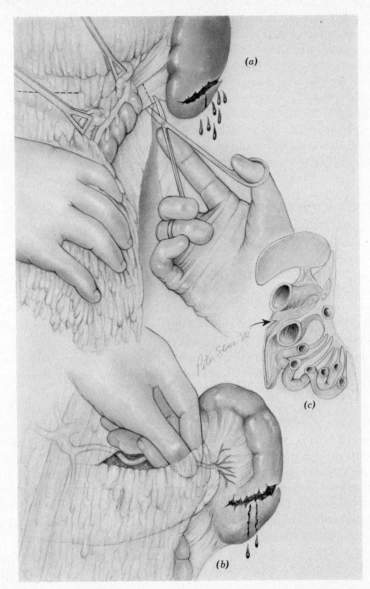

Figure 40. Splenectomy. (*a*) Laceration of the spleen during detachment of the splenocolic ligament. (*b*) Opening the lesser sac and applying pressure to the splenic vessels at the tail of the pancreas, to control massive hemmorhage. (*c*) Entering the lesser sac.

Management of Complications

1. *Hemorrhage.* Good hemostasis of the appendiceal artery will prevent hemorrhage. Bleeding discovered postoperatively should be corrected immediately by laparotomy and ligation of blood vessels.
2. *Intraabdominal Abscess.* The most common place for the formation of an abscess is around the stump (75). A periappendiceal abscess sometimes

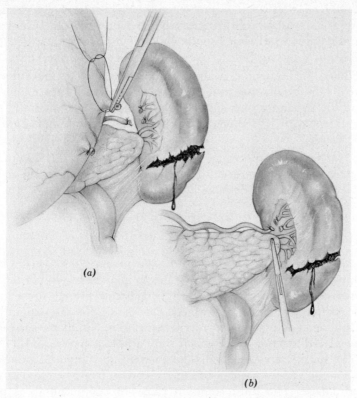

Figure 41. Splenectomy. (*a*) The wall of the stomach inadvertently ligated, which will result in a fistula. (*b*) The inclusion of pancreatic tissue, which may result in a fistula.

involves loops of small bowel and pelvic organs. Such a diagnosis should be suspected when right lower quadrant tenderness, leukocytosis, and fever occur 5 days after the operation. The abscess usually extends downward toward the pelvis and produces pelvic pain. The diagnosis is made by abdominal palpation or by pelvic exam. If the abscess is large and is protuding between the cul-de-sac and the rectum, a drainage through a colpotomy is adequate treatment. If the abscess is in the periappendiceal area, drainage through an abdominal incision should be performed immediately.

The other site of abscess formation is the subphrenic area. An abscess here results from complications of appendicitis or other intraabdominal gastrointestinal surgery. This abscess is usually insidious and difficult to diagnose. The patient may do very well after gastrointestinal abdominal surgery but, suddenly, between the seventh and fourteenth day, exhibit a high fever and an elevated white cell count. Occasionally, pain will develop about the twelfth rib posteriorly; sometimes a muscle spasm is present. The diagnosis of subphrenic abscess is made by a flat plate roentgenogram of the abdomen, showing the elevation of the right hemidiaphragm. A gallium scan can also be helpful in making the diagnosis.

As soon as the diagnosis of subphrenic abscess is made, the abscess should be drained by a subcostal incision. When the abscess is loculated, each one of the cystic areas must be ruptured and drained immediately. Drains are left in place and lavage is performed in the abdominal cavity with large amounts of warm isotonic solution. Liberal use of antibiotics is indicated.

3. *Fecal Fistula*. Infrequently, a fecal fistula develops in the stump of the appendix. It is usually due to inadequate ligation with suture material. The stump of the appendectomy should be inverted carefully. Usually, conservative treatment with I.V. fluids, gastrointestinal suction, and antibiotics will heal the fistula.

4. *Intraluminal Colonic Hemorrhage*. After appendectomy, intraluminal colonic hemorrhage occurs very rarely. It is caused by bleeding at the level of the amputated area after inadequate ligation of blood vessels.

GASTROSTOMIES

Gastrostomies may be necessary in gynecologic oncology because of obstruction of the jejunum caused by the growth of a tumor in an enlarged periaortic lymph node. Gastrostomies can also be used in gastrointestinal diversions when nasogastric suction cannot be performed. Preoperatively, the patient's stomach should be emptied completely, to prevent aspiration. Number 2 silk pursestring sutures are placed around the stomach wall, a hole is made, and a catheter is inserted. The sutures are then tied. The gastric wall should be attached to the tectus fascia in the abdominal wall and the tube should also be fixed carefully for adequate drainage. The most common cause of complications is peritonitis caused by leakage due to poor healing, which is often contributed to by separation of the stomach from the anterior abdominal wall (76).

Acute Gastric Dilatation

Acute gastric dilatation in the absence of an obstruction is usually seen in gynecologic oncology patients who have had major abdominal surgery. This problem, which leads to shock, is most common in patients with advanced ovarian cancer who have required surgical resections. For example, gastric dilatation may occur in patients who have had pelvic exenterations involving removal of the omentum from the greater curvature of the stomach and attachment of the omentum to the perineum. Gastric dilatation also occurs when long intestinal tubes have been used to decompress the small intestine but not the stomach. A gastric tube is usually needed to correct dilatation.

Gastric dilatation is usually a postoperative complication. Anesthesia may play a role by inducing air sucking (77). Nitrous oxide may contribute to the condition because large volumes of the soluble gas are readily diffused into patients, leading to intestinal distention (78). Postoperative oxygen therapy with accompanying intermittent positive pressure breathing may also produce some swallowing of air and lead to distention (78).

There are several nonsurgical causes of dilatation such as trauma and body casts (79). Gastric dilatation is also a complication of diabetic acidosis; it may also occur in diabetics after surgical procedures in the absence of acidosis (77).

Although the pathophysiology of acute gastric dilatation is not fully understood, the problem has been studied by producing gastric dilatation in dogs and then measuring their blood pressure, inferior vena cava pressure, and cardiac output (80, 81). These studies concluded that arterial hypotension results from decreased venous return and that shock is secondary to mechanical obstruction of the inferior vena cava by the distended stomach, although the hemodynamic alteration can also be explained as a reflex mechanism of the splanchnic nerves (82). Shock can also occur in acute gastric dilatation by splanchnic pooling of blood, hypoxia, and metabolic acidosis. A large amount of fluid accumulates in the upper gastrointestinal tract and produces shock from hypovolemia. Suggested pathophysiologic mechanisms of acute gastric dilatation are shown in Figure 42.

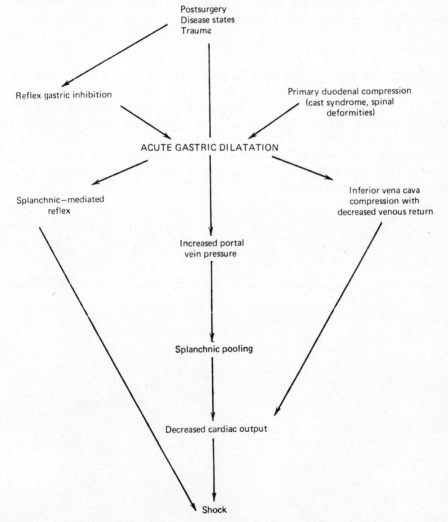

Figure 42. Suggested pathophysiologic mechanisms of acute gastric dilatation. (From Clearfield and Stahlgen, 1974, p. 1115.)

Diagnosis

Unrecognized acute gastric dilatation can produce severe complications, including rupture of the stomach and death (77, 83, 84). Pain is rarely severe. If this condition continues, bile-stained or brownish vomitus appears, followed by tachycardia, sweating, decreased urinary output, and shock. The abdomen may be distended, especially in the upper left quadrant, and exhibit hyperresonance on percussion; the rest of the abdomen may be soft and free from pain. Bowel sounds may be present, especially if a long intestinal tube is in place, making diagnosis very difficult. Dehydration because of persistent vomiting, decreased cardiac output, and acid-base imbalance may contribute to the clinical picture. If the condition is not treated promptly, aspiration pneumonia may develop, leading to death of the patient.

The diagnosis is confirmed by a roentgenogram of the abdomen that shows a massive amount of air and fluid in the stomach.

Treatment

Suction by a nasogastric tube must be performed at the slightest suspicion of gastric dilatation (Fig. 43). Fluid and electrolytes should be replaced expeditiously to treat dehydration and to correct the acid-base balance (84). If an intestinal tube has already been introduced, it does not prevent or solve the problem of gastric dilatation because the tube removes fluid and gas from the small intestine but not from the stomach; a second tube in the gastric cavity is necessary. With the introduction of the second tube, a large amount of air and water can be quickly expelled.

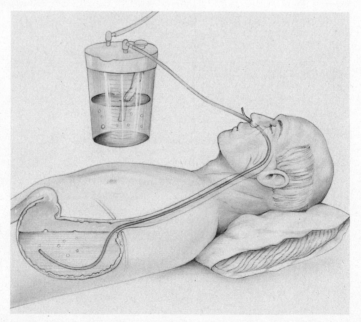

Figure 43. Distention of the stomach due to gastric dilatation may produce shock. Suction of the gastric contents is necessary to prevent aspiration, pneumonia, and death.

The diagnosis of gastric dilatation is difficult, especially in patients with extensive surgery such as pelvic exenteration, because a variety of complications require the establishment of a differential diagnosis. Acute gastric dilatation must be clearly differentiated from bowel obstruction, for which the treatment is surgical.

REFERENCES

1. Barnett WO: Complications of small intestine surgery, in Artz CP, Hardy JD (eds): *Management of Surgical Complications,* ed 3. Philadelphia, WB Saunders Co, 1975, p 472.

2. Heifetz, CJ: A technic for open end-to-end intestinal anastomosis. *Surg Clin North Am* 30:1481, 1950.

3. Chassin JL, Rifkind KM, Susman B, et al: The stapled gastrointestinal tract anastomosis: Incidence of postoperative complications compared with the sutured anastomosis. *Ann Surg* 188:689, 1978.

4. Photopulos GJ, Delgado G, Fowler WC, et al: Intestinal anastomoses after radiation therapy by surgical stapling instruments. *Obstet Gynecol* 54:515, 1979.

5. Hamilton JE: Reappraisal of open intestinal anastomoses. *Ann Surg* 165:917, 1967.

6. Warwick R, William PL: Angiology, in *Gray's Anatomy,* ed 35 (Brit). Philadelphia, WB Saunders Co, 1973, p 588.

7. Steichen FM: The use of staplers in anatomical side-to-side and functional end-to-end enteroanastomoses. *Surgery* 64:948, 1968.

8. Steichen FM: Clinical experience with autosuture instruments. *Surgery* 69:609, 1971.

9. Waugh DE: A new technique for gastrotomy. *Surgery* 70:368, 1971.

10. Doherty C, Fleming R: Restoration of the alimentary tract after total gastrectomy using autosuture staplers. *Am J Surg* 131:629, 1976.

11. Ravitch MM, Steinchen FM: Technics of staple suturing in the gastrointestinal tract. *Ann Surg* 175:815, 1972.

12. Wheeless CR: Avoidance of permanent colostomy in pelvic malignancy using the surgical stapler. *Obstet Gynecol* 54:501, 1979.

13. Reynolds W: Low anterior resection using an automatic anastomosing instrument. *Am J Surg* 124:433, 1972.

14. Ravitch MM: The use of stapling instruments in surgery of the gastrointestinal tract, with a note on a new instrument for end-to-end low rectal and oesophagojejunal anastomoses. *Aust NZ J Surg* 48:444, 1978.

15. Fain SN, Patin CS, Morgenstern L: Use of a mechanical suturing apparatus in low colorectal anastomosis. *Arch Surg* 110:1079, 1975.

16. Arrants JE, Locklair PR: Staple closure of atriotomy incision. *Ann Thorac Surg* 18:638, 1974.

17. Scott, RN, Faraci RP, Hough A, et al: Bronchial stump closure techniques following pneumonectomy: A serial comparative study. *Ann Surg* 184:205, 1976.

18. Heney NM, Dretler SP, Hensle TW, et al: Autosuturing device in intestinal urinary conduits. *Urology* 12:650, 1978.

19. Johnson DE, Fuerst DE: Use of auto suture for construction of ileal conduits. *J Urol* 109:821, 1973.

20. Delgado G: Use of the automatic stapler in urinary conduit diversions and pelvic exenterations. *Gynecol Oncol* 10:1, 1980.

21. Goligher JC, Lee PWR, Lintott DJ: Experience with the Russian model 249 suture gun for anastomosis of the rectum. *Surg Gynecol Obstet* 148:517, 1979.

22. Barnett WO: Mechanical small bowel obstruction. *Am Pract Dig Treat* 11:389, 1960.

23. Barnett WO, Petro AB, Williamson JW: A current appraisal of problems with gangrenous bowel. *Ann Surg* 183:653, 1975.

24. Zollinger RM, Nick WV, Sanzebacher LJ: Ulcerogenic and diarrheogenic endocrine tumors, in Bockus HL (ed): *Gastroenterology.* Philadelphia, WB Saunders Co, 1974, vol 2, p 854.

25. Noble TB Jr: Plication of the small intestine. *Am J Surg* 45:574, 1939.

26. Weckesser EC, Lindsay JF Jr, Cebul FA: Plication of small intestine for obstruction due to adhesions—Noble procedure. *AMA Arch Surg* 65:487, 1952.

27. White RR: Prevention of recurrent small bowel obstruction due to adhesions. *Ann Surg* 143:714, 1956.

28. Singleton AO Jr, Rowe EB: Peristalsis in reversed loops of bowel. *Ann Surg* 139:853, 1954.

29. Smith JP, Golden PE, Rutledge F: The surgical management of intestinal injuries following irradiation for carcinoma of the cervix, in *Cancer of the Uterus and Ovary,* Symposia of the Annual Clinical Conferences on Cancer sponsored by the University of Texas M. D. Anderson Hospital and Tumor Institute at Houston. Chicago, Year Book Medical Publishers Inc, 1969, p 241.

30. Louw JH: Embryology and developmental anomalies, in Bockus HL (ed): *Gastroenterology.* Philadelphia, WB Saunders Co, 1976, p 3.

31. Murray C: Excision of Meckel's diverticulum, in Rob C, Smith R, Morgan CN (eds): *Operative Surgery,* ed 5. Philadelphia, JB Lippincott Co, 1969, p 558.

32. Edmunds LH, Williams GM, Welch CE: External fistulas arising from the gastrointestinal tract. *Ann Surg* 152:445, 1960.

33. MacFadyen BV Jr, Dudrick SJ, Ruberg RL: Management of gastrointestinal fistulas with parenteral hyperalimentation. *Surgery* 74:100, 1973.

34. Dudrick SJ, Duke JH Jr: Parental nutrition—Intravenous hyperalimentation, in Bockus HL (ed): *Gastroenterology.* Philadelphia, WB Saunders Co, 1976, p 395.

35. Bowlin JW, Hardy JD, Conn JH: External alimentary fistulas. *Am J Surg* 103:6, 1962.

36. Welch CE, Hedberg SE: Complications in surgery of the colon and rectum, in Artz CP and Hardy JD (eds): *Management of Surgical Complications,* ed. 3. Philadelphia, WBSaunders Co, 1975, p 633.

37. Allen AW, Welch DC: Cecostomy. *Surg Gynecol Obstet* 73:549, 1941.

38. Dolan PA, Caldwell FT, Thompson CH, et al: Problems of colostomy closure. *Am J Surg* 137:188, 1979.

39. Bacon HE, Herabat T, Tse GN, et al: Is colostomy a necessary complement to elective left colonic resection? *Dis Colon Rectum* 16:29, 1973.

40. Hines JR, Harris GD: Colostomy and colostomy closure. *Surg Clin North Am* 57:1379, 1977.

41. Turnbull RB, Weakley FL: *Atlas of Intestinal Stomas.* St. Louis, The CV Mosby Co, 1967.

42. Sana SP, Rao N, Stephenson SE: Complications of colostomy. *Dis Colon Rectum* 16:515, 1973.

43. Burns FJ: Complications of colostomy. *Dis Colon Rectum* 13:448, 1970.

44. Prian GW, Sawyer RB, Sawyer KC: Repair of peristomal colostomy hernias. *Am J Surg* 130:694, 1975.

45. Rodkey GV, Welch CE: Diverticulitis and diverticulosis of the colon, in Turrell R (ed): *Diseases of the Colon and Anorectum,* ed 2. Philadelphia, WB Saunders Co, 1969, vol 2, p 718.

46. Goligher JC: Treatment of carcinoma of the colon, in Goligher JC (ed): *Surgery of the Anus, Rectum and Colon,* ed 2. Springfield, Ill., Charles C Thomas Publisher, 1972, p 592.

47. Yakimets WW: Complications of closure of loop colostomy. *Can J Surg* 18:366, 1975.

48. Yajko RD, Norton LW, Bloemendal L, et al: Morbidity of colostomy closure. *Am J Surg* 132:304, 1976.

49. Finch DRA: The results of colostomy closure. *Br J Surg* 63:397, 1976.

50. Tilson MD, Fellner BJ, Wright HK: A possible explanation for postoperative diarrhea after colostomy closure. *Am J Surg* 131:94, 1976.

51. Ulin AW, Grotzinger PJ, Shoemaker WC: Experimental closed loop obstruction of the entire colon. *AMA Arch Surg* 71:775, 1955.

52. Gatch WD, Trusler HM, Lyons RE: Effects of gaseous distention of obstructive bowel. Incarceration of the intestine by gas traps. *AMA Arch Surg* 14:1215–19, 1927

53. Roberts SS, Minton JP, Zollinger RM: Obstruction of the large bowel: Closed loop obstruction in the colon, in Turrel R (ed): *Diseases of the Colon and Rectum,* ed 2. Philadelphia, WB Saunders Co, 1969, vol 2, p 667.

54. Wangensteen OH: *Intestinal Obstruction,* ed 3. Springfield, Ill., Charles C Thomas Publisher, 1955.

55. Lowmen RM, Davis L: An evaluation of cecal size in impending perforation of the cecum. *Surg Gynecol Obstet* 103:711, 1956.

56. Douglas DR: Operations for volvulus of the large bowel, in Rob C, Smith R (eds): *Abdomen and Rectum and Anus.* Philadelphia, JB Lippincott Co, 1969, p 676.

57. Gerwig W Jr: Volvulus of the colon. *Arch Surg* 60:721, 1950.

58. Alexander-Williams J: Fistula-in-ano: Management of Crohn's fistula. *Dis Colon Rectum* 19:518, 1976.

59. Hanley PH, Ray JE, Pennington EE, et al: Fistula-in-ano: A ten year follow-up study of horseshoe-abscess fistula-in-ano. *Dis Colon Rectum* 19:507, 1976.

60. Mattingly RF: *Te Linde's Operative Gynecology,* ed 5. Philadelphia, JB Lippincott Co, 1977.

61. Goligher JC: Fistula-in-ano, in Goligher, JC (ed): *Surgery of the Anus, Rectum and Colon,* ed 2. Springfield, Ill., Charles C Thomas Publisher, 1972, p 201.

62. Wheelock, FC Jr, Toll G, McKittrick LS: An evaluation of the anterior resection of the rectum and low sigmoid. *N Engl J Med* 260:526, 1959.

63. Hedberg, SE, Welch CE: Complications following surgery of the colon. *Surg Clin North Am* 43:775, 1963.

64. Goligher JC: Resections with restoration of continuity for rectal and recto-sigmoid cancer, in Rob C, Smith R, Morgan CN (eds): *Operative Surgery, Abdomen and Rectum and Anus.* Philadelphia, JB Lippincott Co, 1969, p 798.

65. Welch CE: The colon and rectum, in Kinney, JM (ed): *Manual of Preoperative and Postoperative Care,* ed 2. Philadelphia, WB Saunders Co, 1971, p 411.

66. Goligher JC: Treatment of carcinoma of the rectum, in Goligher, JC (ed): *Surgery of the Anus, Rectum and Colon,* ed 2. Springfield, Ill., Charles C Thomas Publisher, 1972, p 710.

67. Becker DW Jr, Massey FM, McCraw JB: Musculocutaneous flaps in reconstructive pelvic surgery. *Obstet Gynecol* 54:178, 1979.

68. Morley G, Lindenauers W, Martin S, et al: Vaginal reconstruction following pelvic exenteration: Surgical and psychological considerations. *Am J Obstet Gynecol* 116:996, 1973.

69. Brunschwig A: Cancer of the cervix. Surgery for recurrences, in Barber HR, Graber EA (eds): *Gynecological Oncology.* Proceedings of the symposium held at the Lenox Hill Hospital in New York. Baltimore, Williams and Wilkins, 1970.

70. Rutledge F: Management: Stages III and IV, carcinoma of the cervix, in Rutledge F, Boronow RC, Wharton JT (eds): *Gynecologic Oncology.* New York, John Wiley & Sons, 1976, p 59.

71. Rutledge F: Management: Treatment failures in carcinoma of the cervix, in Rutledge F, Boronow RC, Wharton JT (eds): *Gynecologic Oncology,* New York, John Wiley & Sons, 1976, p 81.

72. Hunt HA: Splenectomy, in Rob C, Smith R, Morgan CN (eds): *Operative Surgery, Abdomen and Rectum and Anus.* Philadelphia, JB Lippincott Co, 1969, p 254.

73. Jordan GL: Complications of pancreatic and splenic surgery, in Artz CP, Hardy JD (eds): *Management of Surgical Complications,* ed 3. Philadelphia, WB Saunders Co, 1975, p 563.

74. Martin JD, Cooper MN: Complications of splenectomy. *South Surg* 16:1047, 1950.

75. Altemeier WA, Culbertson WR: Complications of appendectomy, in Artz CP and Hardy JD (eds): *Management of Surgical Complications,* ed 3. Philadelphia, WB Saunders Co, 1975, p 587.

76. Johnson HD: Gastrostomy, in Rob C, Smith R, Morgan CN (eds): *Operative Surgery, Abdomen and Rectum and Anus.* Philadelphia, JB Lippincott Co, 1969, p 62.

77. Clearfield HR, Stahlgren LH: Acute dilations, injuries and rupture of the stomach, in Bockus HL (ed): *Gastroenterology.* Philadelphia, WB Saunders Co, 1974, vol 1, p 1115.

78. Foldes FR, Kepes ER, Ship AG: Severe gastrointestinal distention during nitrous oxide and oxygen anesthesia. *JAMA* 194:244, 1965.

79. Rimer DG: Gastric retention without mechanical obstruction. *Arch Intern Med* 117:287, 1966.

80. Engler HS, Kennedy TE, Ellison LT, et al: Hemodynamics of experimental acute gastric dilatation. *Surg Forum* 16:329, 1965.

81. Passi RB, Kraft AR, Vasko JS: Pathophysiologic mechanisms of shock in acute gastric dilation. *Surgery* 65:298, 1969.

82. Williams JS: Hemodynamic alterations in acute gastric dilation in the dog. *Surg Forum* 16:335, 1965.

83. Evans DC: Acute dilatation and spontaneous rupture of the stomach. *Br J Surg* 55:940, 1968.

84. Gillesby WJ, Wheeler JR: Acute gastric dilatation. *Am Surg* 22:1154, 1956.

5

Complications Related to the Radiated Gastrointestinal Tract

Julian P. Smith

Irradiation is frequently used in the treatment of pelvic malignancies, both in the United States and abroad. The first description of a radiation injury of the intestines, by Walsh (1), followed the discovery of x-rays by Roentgen by only 2 years; however, bowel injuries from irradiation were relatively uncommon until the introduction of supervoltage x-ray machinery, which came into wide use in the early 1950s. Before the advent of supervoltage therapy, the appearance of radiodermatitis protected patients from high doses of external radiation therapy that could cause injuries to the visceral structures in the pelvis.

The site and type of radiation injuries are dependent upon the manner in which irradiation therapy is given. Intracavitary brachytherapy to the uterus and cervix tends to cause radiation injuries to the adjacent bladder and rectum. Although external irradiation therapy may cause injuries to these structures, this type of therapy may injure the small intestine also.

Irradiation therapy is the principal treatment of invasive carcinoma of the cervix, both in the United States and throughout the world; and it is in this group of patients with cervical carcinoma that we most frequently see severe injuries to the abdominal and pelvic viscera requiring surgery.

During the last 10 years, many institutions have been performing exploratory celiotomies on patients with advanced cancer of the cervix, to determine the extent of their cancer, and then giving these patients irradiation to fields that cover the known areas of metastasis. The use of para-aortic irradiation in patients with metastases to the para-aortic area has caused injuries to the jejunum, duodenum, and even the stomach. Radiation injuries to these structures were uncommon before this type of irradiation.

The most common site of injury from pelvic irradiation for gynecologic cancer is the large intestine, the rectum being the most common site of injury. The small intestine is less commonly injured in standard irradiation; however, with the use of larger doses of whole-pelvis irradiation and with the use of extended-field treatment, which may extend to the bifurcation of the aorta or to the diaphragm, the number of injuries to the small intestine is increasing. Injuries to the small intestine offer a greater challenge to surgeons, and the proper treatment of these injuries is the subject of considerable controversy among surgeons. Most of this controversy concerns whether injured segments should be resected or bypassed.

During irradiation therapy there may be loss of the clonogenic mucosal cells in the intestinal crypts and decreased production of mucus. With the decrease in mucus, the mucosa is more vulnerable to digestion by the digestive enzymes. Digestion of the intestinal mucosa leads to ulceration and inflammatory changes in the submucosal tissues. The initial injury of the intestine that is seen after irradiation often has the appearance of acute inflammation, with edema and hyperemia. Depending on the time interval between the irradiation and the discovery of the injury, and the dose of irradiation to the intestine, patients may have evidence of endarteritis and thrombosis in the smaller vessels. These conditions may lead to mucosal changes with areas of infarction and ulceration. Regardless of the pathologic changes, healing occurs through fibrosis.

After the acute changes have subsided, progressive, obliterative endarteritis with edema and fibrosis leading to thickening of the intestinal wall may develop in these patients. The bowel serosa may appear pale gray, and the mesentery frequently shows similar changes plus edema and fibrosis. Also, the mesentery is often shorter and thicker than normal.

The irradiated intestine frequently shows a loss of villi and fixation of the mucosa to the underlying submucosa. In the areas in which the mucosa is ulcerated, there may be severe scarring and the muscle layers may appear to be replaced with fibrous connective tissue. Commonly, inflammatory cells are seen in the submucosa.

The use of total parenteral nutrition (TPN) has improved the treatment of patients with irradiation injuries to the pelvic and abdominal viscera. The use of TPN is indicated in all patients who have lost weight and who are in a catabolic state due to their injury. The improved healing is so dramatic that this type of nutritional support should be considered in the preoperative and postoperative care of all patients who require surgery because of this type of injury. This improvement in care will necessitate a reappraisal of our surgical management of irradiation injuries in the near future.

INJURIES TO THE SMALL INTESTINE

The common injuries to the small intestine caused by irradiation include stricture, perforation, fistula formation, and rarely, hemorrhage. These injuries lead to abdominal pain, intestinal obstruction, chronic malnutrition, and weight loss. The management of patients with injuries to the small intestine, secondary to irradiation, will depend on many factors, including the severity of symptoms; however, some generalizations can be made about the treatment of this group of patients.

The diagnosis of injury to the small intestine is largely clinical. Abdominal x-rays wth the patient in the supine, upright, or lateral decubitus position may be helpful in verifying the diagnosis of obstruction or in following patients who are being observed for an injury; but contrast x-rays of the small intestine are seldom beneficial, especially if they are peformed when the patient is improving or asymptomatc. All patients who are being prepared for small bowel surgery should have a barium enema beforehand if their conditions allow. A severe constriction of the colon may be overlooked if the patient has had evidence of small intestinal injury. This constriction may lead to failure of an anastomosis in the small intestine if it is not recognized, because of the retrograde pressure on the intestine proximal to the stricture.

Small intestinal injuries caused by irradiation are similar clinically to inflammatory lesions of the small intestine. They produce similar symptoms, are found in the same sites, and may produce similar x-ray findings. Because of this similarity, the general surgeon with limited experience in the care of patients with intestinal injuries from irradiation may treat these patients the same. But the small intestinal injury from irradiation requires more prompt and aggressive surgical management, and the diagnosis is more grave. Intestinal obstructions secondary to regional enteritis may be treated expectantly, but obstructions from irradiation require early surgical correction and seldom should be treated conservatively.

All patients who have evidence of intestinal obstruction after irradiation therapy to the pelvis should be admitted to the hospital for observation. Patients with significant obstruction should be put on NPO and given intravenous fluids. If a patient has significant small intestinal dilatation with cramping and vomiting despite being on NPO, a long intestinal tube should be inserted and attempts made to pass the tube to the area of obstruction. Many of the patients who respond quickly to this conservative management will benefit from conservative treatment: a medical regimen consisting of a low-residue, bland diet; psyllium hydrophillis mucilloid twice a day; and anticholinergic drugs such as propantheline bromide, 15 mg, one-half hour before meals and at bedtime.

Patients who have had previous symptoms of obstruction and who have not improved with a medical regimen or patients who have had previous episodes of partial obstruction and who have had 5,000 rads or more of whole-pelvis irradiation should have surgery without further temporizing. If these patients have had significant weight loss, they may benefit from a short period of TPN 7–10 days before surgery. The length of time for which it is safe to watch patients who have had pelvic irradiation is dependent on the doses of radiation that they have received. Those who have received less than 5,000 rads may be watched for several episodes of partial obstruction; however, if the patient has received 5,000 rads or more, she should not be observed for more than one episode of obstruction. Those who have had more than 6,500 rads of whole-pelvis irradiation should have surgery with their first episode of partial obstruction if it is severe enough to necessitate admission to the hospital.

In a review of 71 patients who had surgery because of a small intestinal injury secondary to irradiation at the University of Texas System Cancer Center, M. D. Anderson Hospital and Tumor Institute in Houston, Texas, the radiation injuries were not related to race, age, or clinical stage of disease but were related to the doses of whole-pelvis irradiation that the patient received. Most of the patients received at least 4,000 rads of whole-pelvis irradiation.

Only 6 of the 71 patients had significant symptoms of radiation enteritis during their treatment. More than half of the patients had had no previous medical complications; however, previous pelvic surgery was very common. Fifty-four of the 71 patients had had a prior abdominal operation. Only 8 of 71 patients who had small intestinal injuries requiring surgery weighed 150 lb or more (Table 1). Fifty-three of the 71 patients had lost more than 10 lb before the small bowel injury was recognized.

Radiation injuries may occur anytime after radiation therapy—as long as 32 years later; however, only in two patients in this series of 71 patients with small bowel injuries did an injury develop more than 6 years after their treatment. In 48% of the patients the injuries developed within 1 year after completion of treatment, and in 74% within 2 years (Table 2).

The most frequent physical finding in patients who require surgery is either partial or complete intestinal obstruction, and this was found in 62 of the 71 patients who had small bowel injuries requiring surgery (Table 3).

The surgical procedures that should be performed in patients who have small intestinal obstructions from radiation is the subject of some controversy (2–6) (Fig. 1). General surgeons who have had experience in treating inflammatory

Table 1. Weight on Admission of Patients with Small Bowel Injuries

Weight (lb)	Number of Patients
55–99	18
100–149	45
150–199	7
200–249	1
Total	71

Table 2. Time from Radiation to Small Bowel Obstruction

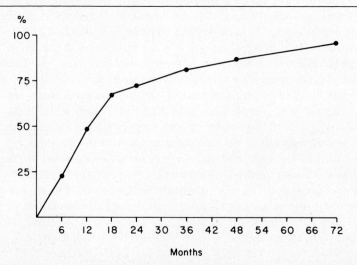

Table 3. Physical Findings Before Surgery

Complication	Number of Patients
Partial obstruction	47
Complete obstruction	15
Perforation with peritonitis	4
Enterovaginal fistula	4
Enterovesical fistula	1
Total	71

diseases of the intestines frequently favor resection of the damaged loop of intestine (5, 6), whereas gynecologic oncologists (2–4) generally favor bypass of the obstructed loop of intestine. Obviously, each patient must be assessed individually. Patients who have necrosis of the intestinal wall with impending perforation or patients who have severe injuries to the intestines as a result of dissection during surgery should have the involved loop of intestine resected and

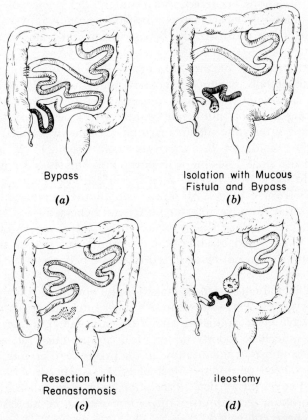

Bypass

(a)

Isolation with Mucous
Fistula and Bypass

(b)

Resection with
Reanastomosis

(c)

ileostomy

(d)

Figure 1. Operations for radiation injuries of the ileum. (a) A simple bypass of the damaged area of intestine; (b) A bypass of the damaged area of intestine with isolation of this segment from the intestinal tract; (c) Resection of the injured area of intestine; (d) Diversion of the intestinal tract proximal and distal to the injured area of intestine.

the bowel continuity restored by the distal segment of the intestine being joined to either the ascending or transverse colon as an end-to-end, end-to-side, or possibly, side-to-side anastomosis. Under these circumstances end-to-side anastomosis is usually satisfatory.

The surgeon with experience in the management of patients with small intestinal injuries will refrain from dissecting agglutinated loops of intestine out of the pelvis and will choose the simplest procedure to relieve the patient's injury. This procedure will consist of bypass of the involved loops of the intestine with a side-to-side anastomosis of the distal intestine to the ascending colon or transverse colon. In a review of the world's literature on this subject by Swan et al., (2) the author found that operative mortality was twice as great in the group who had resection of their injured small intestine as it was in the group who had a bypass to this area—21% mortality for the resected group and 10% mortality for the bypass group. He found that intestinal anastomotic dehiscence occured in 36% of the resected group and in only 6% of the bypass group.

Among the 71 patients with small intestinal complications in the author's series, 37 patients had bypass procedures and 21 had resection of the injured intestine. One-third of those who had resection died in the postoperative period compared with 21% of the bypassed group. Most of the deaths of the patients who had the resections occurred as a result of dehiscence of the intestinal anastomosis leading to local abscess formation and/or reobstruction of the intestine. Most of the deaths in the bypass group were the result of medical complications.

Patients with necrosis of the intestinal wall, patients with enterovaginal fistulas, and occasionally, patients with enterocutaneous fistulas will benefit from a procedure that isolates the loop of injured intestine from the intestinal tract without resecting this loop and creates either one or two mucous fistulas from the divided loops of intestine and an anastomosis of the proximal intestine either to the ascending colon or the transverse colon (Fig. 1). If a patient has perforation of the small intestine with peritonitis, she should have a proximal ileostomy performed. Only rarely, when the infection is well localized and the patient is free from evidence of sepsis, should the perforated intestine be resected or isolated from the intestinal tract and bypassed.

The operative procedure should be as conservative as possible. Obviously, intestine that is entwined in complicated agglutinated masses should be left undisturbed and should not be dissected from the pelvic walls or the depths of the pelvis.

When possible, patients should be taken to the operating room electively and not as an emergency. Perforation of the small intestine or sigmoid colon in patients who have been irradiated carries an extremely poor prognosis. Since irradiated intestine heals poorly under ideal circumstances, it is foolhardy to attempt an anastomosis of the intestine in the presence of an intestinal perforation with generalized peritonitis. Most of these patients will require either a proximal ileostomy with an ileal perforation or a proximal colostomy with a sigmoid perforation. A definitive operation should be deferred until the peritonitis has been controlled.

The surgical techniques involved in anastomosis of the intestine in patients who have suffered irradiation injuries should be meticulous. Great care should be exercised in handling the intestine. The two pieces of bowel that are to be joined should be isolated from the rest of the abdominal cavity with moist laparotomy pads, to prevent soilage of the rest of the peritoneal cavity. When possible, the intestines should be prepared before surgery by passing a long tube, such as a Dennis tube (Argyle), into the small intestine as close to the injured area as possible. This procedure allows decompression of the proximal intestine and protects the anastomosis from intestinal contents until healing has occurred. It also splints the proximal bowel and is useful in preventing complex adhesions, which may lead to postoperative obstruction.

The two pieces of intestine that are to be joined in the anastomosis should be clamped both proximally and distally with atraumatic rubber-shod clamps, and the intestinal contents should be carefully suctioned from each loop of intestine as it is opened. The intestine should be sutured together with a two-layer closure. The first layer is an absorbable suture material such as chromic catgut or one of the newer polyglycolic suture materials. The second layer should be a nonabsorbable material such as cotton, silk, or one of the new synthetic materials. The first layer of the anastomosis should be a watertight closure of the intestine. Interrupted sutures are preferable to continuous sutures because of the compromised blood supply in the irradiated intestine. Sutures should be placed through the entire thickness of the intestinal wall and tied so that the knots are inside the lumen, inverting the intestinal wall (Fig. 2). The second layer of nonabsorbable suture relieves tension from the first layer. It should be placed in such a manner that it does not constrict the blood supply to the inner layer but produces a second watertight layer closure.

When a loop of intestine has been resected, the defect of the mesentery should be closed with fine, nonabsorbable sutures that pierce only the peritoneum and will not interfere with the underlying blood vessels in the mesentery. The abdomen should be generously lavaged after the anastomosis has been completed. The surgeon should change gloves, and the instruments that have been used in the anastomosis should be removed from the operative field. The patient should receive preoperative and postoperative broad-spectrum antibiotics that will be effective against the organisms commonly found in the intestinal tract, and the antibiotics should be continued for a minimum of 5 days after surgery. The new aminoglycosides, such as gentamycin or tobramycin, combined with a second antibiotic, such as ampicillin or chloromycetin, are satisfactory for these patients.

After surgery is completed, the intestine should be put at rest by suction to the long intestinal tube until gastrointestinal function is reestablished. The patient should receive TPN for approximately 21 days or a period long enough to allow satisfactory healing of the intestinal anastomosis, before the anastomosis is tested with normal intestinal contents. After TPN has been started and intestinal functions have returned, the long intestinal tube may be clamped for 24 hours and then removed if the patient is free from cramping, nausea, and vomiting.

In patients who exhibit evidence of sepsis with an intra-abdominal abscess or peritonitis, stress ulcers frequently develop. If blood is found in the intestinal tube, the patient should receive cimetidine, 300 mg every 6 hours, I.V. If bleeding continues or increases, the patent should receive antacid solutions orally at 1- or 2-hour intervals; the stomach contents should be tested for pH before the antacids are repeated.

The abdominal wall should be closed with a mass suture technique such as the

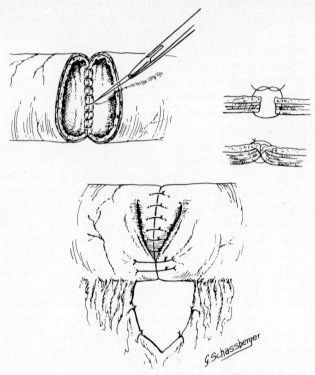

Figure 2. *Bowel Anastomosis.* (Upper) Sutures should be placed through the entire thickness of the intestinal wall and tied so that the knots are inside the lumen, inverting the intestinal wall. (Lower) The second layer of nonabsorbable suture relieves tension from the seromuscular layer.

Smead-Jones closure, by means of a permanent nonreactive suture such as proline or stainless steel wire. If the bowel has not been prepared with antibiotics before surgery, the subcutaneous tissues should be left open and closed 5 or 6 days after surgery as a delayed closure. Patients in whom wound infections develop should have their wounds opened early to prevent disruption of the fascia by necrotizing infections, which may lead to subsequent enterocutaneous fistulas.

If an intra-abdominal abscess is found after surgery, it should be drained, if possible, without exploration of the abdominal cavity. Pelvic abscesses should be drained through the vagina, when possible. Postoperative fever should be investigated by careful physical examinations, blood and urine cultures, and x-rays of the chest and abdomen. If Bacteroides are found in the bloodstream, an intra-abdominal abscess should be suspected. If an obvious site of infection is not found, the patient should be reexplored for the possibility that an undiagnosed abscess is present.

Postoperative complications such as frequent, loose stools and/or diarrhea can usually be managed medically. A low-residue, bland diet; an anticholinergic drug, such as propantheline, 15 mg, one-half hour before meals and at bedtime; and codeine, 15–60 mg, every 6 hours are usually effective in controlling diarrhea. Some patients will benefit from the use of cholestyramine, 9 gm, one to three times per day. Improvement may not occur until 1–6 months after surgery. If the terminal ileum has been resected or bypassed, vitamin B_{12} should be given monthly. Other complications of short bowel syndrome such as nephrolithiasis or peptic ulcer are seldom seen after small intestinal surgery for radiation injuries. The blind loop syndrome requiring antibiotics is uncommon.

INJURIES TO THE LARGE INTESTINE

Radiation injuries to the large intestine include rectovaginal fistulas, proctosigmoiditis, rectosigmoid obstruction, rectosigmoid perforation, and fistula formation with other pelvic viscera. In a series of 72 patients with large intestinal injuries secondary to radiation reported by Smith et al. (3), rectovaginal fistulas were the most common injury, followed by proctosigmoiditis and rectosigmoid obstruction (Table 4). In 18 of the 30 patients in whom rectovaginal fistulas developed a vesicovaginal fistula also developed (60%). Most of these patients had vaginal vault necrosis before their fistulas appeared. Patients with vaginal vault necrosis should be treated with hydrogen peroxide and water douches (1:3), two or three times each day, to arrest the necrotizing process, which may progress to either rectovaginal or vesicovaginal fistulas.

In two of the patients a rectovaginal fistula healed after a diverting colostomy was performed. A simple closure of the rectovaginal fistula after a diverting colostomy is only occasionally successful. In only three of nine patients were fistulas closed successfully this way. If nonirradiated tissue, such as the ischiocavernosus muscle and its surrounding fat pad, the gracilis muscle, or a myocutaneous flap from the leg employing the gracilis muscle and the overlying skin, is introduced into the vagina to reinforce the closure, a higher percentage of success can be expected.

Bricker and Johnston (7) have described a rather unusual method of closing rectovaginal fistulas by dissecting the fistula from the vaginal wall and then dividing the proximal sigmoid colon from the descending colon and folding this over the fistula to increase the caliber of the rectum and to close the defect. (The patients who underwent this procedure all required a prior diverting colostomy.) After the fistula closure has healed, the proximal colon from the colostomy is brought down and joined to the sigmoid colon. Marks (8) has described a

Table 4. Colon Injuries

Injury	Number of Patients
Rectovaginal fistula	30
Proctosigmoiditis	18
Obstruction	17
Perforation	5
Other fistulas	2
Total	72

combined transabdominal-transsacral procedure in which the segment of rectum with the rectovaginal fistula is resected. The proximal colon, which has not been irradiated, is brought down and anastomosed to the very short segment of remaining rectum, a transsacral approach being used to this area. It is necessary that all patients have a diverting colostomy at the time of the initial surgery, and this colostomy is closed after the anastomosis between the descending colon and the distal rectum has healed satisfactorily.

Most patients who have proctosigmoiditis with rectal bleeding can be managed conservatively with a low-residue diet, anticholinergic drugs, and a stool softener, such as psyllium hydrophillic mucilloid. The surgeon will have to decide when a patient should have a colostomy because of rectal bleeding. Many patients will refuse a colostomy until they have received 30−50 pt of blood. In this series of 18 patients who had severe proctosigmoiditis, 16 had diverting colostomies and the bleeding was controlled in 14 of 16 patients; however, no patients required further surgical procedures because of rectal bleeding. Most of these colostomies can be closed when the patient has been free from bleeding for 4−6 months.

Stricture of the rectosigmoid secondary to irradiation is the third most common injury to the colon. Among the 17 patients with rectal strictures, 14 were treated with colostomies and 3 were treated with resections without a diverting colostomy. Two of the resections were satisfactory, but one patient experienced multiple complications that eventually led to her death. Many of the patients with stricture of the rectosigmoid will improve enough to have their colostomies closed later. The colostomies for rectal injuries were about equally divided between transverse colostomies and descending colon colostomies; most were simple loop colostomies.

Necrosis of the rectosigmoid colon with perforation is an uncommon but catastrophic complication. This complication frequently leads to generalized peritonitis. Among a group of five patients with perforation of the rectosigmoid, only two survived, one who had a small perforation and localized peritonitis and one who had generalized peritonitis. Patients with perforations should be treated with vigorous lavage of the entire peritoneal cavity and should receive high-dose systemic antibiotics to treat all the organisms that could be present. A drain is inserted into the area of abscess formation through the vagina, when possible. If generalized peritonitis is present, some consideration should be given to irrigating the abdominal cavity with antibiotic solution introduced through irrigation catheters placed through the abdominal wall. If the abdominal cavity is irrigated with antibiotic solution, only drugs such as the synthetic penicillins or one of the cephalosporins with a wide range of safety should be used. The aminoglycosides should not be given intraperitoneally unless the serum levels are monitored carefully.

All the patients with sigmoid perforations were treated with diverting colostomies. The Hollister plastic bridge has simplified the construction of colostomies in this group of patients (Fig. 3). The colostomy is opened in the operating room, and the proximal end is matured to the skin by folding the bowel wall on to itself. The distal end is simply attached to the skin. In time, this procedure leads to retraction of the distal limb so that it is barely visible. The newly opened colostomy is covered with a 4½-inch karaya-gum ring colostomy bag in the operating room.

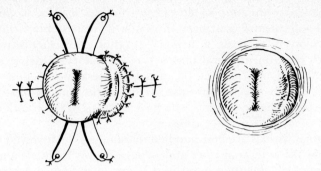

Figure 3. *Colostomy.* The Hollister plastic bridge has simplified the construction of colostomies.

FISTULAS

Fistulas from the small intestine to the colon, to the bladder, to the skin, or to the vagina may develop after surgery, recurrent cancer, or necrosis of the intestinal wall, but occasionally they occur without these antecedent causes. Although enterocutaneous fistulas secondary to surgery in nonirradiated patients will frequently heal if TPN or, occasionally, tube feeding with a low-residue diet supplement is employed, radiation injuries seldom heal with this conservative treatment (9, 10). In most instances, the involved segment of intestine must be resected and the proximal, healthy intestine joined to the ascending colon in either an end-to-side or side-to-side anastomosis. Occasionally, there is an inflammatory reaction present with a conglomerate mass of multiple loops of bowel. The involved intestine and the fistula must be isolated from the intestinal tract (Fig. 1). It is extremely important that the intestine with the fistula be divided from the intestinal tract both proximally and distally. Although the ileocecal valve in nonirradiated patients may be competent and prevent retrograde spillage of intestinal contents through an enterocutaneous fistula in the terminal ileum, in patients who have had irradiation, the ileocecal valve is seldom competent; if the fistula is in the distal ileum, spillage of intestinal contents from the cecum through the ileocecal valve and then into the fistula is the rule rather than the exception.

Enterocutaneous fistulas from the colon to the skin are uncommon secondary to irradiation. These fistulas from the cecum or the transverse colon may be treated conservatively and spontaneous closure anticipated if there is no evidence of distal obstruction of the colon. Enterocutaneous fistulas of the sigmoid colon to the abdominal wall will seldom heal spontaneously and will require resection and/or a diverting proximal colostomy.

Enterovesical fistulas are, fortunately, relatively uncommon but may be extremely difficult to manage. In almost every instance, the involved loop of the intestine should be resected, if the patient's condition allows, and the bladder closed primarily. Patients with sigmoid vesical fistulas will usually require diverting colostomies, and in most patients this will be the definitive treatment because of the multiple pelvic abscesses secondary to the sigmoid vesical fistula. In an occasional patient, it is possible to resect the involved segment of sigmoid colon with an end-to-end anastomosis and protecting proximal colostomy. The occasional patient with complicated pelvic abscesses leading to necrosis of the bladder wall will require a urinary diversion in which either the jejunum or transverse colon is used as a urinary conduit. In patients with a severe inflammatory reaction, ureteral obstruction secondary to pelvic necrosis, and cellulitis, nephrostomies may be beneficial or lifesaving. A new technique in which an adhesive is injected into the ureters at the time of bilateral nephrostomy may be beneficial to patients who have necrosis of the bladder from pelvic cellulitis.

Enterovaginal fistulas are best handled by isolating the involved loop of small intestine from the intestinal tract and bypassing this isolated loop proximally (Fig. 1). If only a small loop of intestine is involved, a single mucous fistula from the most distal end of the isolated loop of intestine is usually satisfactory. Only rarely should the loop of intestine that is adherent to the apex of the vagina be resected. If this loop is resected, frequently another loop will become adherent in the same area, and if the inflammatory changes that caused the original fistula are still present, a fistula may occur in the next loop of intestine that becomes adherent.

RADIATION CYSTITIS

Radiation cystitis can be extremely distressing. Severe hematuria can usually be controlled by irrigating the bladder through a three-way catheter, using either 0.5% or 1.0% acetic acid solution. Other irrigation solutions that may be helpful include hydrocortisone solutions or potassium permanganate, 1–10,000. It is extremely important to evacuate all clots in the bladder before attempting to irrigate it. Vigorous irrigation of the bladder with an Ellik syringe will often remove clots. Occasionally, a patient whose hematuria continues despite irrigation through a three-way catheter will benefit from irrigation of the bladder through a suprapubic catheter and simultaneous drainage of the bladder through a urethral catheter. Irrigating the bladder with cold saline solution or instilling cold saline solution in a condom tied to a straight French catheter inside the bladder may be of some benefit in controlling bleeding. In patients with severe bleeding, condom tied to a French catheter inside the bladder may be inflated with air to approximate the diastolic blood pressure. Freezing the bladder mucosa with a cold solution of alcohol inside a condom may rarely be of benefit to patients with severe hematuria who have not responded to other forms of treatment.

After the bladder has stopped bleeding, the patient should receive methenamine mandelate (Mandelamine) and/or ascorbic acid for several weeks.

Only rarely should a patient have a urinary conduit because of hematuria. Rarely, a patient with severe hematuria and a large clot in the bladder will develop necrosis of the bladder wall leading to perforation of the bladder and generalized peritonitis. These patients should have bilateral nephrostomies, abdominal exploration and removal of the blood clots in the bladder, and closure of the bladder defect. The pelvis should be drained through the vagina.

An occasional patient with severe radiation cystitis will have ulceration of the bladder mucosa with intractable pain. These patients may benefit from irrigation of the bladder with dimethylsulfoxide.

PELVIC PAIN

Chronic pelvic pain from radiation necrosis is an extremely difficult problem. Vaginal vault necrosis can be treated with oxidizing douche solutions such as half-strength Dakin's solution or hydrogen peroxide mixed with water (1:3), two to four times per day. Patients who have extensive pelvic necrosis with vesicovaginal and rectovaginal fistulas should be treated with a diverting colostomy and urinary conduit followed by vigorous cleansing of the pelvic cavity with half-strength Dakin's solution or hydrogen peroxide solution. Most patients who do not have obvious pelvic necrosis with involvement of the rectum and/or vagina will have another cause of their pelvic pain, such as recurrent cancer involving the sacral nerves. It may be difficult to establish this diagnosis. Occasionally, these tumors are recurrent in areas of severe fibrosis and will grow slowly over a long period of time before the diagnosis of recurrent cancer is made.

DECUBITUS ULCERS

Sacral decubitus ulcers in debilitated patients who have other problems such as recurrent cancer or radiation necrosis of the pelvis are extremely difficult to manage and will tax the ingenuity of the nurses and the physicians who care for these patients. These patients are often receiving large doses of narcotics and may be very resistant to efforts to keep them from lying on their backs or sides. Small decubitus ulcers may be treated by covering them with karaya gum and changing the karaya frequently. Larger ulcers require debridement both surgically and mechanically. Multiple irrigation solutions such as Dakin's solution, hydrogen peroxide solution, and mixtures of zinc peroxide in carboxymethylcellulose have been used in the care of these wounds. Honey or sugar has also been reported to be beneficial in the treatment of decubitus ulcers. The CO_2 laser may be helpful in some patients. This instrument allows the operator to limit the amount of tissue that is removed. Rarely will it be possible to clean a decubitus ulcer over the sacrum and to skin-graft the injured area either with a flap of adjacent skin or a split-thickness skin graft if the area has been irradiated. Radiation ulcers of the skin of the abdominal wall, however, are more amenable to this kind of treatment.

REFERENCES

1. Walsh D: Deep tissue traumation from roentgen ray exposure. *Br Med J* 2:272, 1897.
2. Swan RW, Fowler, WC Jr, Boronow RC: Surgical management of radiation injury to the small intestine. *Surg Gynecol Obstet* 142:325–327, 1976.
3. Smith JP, Golden PE, Rutledge FN: The surgical management of intestinal injuries following irradiation for carcinoma of the cervix, in *Cancer of the Uterus and Ovary*. University of Texas M.D. Anderson Hospital and Tumor Institute at Houston, Year Book Medical Publishers Inc, 1969, p 241.
4. Wheeless CR Jr: Small bowel bypass for complications related to pelvic malignancy. *Obstet Gynecol* 42:661–666, 1973.
5. DeCosse JJ, Rhodes RS, Wentz WB, et al: The natural history and management of radiation induced injury of the gastrointestinal tract. *Ann Surg* 369–384, 1969.

6. Palmer JA, Bush RS: Radiation injuries to the bowel associated with the treatment of carcinoma of the cervix. *Surgery* 80:458–464, October 1976.

7. Bricker EM, Johnston WD: Repair of postirradiation rectovaginal fistula and stricture. *Surg Gynecol Obstet* 148:499–506, April 1979.

8. Marks G: Combined abdominotranssacral reconstruction of the radiation-injured rectum. *Am J Surg* 131:54–59, 1976.

9. MacFadyen, BV Jr, Dudrick SJ, Ruberg RL: Management of gastrointestinal fistulas with parenteral hyperalimentation. *Surgery* 74:100–105, July 1973.

10. Reber HA, Roberts C, Way LW, et al: Management of external gastrointestinal fistulas. *Ann Surg* 188:460–467, October 1978.

6
Complications of Ureteral Surgery in the Nonradiated Patient

Karl C. Podratz

Neil S. Angerman

Richard E. Symmonds

Continued technologic and therapeutic advances, particularly in physiologic and biochemical monitoring, postsurgical adjuvant radiotherapy and chemotherapy, parenteral nutritional support, and microbial control, have allowed the gynecologist additional freedom in attempting to control pelvic malignancies. Extensive debulking procedures for ovarian neoplasms that were previously designated "unresectable," extended radical hysterectomy, and the various exenterative procedures for control of primary and recurrent cervical carcinoma have become first-line methods of treatment for the pelvic surgeon dealing with a high volume of tumors. Inherent in the successful execution of these extirpative techniques is the frequent need for partial resection of the gastrointestinal and urinary tracts. Therefore, the well-trained gynecologist must have complete knowledge of normal pelvic anatomy (and common variants), an understanding of the natural history of the disease processes, comprehension of the basic principles of intestinal and urologic surgery, and experience with the techniques required to restore the continuity of the gastrointestinal and urinary tracts.

Deliberate transection or partial resection of one or both ureters in the nonradiated patient is seldom associated with untoward sequelae if appropriate ureteroplasty with adequate drainage is performed. Likewise, inadvertent ureteral injuries recognized and repaired intraoperatively have a low associated morbidity. Unfortunately, many surgically related ureteral injuries are not appreciated at the time of operation and become manifest during postoperative convalescence, and others remain silent and often progress to renal dysfunction and atrophy. Although the exact incidence of this problem is difficult to determine, various authors estimate that ureteral injury accompanying "routine" gynecologic procedures for benign disease ranges from 0.3% to 3% (1–3). The reported association of ureteral trauma with radical pelvic surgery is highly variable and depends on the type of procedure; an incidence as high as 19% has been reported with radical vaginal hysterectomy (4). Although similarly inflated rates are often quoted for radical abdominal hysterectomy, several recent reports have not substantiated these claims (5–8). During the past 20 years, 423 radical hysterectomies were performed at the Mayo Clinic in nonradiated patients; only 6 (1.4%) ureteric fistulas occurred (8).

Despite considerable variation in the rate of associated ureteral injury, the risk of potential damage to the ureters exists during any form of pelvic surgery. Therefore, the anatomy of the ureters and their relationship to adjacent structures, the various types and predisposing causes of ureteral injuries, and the many techniques available for ureteral repair should be periodically reviewed by the gynecologist, particularly when experience with ureteral manipulation is limited.

URETERAL ANATOMY

Anatomic Relationships

The ureters are muscular conduits from 25 to 30 cm long that actively transport urine from the kidneys to the bladder. They are arbitrarily divided into abdominal and pelvic portions. Each ureter leaves the renal pelvis at or near the hiatus beneath the renal vessels and descends in the retroperitoneal adipose tissue anterior to the psoas muscles. Proximally, the ureters are incorporated by Gerota's fascia (a thin condensation of perinephric fascia), which extends inferiorly from the kidney; more distally, the ureters are intimately associated with the retroperitoneum and usually remain attached to it during mobilization. The abdominal ureters course downward and medially on the psoas muscles, which separate them from the tips of the transverse processes of the lumbar vertebrae. At the level of L-III, they are crossed by the ovarian vessels, which are located first medial and then lateral to the ureters. The duodenum overlies the right ureter at its origin, and the right colic and ileocolic vessels and distal ileum overlie this ureter in its abdominal course. The left ureter is crossed by the left colic vessels and passes posterior to the sigmoid colon and its mesentery as it approaches the pelvis, so that the pelvic ureter is located lateral to the sigmoid colon.

The right ureter enters the pelvis by coursing over the external iliac artery, whereas the left ureter crosses anterior to the common iliac artery. The ureters then run posterolaterally, turning medially at the level of the ischial spines, where they lie in the fibrous adipose tissue posterior to the ovarian fossae. The ureters continue medialward and forward along the lateral aspect of the uterine cervix. At this level, the uterine arteries accompany the ureters for about 2.5 cm. The arteries then cross over the ureters and ascend between the two layers of the broad ligament to the uterus. At this level, the ureters are located about 2 cm from the lateral aspect of the cervix.

Finally, when the ureters enter the bladder, they run obliquely for about 2 cm through the bladder muscularis and open by slitlike apertures into the cavity of the viscus at the lateral angles of the trigone. When the bladder is distended, the ureteral openings are about 5 cm apart. When the bladder is empty, the interureteric distance is about 2.5 cm. The abdominal and pelvic courses of the ureters are shown in Figures 1 and 2.

Blood Supply

The arterial blood supply to the ureter is segmental, with contributions from aorta and the renal, ovarian, common iliac, internal iliac, uterine, vesical, and vaginal arteries. These segmented branches divide into ascending and descending parts when they reach the fibrous sheath of the ureter and anastomose freely within this sheath with other segmental branches from above and below.

Although the entire ureter is well vascularized in this manner, the midportion of the ureter usually has a less extensive blood supply than does the renal pelvis or pelvic ureter (Fig. 2). The most constant vessel supplying the pelvic ureter is the uterine artery, which, together with the vesical arteries, communicates with the ureter on its lateral aspect; therefore, during dissection below the midpelvis,

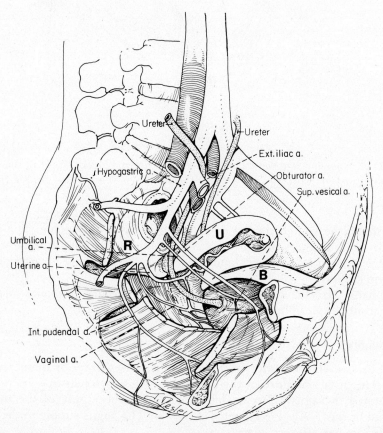

Figure 1. The gross anatomic relationships of the ureters and adjacent structures. R = rectum; U = uterus; B = bladder.

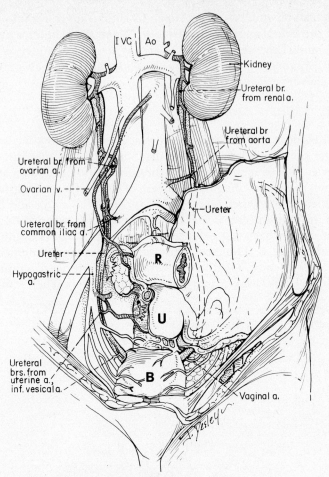

Figure 2. A schematic representation of the major arterial blood supply of the ureters. IVC = inferior vena cava; Ao = aorta; R = rectum; U = uterus; B = bladder.

vessels should be ligated medial to the ureter whenever feasible. The venous return from the ureters includes a series of plexuses that anastomose with the inferior vena cava on the right and the veins accompanying its arterial blood supply on the left.

Lymphatic vessels course in close proximity to the ureteral veins and drain into adjacent lymph nodes.

Nerve Supply

Nerve fibers reach the ureter from adjacent plexuses (inferior mesenteric and pelvic). The distal one-third of the ureter contains nerve cells that are probably incorporated in vagus efferent chains. The afferent supply of the ureter is contained in the T-XI, T-XII, and L-I nerves. The vagus supply to the ureter probably also has afferent components.

Anatomic Variations

The most frequent ureteral anomaly is duplication, which exists in approximately 0.6% of patients. Duplicate ureters usually share a common vascular sheath that becomes a more prominent investing fascia at the level of the uterine artery and consequently causes more fixation of the ureter and its blood supply. Therefore, ureteral separation during dissection at this level may lead to devascularization and necrosis. In addition, variations in the ureteral blood supply can result in a paucity of vessels to the ureter above the midpelvis, a condition that predisposes to easy ureteral devascularization when long segments of ureter require skeletonization for adequate tumor extirpation.

URETERAL EVALUATION

Excretory Urography

When pelvic examination suggests that either a benign or a malignant pathologic condition is present, the anatomic and functional states of the ureters merit close evaluation. The most useful noninvasive technique for visualizing the urinary tract is excretory urography; its roles as a prognostic indicator in the staging of cervical carcinoma and as a means of detection of recurrent disease are well recognized. The observation of partial obstruction, marked displacement, or excessive distortion of the collecting system is generally associated with ureteral impingement by either endometriosis or neoplasms of ovarian or uterine origin. Preoperative documentation of such ureteral aberrancies is frequently useful in staging and planning treatment of these disease entities.

However, it is not our intention to encourage the indiscriminate use of this valuable diagnostic method. To the contrary, "routine" urography before uncomplicated pelvic surgery is not cost-effective and does not aid the surgeon in identifying the ureters at the time of operation. The preoperative urographic demonstration of normal ureteral anatomy and function does not allow the gynecologist to forgo direct visualization and palpation of the ureters during the surgical exercise.

Ureteral Catheters

The value of preoperative placement of ureteral catheters to facilitate intraoperative recognition of the ureters has been debated for decades. Although we are not opposed to selective use of preliminary ureteral stenting (particularly during transvaginal surgical manipulation close to the ureterovesical junction), the inherent shortcomings of this practice as applied to all routine major gynecologic procedures have recently been addressed by Symmonds (3). Advocates of preoperative catheterization maintain that by serving as useful guides during pelvic dissection, stents minimize ureteral trauma. However, an intubated ureter rarely alters the indications or extent of deliberate segmental resection; and the inadvertent injuries are usually associated with the so-called simple hysterectomy. Since the practicality of routine preoperative passage of ureteral catheters is not tenable, we submit that visualizing or palpating (or both) the ureters from pelvic brim to bladder insertion during "routine" hysterectomies greatly aids ureteral mobilization in patients with unfavorable pathologic conditions and reduces the need for preliminary catheter placement. Furthermore, the use of sharp dissection for difficult ureteral exposure is undoubtedly less traumatic in the absence of a stenting device. Finally, should ureteral catheterization become desirable intraoperatively, insertion of a catheter can be expeditiously accomplished through an extraperitoneal cystotomy.

Ureteral Exposure

Accurate atraumatic ureteral dissection, intraoperative recognition of ureteral injuries, and precise ureteral reconstruction can be accomplished with facility when adequate exposure of the ureters and adjacent pelvic structures can be secured throughout the operation. Unfortunately, such exposure is frequently forfeited at the start of the procedure by an inappropriately chosen abdominal incision. Too often, the priority afforded cosmesis results in inadequate vertical or transverse incisions that jeopardize pelvic exposure, surgical technique, and final results. The frequency with which the Pfannenstiel or low transverse incision is employed is generally inversely related to the surgeon's training and experience and is to be condemned in the management of pelvic neoplasia, extensive endometriosis, and chronic pelvic inflammatory disease. Such practice only predisposes to incomplete resection of the diseased area, blind clamping and suturing for hemostasis, and the ureteral injuries to be discussed later in this chapter. In general, a vertical incision extending from the symphysis pubis to or around the umbilicus provides the necessary exposure of both pelvic and lower abdominal structures.

After the pelvic pathologic condition has been inspected, the ureter or ureters should be identified by direct visualization or palpation. The peritoneum lateral to the infundibulopelvic ligament (and above the disease process) can be incised either with or without ligation of the round ligament, and the avascular space of the broad ligament can be entered for direct visualization and palpation of the ureter from the pelvic brim (or above) down to and frequently beyond the uterine artery. With the index finger behind the lateral vaginal fornix and the thumb over the area of the bladder pillar, the ureteral course below the uterine vessels can readily be determined by direct palpation. If additional clearance is required, the ureter can be mobilized from beneath the uterine artery and, if necessary, the latter can be sacrificed without influencing morbidity. This identification process requires only seconds to accomplish while fulfilling the basic surgical principle of exposing all adjacent structures that are potentially subject to operative trauma. It does not involve significant mobilization of the ureter from its attachment to the pelvic peritoneum except when necessitated by disease. Thus, there is minimal risk of damage to the ureteral sheath and its corresponding blood supply.

If neoplasia and benign scarification or fibrosis are present, sharp dissection of the involved ureter is preferable; vascular atraumatic forceps and vein retractors (rather than tapes, Penrose drains, and so forth) are used to manipulate the ureter. Likewise, proper pelvic toilet—including meticulous hemostasis, clean reperitonealization, extraperitoneal drainage with lymphatic interruption, and primary vaginal closure—and correct use of ureteral stents, Foley catheters, antimicrobial agents, and perianastomotic drains minimize postoperative morbidity.

URETERAL INJURIES

The progression of neoplasia or ureteral compromise resulting from various methods of treatment can cause alterations in lower urinary tract function that have the potential for subsequent renal impairment. Early recognition of these causative factors can generally avert, or at least minimize the extent of, ureteral dysfunction. The management of surgically related ureteral damage frequently depends on the interval from injury to recognition; therefore, the anatomic or functional alterations can be classified according to the time of recognition, namely, intraoperative and postoperative ureteral injuries.

Intraoperative Ureteral Injuries

The prevention and recognition of surgically related ureteral trauma depends on complete spatial familiarity of the ureter to adjacent structures (discussed previously) and an appreciation of the common sites frequently associated with ureteral injuries. The sites at risk include (1) the pelvic brim, where the ureter and gonadal vessels are in intimate association anterior to the common iliac vessels and are subject to trauma during ligation of the infundibulopelvic ligament and pelvic reperitonealization, (2) the base of the broad ligament, where blind ligation of the ligamentous and vascular pedicles or indiscriminate attempts at hemostasis can result in ureteral compromise, and (3) the intravesical ureter, which is prone to injury during extended bladder mobilization, repair, and hemostasis and during vaginal cuff closure. Visualization or palpation of the ureters from the pelvic brim to bladder insertion during sharp dissection with appropriate traction and countertraction through a generous abdominal incision minimizes inadvertent intraoperative trauma.

Conditions associated with an increased incidence of ureteral compromise can generally be anticipated after a thorough preoperative evaluation and can be identified at exploration before dissection. The necessity of adequate cytoreductive surgery with ovarian neoplasia and the procurement of wide margins of clearance with cervical carcinoma predispose the pelvic ureter to intraoperative injury. Not infrequently, difficulties of ureteral mobilization and dissection are compounded by unfavorable benign conditions, such as endometriosis, chronic inflammatory reactions, and interligamentous lesions. The most common ureteral injuries recognized intraoperatively are sheath trauma, needle perforation, crushing, ligation, and transection.

Needle Perforation and Ureteral Sheath Trauma

The most common form of ureteral injury encountered by the gynecologist is the disruption of the ureteral sheath during its pelvic mobilization. The ureter below the midplane of the pelvis requires frequent manipulation to assure its integrity and, therefore, is also most vulnerable to sheath trauma. Endometriosis, pelvic infection, and postsurgical changes commonly induce fibrosis and scarification at the base of the broad ligament; the results are difficulties with ureteral dissection and an increase in the risk of sheath compromise. Likewise, the tunneling and lateral displacement of the distal portion of the ureter during Wertheim hysterectomy can lead to segmental damage. Partial disruption of the ureteral sheath results in a corresponding interruption of the longitudinal blood supply. However, vascularly compromised segments, if damage is partial and limited, are well tolerated in the nonradiated pelvis. Treatment likewise depends on the extent of sheath damage, with particular reference, again, to the accompanying blood supply. With minor localized segmental trauma (including needle perforation), no treatment except careful inspection is usually necessary, whereas with more extended damage, retrograde placement of a ureteral stent to minimize the effects of transient edema, ascending infection, and stricture formation is desirable. In contrast, when the size of the injury suggests devitalization, excision or shunting of the damaged section and restoration of lower tract continuity by either ureteroureterostomy or ureteroneocystostomy (procedures to be described) are preferable.

Crushed and Ligated Ureters

When the ureter is inadvertently crushed, prompt removal of the crushing instrument generally constitutes sufficient therapy without unexpected sequelae. The extent of ureteral damage undoubtedly depends on the size of the crushed area (related to clamp size) and how much time elapses before the injury is recognized. Revascularization of the blanched region and propagation of peristalsis through the traumatized segment after release of the clamp signify minimal ureteral damage. However, if injury is more extensive—as judged by a prolonged crushing interval, a widely traumatized segment, or sluggish ureteral function—stenting of the involved ureter for about 10 days is recommended. If inspection shows sufficient ischemia to suggest the likelihood of subsequent necrosis, complete excision of the crushed region must be considered; after excision, either direct ureteral anastomosis or vesical reimplantation can be performed.

Although management of the ligated or kinked ureter is similar to the treatment of crush injuries, this entity is less often recognized during the operation and is generally first noticed during convalescence as symptoms become apparent. In addition to the ureter, the occlusive ligature usually contains other soft tissue structures that minimize the shearing forces of the suture and thus preserve vascular and functional integrity. Except under rare circumstances (prolonged ligation, irradiated pelvis, and so forth), simple deligation and meticulous hemostasis are sufficient to restore full function.

Ureteral Transection

During treatment of various gynecologic malignancies and, occasionally, benign pelvic processes, transection or segmental excision of one or both ureters may be necessary. Detailed preoperative evaluation of the extent of neoplastic involvement and its urographically delineated relation to the ureters generally allows the surgeon to reliably predict when ureteral reanastomosis, substitution, or diversion may be required. Less predictable is the degree of fibrosis from antecedent surgery, infection, or endometriosis; fibrosis predisposes to devitalization during ureteral dissection and frequently necessitates resection and reconstruction. Restoration of lower urinary tract unity requires familiarity with the various methods of repair (subsequently described in detail). Selection of the technique is based on several factors, as previously discussed by Symmonds (3); however, the level of transection and the extent of the ureteral defect are the major determinants. Other variables are causative and coexisting pathologic conditions; the patient's physical state; the prognosis; the condition of the bladder, ureter, and adjacent pelvic structures; and the experience of the surgeon.

Although management of the transected ureter is dictated by the individual circumstances, the most important factors governing repair of the injury are the site and the extent of the ureteral defect. Although exceptions are not uncommon, several generalizations about choice of restorative techniques can assist in selection in the nonirradiated patient. Generally, transections below the midplane of the pelvis can readily be repaired by an end-to-side ureteroneocystostomy; similar defects above the midpelvis are correctable by a vesicopsoas hitch procedure or an end-to-end ureteroureterostomy. When partial ureterectomy and extirpation of the distal collecting system are necessary, ureteral substitution (bladder flap isolation or ileointerposition) and urinary diversion (intestinal conduit), respectively, are usually indicated. However, if immediate repair is contraindicated because of coexisting disease or the surgeon's unfamiliarity with the methods of repair, temporary external urinary diversion by either cutaneous ureterostomy or catheter ureterostomy should be considered. We recommend the latter, which simply involves retrograde placement of a ureteral stent and its distal exteriorization through the abdominal wall. Because initial ureteral mobilization is not required, this approach minimizes scarification and thereby facilitates ureteral dissection and mobilization during delayed definitive repair.

POSTOPERATIVE URETERAL INJURIES

As an aid in discussion of diagnostic evaluation and definitive treatment, ureteral injuries discovered after surgical manipulation are subclassified as those recognized during early convalescence and those found after surgical dismissal.

Early Recognition

Most ureteral injuries not recognized at the time of operation become manifest during the early convalescent period. A smaller number surface after a delayed interval, and an even smaller group remain silent despite eventual loss of kidney parenchyma. The most obvious clinical presentation of ureteral trauma is postoperative anuria, which unfortunately is often confused with a prerenal process. Lack of urine formation after pelvic manipulation should immediately alert the surgeon to the possibility of bilateral ureteral injury. Other causes of anuria are unilateral ureteral disruption of a solitary (anatomic or functional) renal unit or reflex urinary suppression of the contralateral but previously normal functioning kidney. However, more commonly, the unrecognized unilateral injury does not significantly alter urine output but appears as fever, chills, abdominal or flank pain or tenderness, or urinary leakage from the vaginal or abdominal incision. Likewise, creatinine elevation, prolonged ileus, abdominal distention, ascites, and an abdominal mass are more subtle signs compatible with ureteral disruption.

When the postoperative clinical findings suggest ureteral injury, excretory urography and cystoscopy with ureteral catheterization generally aid in defining the nature and level of the insult. Urographic findings indicative of trauma may include hydronephrosis, nonvisualization, delayed excretion, extravasation, and ureteral narrowing, and except when bilateral trauma occurs, a normal, functioning contralateral ureterorenal unit is generally visualized. Although ureteral trauma is usually demonstrable by excretory urography, the site of injury is often not localized, as can easily be understood with delayed urinary excretion or nonvisualization of the affected unit. Under these circumstances, cystoscopy with retrograde ureteral catheterization can aid in defining the level of compromise and, often, the cause, both of which may be beneficial in the selection and execution of subsequent treatment. If passage of the ureteral catheter is uninhibited, either minimal ureteral damage (such as perforation) or extraluminal placement suggestive of transection can be expected; it is verified by extravasation after instillation of a contrast medium. More commonly, passage of the catheter is impeded by ligature obstruction or acute angulation, and caution must be exercised to avoid additional trauma by overly zealous attempts at catheter probing. Injection of contrast material outlines the distal ureter as the medium flows back into the bladder. Occasionally, an obstructing bulb catheter better delineates the site of injury and differentiates periureteral edema, partial obstruction, and extravasation.

The management of ureteral injury recognized during early convalescence must be individualized. It is influenced by the patient's physical status, the type of trauma identified, and the interval since surgery. The successful passage of a ureteral catheter to the renal pelvis suggests partial transection, perforation, or partial obstruction (from periureteral edema, ureteral tenting, or incomplete ligation) and may constitute definitive therapy. The catheter is left in situ for 10–14 days, functioning as a urinary conduit through the traumatized area, to allow resolution of edema and infection, revascularization of the injured tissues, or partial absorption of the compromising suture material. Healing under these circumstances generally occurs spontaneously and with a minimum of sequelae. However, in complete transection or partial necrosis, evaluation of the lower urinary tract to demonstrate extravasation is usually prompted by symptoms. The accompanying chemical irritation and inflammatory response in the area recently operated on necessitate deferment of definitive reconstruction. Proximal urinary diversion by nephrostomy or intubated ureterostomy and, if indicated, drainage of the extravasation site preserve kidney function while one awaits resolution of ureteral and periureteral tissue changes.

Management of the ligated or acutely angulated ureter resulting in complete obstruction continues to be controversial. Many pelvic surgeons maintain that immediate nephrostomy with deligation after several weeks of proximal drainage is the preferred approach, whereas others advocate immediate deligation with retrograde stenting. We prefer the latter approach unless the patient's general or localized pelvic conditions warrant delay of definitive treatment. In contrast, decompression or urinary diversion proximal to the site of obstruction is preferable in the septic, severely azotemic, or otherwise critically ill patient. Although fluoroscopically directed percutaneous placement of decompression catheters is now available, we continue to prefer direct surgical guidance of a diverting catheter through the kidney parenchyma into the renal pelvis by way of the most dependent major calyx. Definitive ureteroplasty is generally delayed for 2–4 months to allow maximal healing of the ureter and adjacent tissues. Occasionally, during this interim period of nephrostomy drainage, ureteral patency is spontaneously reestablished and surgical intervention avoided.

Delayed Recognition

Surgically related ureteral injuries may remain silent for varying periods, and ureteral obstruction or fistula formation may not be recognized until several weeks to months after primary treatment. Although partial or complete ureteral obstruction is occasionally inadvertently discovered during routine follow-up examination in an otherwise asymptomatic patient, nonspecific discomfort localized to the flank, lumbar, or pelvic regions usually prompts the patient to seek medical evaluation. Excretory urography and cystoscopy with retrograde catheterization aid in defining the impairment of renal function as well as the level and degree of ureteral obstruction. The management of postoperative ureteral compromise depends on several factors, including the patient's age, the original surgical pathologic report and prognosis, the interval since surgery, and the cause and degree of ureteral obstruction.

Presumably either intraoperative trauma or postoperative pelvic scarification and fibrosis are the cause of partial or complete ureteral obstruction that occurs within several months after surgery for localized neoplasia or benign disease. Although a trial of limited, cautious observation (awaiting spontaneous resolution) or attempted ureteral dilation may be considered, partial ureteral obstruction causing anatomic or functional alterations is preferably corrected surgically to prevent additional renal deterioration. Likewise, complete ureteral obstruction, including instances in which much time has elapsed since the original procedure, should receive aggressive surgical consideration. Generally, the time of obstruction can only be guessed at; if the obstructing process is secondary to fibrosis, it may be quite recent. Furthermore, the interval between ureteral obstruction and irreparable kidney loss in the human being is unknown; follow-up results of 40 cases reported by Brunschwig and associates (9) suggest that it is highly variable. Ureteral continuity can usually be restored by either direct anastomosis or ureteral substitution. Preliminary nephrostomy is seldom necessary, except when acute pelvic infection, pyelonephritis, or sepsis supervenes. Certainly, a more conservative approach is recommended in the elderly, in patients with multiple medical problems, and in those in whom the original disease entity was prognostically unfavorable.

In a woman, complete or partial ureteral obstruction several months or years after primary treatment for pelvic malignant disease can represent either recurrent cancer or posttreatment fibrosis. Differentiation is often difficult for the gynecologist, and although a recurrent tumor should be the presumed diagnosis, histologic confirmation is mandatory. Frequently, surgical exploration is necessary to exclude recurrent malignancy; and the surgeon should be prepared to restore urinary tract patency if stenosis related to therapy is found or to perform a wide extirpation (probable exenterative procedure) if a resectable tumor is encountered. Corrective surgery requires ureteral anastomosis, substitution, or diversion (procedures described later in this chapter). In contrast, ureteral obstruction when unresectable cancer is present seldom warrants corrective intervention since a silent uremic death is preferable to death from painful metastases. However, early unilateral obstruction with malignant recurrence and accompanying infection or pending sepsis generally requires proximal decompression. Although nephrostomy has been considered the standard procedure for temporary or palliative urinary diversion, the placement of an indwelling, internal ureteral stent (Gibbons or Cook pigtail) should be attempted first, to eliminate the various technical problems and the inconvenience to the patient of nephrostomy drainage.

Urine in the vagina or at the incision margins may be the first sign of ureteral trauma. The time after surgery at which ureterovaginal or ureterocutaneous fistulas become apparent is generally related to the type of ureteral injury. Ureteral transection or ligation appears during early hospitalization; ureteral devascularization with necrosis, during intermediate convalescence; and posttreatment compromise, after a delayed interval. Managing a genitourinary fistula begins with establishing its urinary origin. Lack of staining of an intravaginal tampon after transurethral instillation of methylene blue but staining after intravenous administration of indigo carmine localizes the origin of the fistula to the ureter. Excretory urography and cystoscopy with ureteral catheterization verify the integrity of the contralateral side and identify the site of origin of the fistula. Cautious stenting of the involved ureter should be attempted. If there is no significant obstruction or infection, definitive surgery is preferably delayed for 2–4 months to allow edema and inflammation to be resolved and to promote revascularization and tissue pliability. Not infrequently, this conservative approach to the management of ureteral fistulas is compensated for by spontaneous restoration of lumen integrity and ureteral function, as demonstrated by the urograms in Figure 3.

Definitive correction of persistent ureterovaginal fistulas in the nonirradiated patient can generally be accomplished with minimal difficulty. Ureteroneocystostomy with or without a psoas hitch is usually suitable for restoring lower tract unity. Occasionally, however, ureteral substitution, ureteral diversion, or nephrectomy is indicated. In contrast, ureterovaginal fistula repairs in the previously irradiated pelvis should be delayed longer; often, the surgeon is more restricted in the methods available for fistula repair, as discussed elsewhere.

DIRECT URETERAL ANASTOMOSIS

The management of ureteral injury requiring restoration of urinary tract continuity is based on numerous determinants. The ultimate procedural selection is influenced predominantly by the length of the compromised ureteral

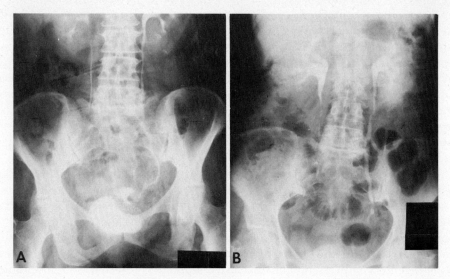

Figure 3. Spontaneous healing of a ureterovaginal fistula. (*a*). An excretory urogram of a patient with a ureterovaginal fistula 49 days after vaginal hysterectomy. (*b*). Urography shows spontaneous reestablishment of urinary tract continuity after 2 months of conservative management.

segment and the level at which the compromise occurred. Most ureteral defects are amenable to correction by direct ureteral anastomosis; ureteroureterostomy and ureteroneocystostomy are suitable for minor defects, while the vesicpsoas hitch and transureteroureterostomy are applicable for larger segmental losses.

Ureteroureterostomy

When the ureter is transected, partially excised, or devitalized during surgical manipulation above the midplane of the pelvis, an end-to-end ureteroureterostomy is generally the corrective procedure of choice. If debridement is liberal, anastomotic tension is avoided, and drainage is adequate, satisfactory healing and normal ureteral and renal function are to be expected. The length of segmental excision or devitalization of the proximal or middle portion of the ureter influences the surgical approach. With increasing segmental losses, additional mobilization of one or both ureters and of the bladder or the kidney (or both) may be necessary. Furthermore, previous pelvic radiation, radical surgery, infection, or endometriosis often produces enough scarification and loss of tissue elasticity to limit severely the feasibility of direct reconstruction. Under such conditions, alternative techniques, as subsequently described, must be used.

Historically, because of high associated morbidity, reconstruction of the transected ureter was performed with much reluctance. Stricture formation, pyelonephritis, urinary extravasation, sepsis, and renal compromise were among the commonly encountered complications after attempts at primary anastomosis. Early postoperative studies noted proximal dilatation and frequent extravasation resulting in inflammation, scarification, and eventually, stricture formation, infection, and loss of kidney parenchyma. Dissociation of the myoelectric activity at the anastomotic junction, disallowing progression of normal peristalsis, was suggested as the underlying physiologic mechanism responsible for the unacceptable morbidity rates. The multiple methods described for ureteral anastomosis attest to the generally unsatisfactory long-term results. However, in 1957, Hamm and Weinberg (10), using a canine model, altered the basic approach by suggesting the use of noncircular anastomosis, proximal ureteral drainage, and perianastomotic drainage. The adoption of these principles by urologic surgeons resulted in a significant reduction of the morbidity rate, and they continue to be of foremost importance to contemporary gynecologic oncologists.

As with all ureteral injuries, repair of the ureter above the midplane of the pelvis begins with the evaluation of the extent of ureteral trauma. The extent of vascular compromise as a result of the surgical injury determines the potential for subsequent ureteral necrosis. As already discussed, the rich longitudinal blood supply traverses the ureteral sheath and can adequately be assessed for viability by observing the degree of blanching when the ureteral and periureteral tissue is gently compressed. The devitalized segment is resected, and, if feasible, all adjacent traumatized tissue is debrided. Seldom does a sharply transected ureter require more manipulation than routine anastomosis. In contrast, partial excision in the course of tumor reduction or blunt surgical trauma necessitates careful visual inspection and adequate debridement to optimize healing. The extent of debridement determines whether an end-to-end ureteroureterostomy is feasible or an alternative procedure is required. With partial resection, varying degrees of ureteral mobilization are generally necessary to assure a tension-free suture line. Occasionally, such mobilization entails inferior displacement of the kidney and proximal portion of the ureter and superior displacement of the bladder (11). Inherent in such mobilization is the disruption of the vascular communications between the ureteral sheath and the aorta and iliac vessels. However, in the nonirradiated pelvis, no significant sequelae are encountered if the integrity of the longitudinal blood supply is not compromised.

After debridement and mobilization, continuity of the ureter is restored in such a fashion as to avoid a circular suture line. We routinely spatulate the transversely debrided ends at opposing 180 degrees, to create an oblique closure (Fig. 4a). The ureters are handled only with atraumatic vascular forceps and vein retractors, and watertight anastomoses are sought with full-thickness, tension-free interrupted sutures of 4-0 or 5-0 chromic catgut. An overly zealous repair employing excessive suture material can result in additional vascular embarrassment wth eventual stricture formation. Seldom are more than six to eight interrupted sutures necessary to effect a watertight repair. An alternative method of anastomosis that further increases the ureteral diameter at the repair site is the Z-plasty technique (Fig. 4b). Occasionally, disproportionate ureteral diameters are encountered as a result of stricture formation or neoplastic obstruction. After resection of the obstructing lesion and proximal decompression, the dilated proximal segment constricts considerably; with spatulation of only the distal portion, an effective anastomosis can be accomplished with relative ease and good long-term results.

Temporary diversion of urine proximal to the anastomosis is necessary to minimize extravasation and, thereby, to limit infection, periureteral fibrosis, and

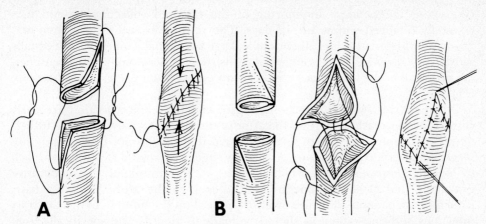

Figure 4. A ureteral anastomosis. (*a*). Opposing spatulation of the debrided ends of the ureter and oblique approximation with interrupted fine catgut. (*b*). Z-plasty technique: parallel oblique ureteral incisions and increased anastomotic diameter.

stricture formation. Equally relevant is the need for adequate retroperitoneal drainage should extravasation or infection (or both) occur postoperatively. We currently prefer to place a ureteral stent for proximal urinary diversion and to evacuate serosanguineous fluid and urine with a retroperitoneal fenestrated suction catheter placed adjacent to, but not in contact with, the anastomosis. A 6F or 8F Silastic catheter is inserted cephalad up to the renal pelvis and, through an extraperitoneal suprapubic cystotomy, is delivered transurethrally for subsequent anchoring to the Foley catheter (Fig. 5). The ureteral stent also allows

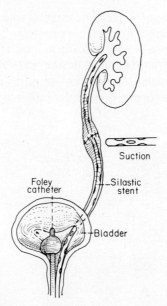

Figure 5. A ureteroureterostomy with an indwelling ureteral stent for splinting repair and proximal internal drainage.

continuous independent monitoring of the repaired collecting system; it is generally removed within 10–12 days. The retroperitoneal drain is removed about 5 days later, after the absence of leakage has been documented. An equally satisfactory alternative is placement of a diverting ureterotomy several centimeters proximal to the anastomosis, either with or without a ureteral stent in place (Fig. 6).

Pyelonephritis, wound infections, sepsis, and urine extravasation are early complications occasionally reported after ureteroureterostomy; stricture formation, hydronephrosis, and progressive renal dysfunction are infrequently observed long-term complications. As already suggested, the therapeutic approach to limiting postoperative morbidity begins with comprehensive preoperative evaluation and close intraoperative adherence to the aforementioned basic principles. In patients who have overt or subtle clinical symptoms of urinary tract infections, judicious attempts should be made to identify and specifically treat the pathogenic organism or organisms. Likewise, adequate debridement, tension-free anastomosis, proximal urinary diversion, perianastomotic drainage, and oblique watertight approximation promote primary stricture-free healing. We routinely use antimicrobial agents before and after the procedure. Also, an excretory urogram is obtained during convalescence if a definitive evaluation of the collecting system is indicated, for example, to document a functionally intact ureter before retroperitoneal drainage is stopped. Recently, Carlton and associates (12), evaluating management of middle and upper ureteral injuries by end-to-end anastomosis, proximal urinary diversion, and drainage, reported that postoperative courses were uneventful in all 25 patients. Excellent long-term follow-up was documented in the 84% having subsequent evaluation.

Ureteroneocystostomy

With intentional resection or inadvertent surgical trauma of the ureter below the midplane of the pelvis, direct ureteral anastomosis can be technically difficult, inaccurate, and accompanied by significant morbidity. Likewise, ureterovaginal fistulas, ureterovesical strictures, and lower ureteral obstructions—common sequelae of radically treated neoplasms—require replacement of the compromised segment. Ureterovesical reimplantation is a reliable procedure for

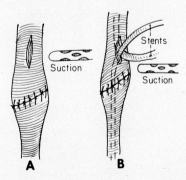

Figure 6. Proximal urinary diversion by a ureterotomy and continuous suction evacuation without (*a*) and with (*b*) ureteral stents.

reestablishing continuity of the distal third of the ureter. When the defect is minimal and the proximal portion of the ureter reaches the bladder, a tension-free ureteroneocystostomy can be readily accomplished. However, if the extent of damage does not permit a tension-free anastomosis, techniques of bladder, ureter, and kidney mobilization should be used to bridge the defect. The vesicopsoas hitch procedure described in detail later in this chapter should be familiar to every gynecologic surgeon; it can replace the pelvic ureter up to and frequently beyond the bifurcation of the iliac vessels. Limitations of this technique are determined by bladder wall integrity; alternative methods are recommended in patients with (1) thick-walled fibrotic bladders due to previous surgery or radiation, (2) urethral obstruction, or (3) atonic bladders.

Ureteroneocystostomy has its greatest application in the treatment of benign congenital vesicoureteral reflux or obstruction; and the successful surgical management in this pediatric age group depends on the use of an effective antireflux anastomosis. Currently, modifications of either the Politano-Leadbetter or Paquin submucosal tunneling technique (13,14) are generally employed to correct symptomatic reflux or obstruction. Although similar procedures are occasionally desired in the gynecologic patient with a tumor, antireflux reimplantation requires an additional 2 or 3 cm of ureter in a setting already selected, to bridge a significant ureteral defect. In adults without preoperative evidence of bladder or ureteral dysfunction, postoperative reflux is significantly less common and is better tolerated than in pediatric patients and seldom leads to progressive renal deterioration (15). Therefore, although antireflux techniques are occasionally employed when apparent ureteral redundancy or preoperative ureteral dysfunction is noted, we prefer a direct end-to-side ureterovesical anastomosis. The successful use of this approach in the treatment of 30 patients with ureterovaginal fistulas has previously been reviewed (16).

When reimplantation is elected for replacement of various segments of the distal portion of the ureter, we prefer a direct transvesical mucosa-to-mucosa anastomosis, as illustrated in Figure 7. For defects of less than 3 or 4 cm, a ureteroneocystostomy can be effectively accomplished with minimal anatomic alteration. The ureter is debrided to secure appropriate vascularity and is mobilized so that a tension-free anastomosis can be constructed. The reflection of the bladder and division of the paravesical peritoneum of the involved side aid in bridging the ureteral defect and allow adequate exposure for extraperitoneal cystotomy. A vertical or curvilinear incision is made on the anterior surface of the bladder, and two fingers are inserted to laterally displace and tent the bladder for aid in selecting the appropriate site for anastomosis. The ureter is spatulated for 0.5–1 cm, and a 3-0 or 4-0 chromic catgut full-thickness suture is placed at the apex of the spatulation. The implantation site, preferably on the posterolateral aspect of the bladder, is incised (0.5–1 cm), and the ureter is delivered with the aid of the previously placed apical suture. Routinely, four to six additional sutures are inserted to complete the anastomosis. The implantation is reinforced with several extravesical sutures that transfix the ureteral adventitia to the bladder muscularis. Additional strength can be derived by anchoring a preserved ureteral-associated peritoneal flap to the bladder wall immediately distal to the anastomosis.

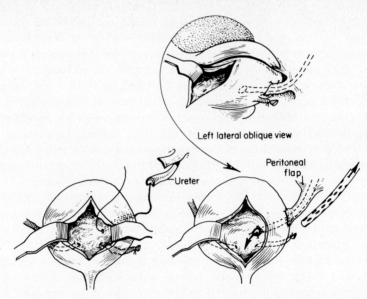

Figure 7. A transvesical ureteroneocystostomy. (From Symmonds RE: Ureteral injuries associated with gynecologic surgery: Prevention and management. *Clin Obstet Gynecol* 19:623, 1976. By permission of Harper & Row, Publishers.)

If an antireflux anastomosis is desired, the bladder muscularis is obliquely incised by repeatedly opening and closing the dissecting scissors until tenting of the bladder mucosa occurs. A right-angled gallbladder forceps (Shallcross) is effectively used to develop a submucosal tunnel, which is incised at an appropriate length. The spatulated ureter is guided through the submucosal defect by a retrograde-placed right-angled forceps, and the anastomosis is secured as described earlier (Fig. 8). Ideally, the intramural ureteral length, usually 2–3 cm, should be approximately four or five times greater than the diameter of the new ureteral orifice.

Stenting of the anastomosis is usually unnecessary with the direct end-to-side reconstruction but is recommended when an antireflux technique (associated with more tissue edema and transient obstruction) is selected. The stent is exteriorized in tandem with either a suprapubic or a transurethral Silastic catheter, and the bladder is closed in the usual two-layered fashion with continuous 3-0 chromic catgut. The ureteral catheters are removed after 10 days, and bladder drainage is discontinued after an additional 2–4 days. The retroperitoneal space is drained by continuous suction evacuation.

Vesicopsoas Hitch

When extensive lower ureteral injuries not correctable by direct ureterovesical reimplantation are encountered, the use of a vesicopsoas hitch procedure in conjunction with ureteroneocystostomy generally restores urinary tract continuity without anastomotic tension (Fig. 9). The technique requires mobilization of the parietal peritoneum from the anteroinferior abdominal wall and retropubic displacement of the bladder. Division of the peritoneum along the

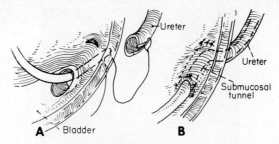

Figure 8. An antireflux ureterovesical anastomosis. (*a*). The ureter is delivered through a 2- to 3-cm submucosal tunnel. (*b*). The spatulated distal end is anastomosed to the bladder mucosa.

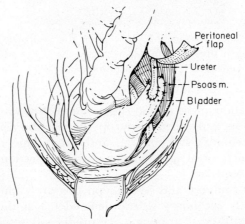

Figure 9. The technique of ureteroneocystostomy with a vesicopsoas hitch.

superior and ipsilateral margins of the bladder, ligation of the obliterated hypogastric artery, and paravesical mobilization allow superior displacement of the usually atonic bladder (anesthetic-induced) to the iliopsoas muscle above the iliac vessels. If additional length is required, management of the contralateral side in a similar fashion allows further vesical mobilization.

The bladder muscularis is anchored to the iliopsoas fascia above the iliac vessels with several interrupted 1–0 chromic catgut sutures; incorporation of the genitofemoral nerve is avoided. The ureterovesical anastomosis and drainage techniques are similar to the methods described previously, except that we prefer an anterior anastomotic site with the posterior vesical fixation. Figure 10 demonstrates the roentgenographic ureterovesical silhouette obtained 11 years after a vesicopsoas hitch procedure was performed in conjunction with a ureteroneocystostomy.

The gynecologist is seldom requested to correct symptomatic ureteral dysfunction resulting from primary urologic disease but generally treats acquired processes in an otherwise normal collecting system. Therefore, when properly selected and accomplished, ureteral implantation restores lower tract unity with minimal morbidity in most patients. For effecting a strong union with few acute and long-term complications, several technical points must be assured, including

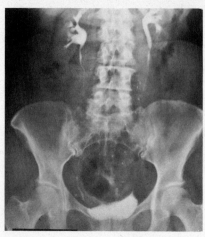

Figure 10. An excretory urogram 11 years after the vesicopsoas hitch procedure. Resection of the midpelvic ureter (4 cm) was required during a cystoreductive operation for recurrent ovarian mucinous cystadenocarninoma.

appropriate mobilization of the ureter, preservation of its vascularity, avoidance of anastomotic tension, and adequate retroperitoneal and bladder drainage. In addition, frequent clinical, biochemical, and urographic reassessments and judicious use of antimicrobial agents promote early detection and resolution of potential untoward sequelae.

Postoperative hydroureter and hydronephrosis are common observations. They are presumably secondary to transient edema at the anastomotic site impeding the normal flow of urine and are predictably resolved within 2 or 3 weeks. More prolonged or progressive dilatation of the proximal collecting system suggests obstruction from another cause. Pathologic causes of obstruction include excessive angulation of the intramural ureter (with submucosal tunneling) and fibrosis or scarification at the ureterovesical junction. With superimposed ureteritis and pyelonephritis, the incidence of stricture formation and renal deterioration increases and prompt proximal diversion should be secured. After satisfactory resolution of the acute process, urographic evaluation determines whether ureteral dilatation will be a feasible alternative to the generally required second major reconstructive procedure. Successful correction of the obstructive process usually entails a repeat ureteroneocystostomy.

Although incorporating an antireflux technique is desirable, ureteral redundancy is a luxury infrequently experienced by the pelvic surgeon performing ureteroneocystostomies for ureteral injuries in adult patients with tumors. Postoperative reflux is usually unacceptable in children with vastly differing surgical indications but is relatively well tolerated in adult women with normal urodynamics before ureteral injury. Therefore, submucosal tunneling is performed when feasible, but extraordinary measures, such as bladder flap isolation, contralateral vesical mobilization, and inferior ureter and kidney displacement, are not entertained simply to create a reflux-free system. Landau (15) demonstrated a 30% incidence of reflux in 39 patients (older than 12 years) with a "fish mouth" type of anastomosis and found only two patients with unsatisfactory long-term results attributable to reflux. Likewise, Lee and Symmonds (16) reported good function with extended follow-up in 27 of 30 patients (three failures unrelated to reflux) who had direct ureteral reimplantation for treatment of ureterovaginal fistula formation. Our intention is not to discourage the incorporation of antireflux maneuvers with ureterovesicoplasty but rather to stress the inappropriateness of selecting more complex surgical procedures or risking anastomotic tension to obtain additional ureteral length for submucosal placement when minimal morbidity is observed with direct anastomosis in the adult patient with a tumor.

Ureteral slough, stricture formation, and fistula formation are less commonly reported complications of ureterovesical reconstruction. The causes of such sequelae are often multifactorial but usually include a compromised vascular supply or urine extravasation with perianastomotic inflammation. Definitive therapy generally requires secondary reimplantation or ureteral substitution.

Transureteroureterostomy

Transureteroureterostomy is a valuable option when extensive ureteral defects cannot be adequately bridged by a vesicopsoas hitch procedure or when ureteral substitutions are not desirable. Frequently cited indications for transureteroureterostomy are loss of large ureteral segments in the upper pelvis as a result of deliberate excision during extirpative surgery for neoplasia, partial uretectomy for stricture formation, and accidental ureteral injuries. The procedure also has merit when surgical or pathologic alterations of the distal portion of the ureter or bladder (or both)—such as disease or irradiation-induced bladder contraction and fibrosis, pelvic sepsis resulting in edematous and friable tissues, and radical resection that includes partial cystectomy—exclude primary single-stage ipsilateral reconstruction. In high-dose pelvic irradiation, retroperitoneal fibrosis, calculus disease, and contralateral reflux or partial obstruction, alternative methods are mandatory.

Although the concept of transureteroureterostomy was suggested nearly a century ago, Hodges and associates (17) reported on the first sizable series in 1963. The procedure continues to be used infrequently, as judged by the collective experiences of British and Irish surgeons (18). Despite about 200 reported cases of successful reconstruction with minimal morbidity, pelvic surgeons have been reticent to use this procedure because of the potential compromise to the recipient ureterorenal unit. Udall and associates (19) addressed this concern in their evaluation of 76 cases and concluded that "apprehension concerning the safety of the recipient ureter seems unwarranted." However, recent reports (20, 21) have documented major complications in the recipient unit, most notably stricture formation at the site of anastomosis requiring major surgical reconstruction. Although we recognize that transureteroureterostomy is an essential procedure within the pelvic surgeon's repertoire, we continue to suggest its use only when other more direct or safer options are not applicable.

The success of the procedure again depends primarily on a good longitudinal blood supply and a tension-free anastomosis. The former is assured by adequate debridement of the insulted ureter and its adventitia and by the use of atraumatic surgical instruments, and the latter can be accomplished with appropriate mobilization. Incision of the lateral peritoneal reflection and medial reflection of the colon and its mesentery allow adequate visualization of the donor ureter for necessary ureteral manipulation (Fig. 11*a*). The peritoneum medial to the recipient ureter is generously incised in such a way that the expected anastomotic site will be above the pelvic brim, to minimize compression and angulation. A generous retroperitoneal tunnel, traversing anterior to the greater vessels in a gradual cephalad course, is formed by gentle blunt dissection. The position of the donor ureter relative to the inferior mesenteric artery is determined by the length of the ureter and the location of the anastomotic site. If placement of the ureter inferior to this vessel results in either anastomotic tension or a nontangential union, a shorter course above the inferior mesenteric artery can be chosen (Fig. 11*b*).

Preferably, to minimize perianastomotic adhesions, the surgeon should not mobilize the recipient ureter and its corresponding prelumbar fat. A 1.5-cm linear ureterotomy is made on the anteromedial aspect of the ureter, and the obliquely matured, spatulated donor ureter is anastomosed in a watertight tangential fashion with interrupted 4-0 chromic catgut (Fig. 11*b*). The value of routine ureteral stenting in transureteroureterostomy is as yet unsettled. Retrograde placement of two 4 F or 5 F Silastic catheters to the level of the renal pelvis can be accomplished with ease through a retropubic cystotomy; the distal segments are exteriorized through the urethra and fixed to the Foley catheter. Before closure of the retroperitoneum, fenestrated suction catheters for evacua-

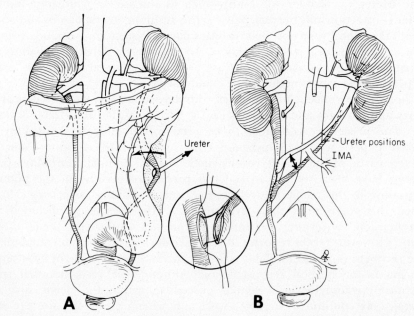

Figure 11. The technique of transureteroureterostomy. (*a*). Medial colonic reflection is done for exposure and mobilization of the donor ureter. (*b*). Alternative retroperitoneal courses of the ureter, with tangential end-to-side anastomosis above the pelvic brim. IMA = inferior mesenteric artery.

tion of serosanguineous fluid and extravasated urine are placed adjacent to, but not in direct contact with, the anastomosis and brought out through the mobilized retroperitoneal space.

Bilateral hydroureter during immediate postoperative convalescence is a common finding, owing presumably to edema at the anastomotic site. Signs of partial resolution of this phenomenon can generally be seen during the immediate postoperative period. In contrast, progression of this process, particularly if urine leakage is present, can result in hydronephrosis, pyelonephritis, or sepsis. In addition to routine use of antimicrobial agents and retroperitoneal drainage, judicious use of temporary proximal diversion by nephrostomy should be considered under such circumstances.

If drainage is appropriate, urinary extravasation is usually resolved spontaneously and without sequelae. However, prolonged urinary drainage or subsequent fistula formation, increasing hydronephrosis, or recalcitrant or recurrent pyelonephritis may indicate impediment of normal urine flow secondary to anastomotic disruption, mechanical obstruction, or stricture formation. The specific treatment of these anomalies is preventive and begins by the securing of a tension-free, well-vascularized primary anastomosis. Although retrograde ureteral catheterization or nephrostomy seldom supplants corrective surgery under these circumstances, diversion generally hastens resolution of local inflammation, infection, and tissue friability. The reparative procedure or procedures are dictated by the operative setting, which may include bladder implantation, recipient ureter reanastomosis, ureteral substitution, or nephrectomy of the donor unit.

URETERAL SUBSTITUTIONS

When the magnitude of the ureteral injury or the accompanying paravesical or paraureteral pathologic condition is not conducive to correction by direct ureteral or vesicoureteral anastomosis, alternative definitive methods must be considered. They include transureteroureterostomy (discussed previously), ureteral substitution, autotransplantation, intentional ureteral ligation, and nephrectomy. The cause of the injury, the age of and long-term prognosis for the patient, and the coexisting functional status of the collecting system are important determinants in proper selection of the procedure. With few exceptions, ureteral substitution—specifically, vesical tubularization—is our procedure of choice when surgical evaluation suggests favorable vesical and proximal ureteral anatomy.

Vesical Tubularization

The successful clinical use of a tubularized full-thickness bladder flap for replacement of a large segment of ureter was first reported by Ockerblad (22) about 50 years after its conception by Casati and Boari (23). The technique has subsequently gained acceptance as a functional alternative when the aforementioned methods are unlikely to bridge, in a tension-free manner, defects of the proximal and middle portions of the ureter. Therapeutically induced ureteral dysfunction requiring circumvention of large fibrotic, poorly vascularized segments of ureter and treatment of pelvic neoplasia necessitating extensive en bloc resection are surgical settings in which the vesical flap is commonly used. The procedure is likewise applicable when a lesser distal (below midpelvis) ureteral defect is noted but vesical mobilization is suboptimal; extensive paravesical dissection during radical surgical manipulation can result in scarification that greatly limits subsequent bladder mobilization for use in the preferred vesicopsoas hitch procedure. If bladder size is adequate and vascularity is appropriate, the vesical flap can be selected under these circumstances to restore distal ureteral continuity. However, alternative methods merit consideration when the conditions just cited are compounded by previous irradiation or operations or by a bladder of minimal capacity.

Our preferred method of bladder flap construction is a modification of the Boari-Ockerblad technique. After appropriate debridement of compromised tissue, the proximal portion of the ureter and the bladder are mobilized in a way similar to that described for the vesicopsoas hitch procedure. The length of bladder wall necessary to bridge the defect adequately without tension is projected. The base of the flap is located on the posterolateral aspect of the bladder, ipsilateral to the injured ureter (Fig. 12). A flap 5–8 cm in length coursing in a gradual spiral over the anterior surface of the bladder is isolated, and the integrity of the blood supply is maintained by securing a widely contoured section of bladder wall. Ideally, the flap apex should be 3 or 4 cm wide and the base width should exceed 5 cm. The spatulated ureter is delivered

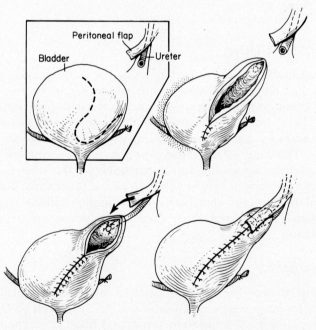

Figure 12. The modified Boari-Ockerblad technique for bladder tubularization. (From Symmonds RE: Ureteral injuries associated with gynecologic surgery: Prevention and management. *Clin Obstet Gynecol* 19:623, 1976. By permission of Harper & Row, Publishers.)

through the incised posterior wall of the flap at a point 1–1.5 cm from the distal margin and is anastomosed in a mucosa-to-mucosa (full-thickness ureter to near-full-thickness bladder wall) fashion. The muscularis is fixed to the iliopsoas fascia, and the vesical incision is closed in two layers, as previously described. The peritoneal flap associated with the ureter is sutured over the incision, to promote a tension-free apposition. Stenting of the anastomosis is not necessary unless a submucosal tunneling technique is used. Continuous retroperitoneal suction evacuation is employed, and Foley catheter drainage allows bladder inactivity for 10–12 days.

The Demel technique (24), a variant of the Boari flap, is a suitable alternative to the procedure just described and has the advantages of requiring less tailoring and having a less precarious blood supply (Fig. 13). The bladder is incised on the lateral aspect of the involved side, and the incision is extended medially through both the anterior and the posterior vesical surfaces. The incision is closed vertically to allow for exaggerated superior displacement of the bladder fundus, which bridges larger ureteral defects. Figure 14 illustrates the roentgenographic appearance of the urinary collecting system several months after ureteral substitution with the preceding technique.

Thompson (25) recently reviewed the long-term results in 30 patients subjected to vesical tubularization and reported a success rate of 92%. The frequency of urinary tract infections, the incidence and effect of ureteral reflux, and general bladder function were evaluated. Despite the frequent occurrence of preoperative urinary tract infections, positive results of urine culture during the postoperative follow-up period were relatively unusual if bladder anatomy was normal. Likewise, ureteral reflux occurred initially in all patients but was well tolerated and did not have any apparent acute or long-term deleterious effects; with extended follow-up, from 40% to 50% did not have continued

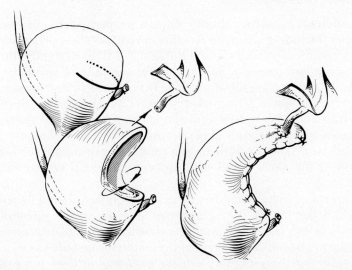

Figure 13. The Demel technique for ureteral substitution. (From Symmonds RE: Ureteral injuries associated with gynecologic surgery: Prevention and management. *Clin Obstet Gynecol* 19:623, 1976. By permission of Harper & Row, Publishers.)

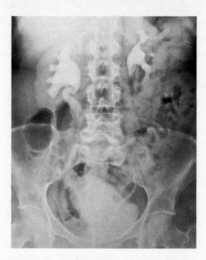

Figure 14. A Demel bladder flap. An excretory urogram 7 months after partial cystectomy and ureterectomy (distal 8 cm) for recurrent cervical carcinoma. A wertheim hysterectomy and bilateral lymphadenectomy for Stage IB squamous cell carcinoma of the cervix with a solitary metastatic right obturator node antedated the procedure by 27 months.

ureteral reflux. Presumably, the graded pressure differential along the vesical flap and the long-term alterations in spontaneous flap modification or ureteral lengthening minimize ureteral reflux. As illustrated by radiologic examination several years after tubularization, the bladder has resumed a relatively normal contour (Fig. 15).

Ureteroileoneocystostomy

The ideal ureteral substitute should display properties characteristic of the normal ureter, including adequate mobility, a rich blood supply, minimal tissue reactivity, peristaltic capabilities, and the absence of vesicoureteral reflux. Except in satisfying the last criterion, an expendable segment of small bowel would appear to be an appropriate substitute. The first attempt at ileal replacement of a diseased ureter was that of Schoemaker in 1909 (26). Presumably, the limitations of urinary tract antisepsis as well as the anticipated biochemical alterations with intestinal reabsorption delayed general approval of this technique. However, after Bricker's successful use of ileum as a conduit for urinary diversion (27), the interposition of the small bowel in the closed collecting system soon gained acceptance.

The treatment of ureteral injuries by ileal substitution should be reserved for cases in which the use of the vesicopsoas hitch or vesical mobilization with tubularization or direct ureteral anastomosis will not adequately restore urinary tract continuity. The indicative surgical presentations include cases in which (1) optimal vesical and ureteral (and kidney) mobilization does not bridge large ureteral defects, (2) extensive pelvic fibrosis and scarring from previous therapeutic manipulation render these pelvic organs relatively immobile without undue risk of additional compromise, and (3) the pelvic segments of both ureters

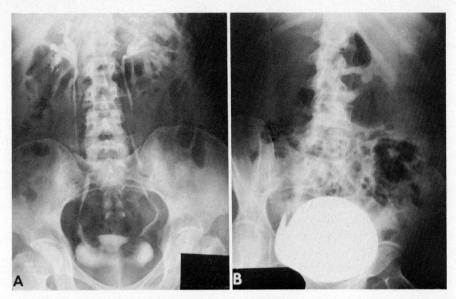

Figure 15. An excretory urogram (*a*) and retrograde cystogram (*b*) 2 years after Boari-Ockerblad vesical tubularization for correction of a ureterovaginal fistula that developed after surgical treatment of endometriosis.

must be replaced. The repair of ureterovaginal fistulas after primary treatment of cervical carcinoma is the most common indication for ureteroileoneocystostomy. Likewise, intentional excision or shunting of a segment of ureter for treatment of neoplasia or stricture formation if the bladder has been subjected to previous irradiation or operations or is inherently small may require consideration of an ileoureter.

The technique for ileal interposition in the urinary collecting system is an extension of the Bricker procedure. By appropriate transillumination, a well-vascularized segment of ileum (15–25 cm) is isolated and the distal 15 cm of small bowel is preserved (Fig. 16*a*). An ileoileostomy is performed in the usual manner to restore bowel continuity, and the mesentery is repaired transversely, to minimize vascular compromise and torsion of the graft pedicle (Fig. 16*b*). The proximal end of the loop is closed in two or three layers, and the ureter or ureters are adequately mobilized and debrided. The spatulated ureter is anastomosed to the antimesenteric side of the bowel (single-layer, full-thickness, mucosa-to-mucosa) with interrupted 3-0 chromic catgut. If the ureteral injury is bilateral, the second ureteroileal anastomosis is located about 2.5 cm distal from the first junctional site. The ureteral-associated peritoneal flap is sutured to the bowel serosa distal to the anastomosis, and the proximal portion of the ileal loop is fixed to the prelumbar fascia, to assure a tension-free union (Fig. 16*c*). The ileovesical anastomosis is generally accomplished in a two-layered manner. Occasionally, if there is an associated large vesicovaginal fistula or other bladder defects, the antimesenteric bowel wall can be spatulated to enlarge the potential anastomotic site and to serve as a bladder "patch." Ideally, the ileal segment is partially extraperitonealized; alternatively, the peritoneum and mesentery are repaired in such a manner as to minimize internal visceral herniation. Stenting is usually not required, but a transurethral Foley catheter of large diameter is necessary to allow adequate drainage of both urine and bowel mucus.

Immediate and long-term postoperative morbidity in several large series of ileal substitutions was recently reported; emphasis was placed specifically on urinary tract infections, vesicoileal reflux, and biochemical alterations (28–31). The overall success of the procedure and the long-term prognosis are significantly influenced by the preoperative renal status. Patients with normal renal function before ileal interposition can readily compensate for intestinal absorption, as judged by the usually normal electrolyte profiles. However, compromised renal function (creatinine levels exceeding 2 or 3 mg/dl) before intestinal substitution is often associated with hyperchloremic acidosis and other electrolyte imbalances during the immediate and long-term postoperative convalescences. Urinary diversion is preferred when preoperative creatinine levels exceed 2–2.5 mg/dl; eventual undiversion is considered if correction of the ureteral pathologic condition successfully reverses renal dysfunction.

Although vesicoileal reflux is usually demonstrable by cystography after ureteroileovesicoplasty, particularly during micturition, radiographic and biochemical analyses suggest that there are no apparent deleterious effects on renal function. Boxer and associates (28) found ileal reflux in 40 of 55 patients subjected to ileal substitution; outcomes were successful in 39 of the 40 cases (97.5%). In contrast, results were satisfactory in only 9 of 15 patients without postoperative vesicoileal reflux; thus, a beneficial role is implied for this type of reflux. Presumably, vesicoileal reflux "dampens" the retrograde pressures to such an extent that minimal ileoureteral reflux occurs and the proximal collecting system is indirectly shielded against pathologic retrograde pressures.

With normal ileal peristaltic activity and bladder dynamics, the incidence of recurrent postoperative urinary tract infection is relatively low. However, continued use of antimicrobial agents and large-caliber transurethral drainage for several weeks is encouraged to prevent urinary sepsis and obstruction of the mucus-laden urine. Production of mucus progressively decreases with increasing time of mucosal exposure to urine and urinary by-products. Intermittent laboratory assessment, including urine cultures and sensitivities, renal function tests, and urography, is recommended but should be done with decreasing frequency in asymptomatic patients.

URETERAL DIVERSION

Surgical management of advanced primary and recurrent pelvic malignancies and of posttreatment complications frequently requires radical resective techniques, including partial ureterectomy and cystectomy. Webb and Symmonds (8) recently reported that the 5-year survival rate was 33% in a series of 198 exenterative procedures performed predominantly for recurrent cervical and vaginal carcinoma and other advanced or recurrent genital, urinary, and colorectal neoplasms. The increasing success and acceptance of this technique reflect the progressive advances, both medical and technical, that have occurred over the past several decades. Possibly, the most significant factor in favorably

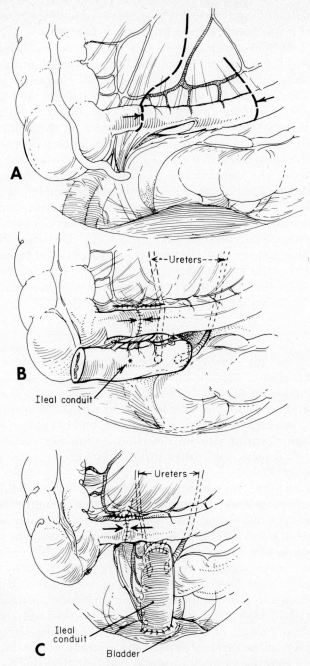

Figure 16. The technique of ureteroileoneocystostomy. (*a*). A well-vascularized segment of ileum is selected. (*b*). Isolation of the ileal segment, ileoileal reanastomosis, and transverse repair of the mesenteric defect are done. (*c*). Urinary tract continuity is restored with ureteroileal and ileovesical anastomoses.

altering the morbidity and mortality associated with this operation was the development of a functional method for urinary diversion.

Ureterosigmoidostomy, with use of either intact or cutaneously diverted bowel, was initially the method of choice for permanent urinary diversion. However, the associated complications, including (1) electrolyte and acid-base imbalances leading specifically to hyperchloremic acidosis, and (2) ascending infections resulting in severe pyelonephritis, contributed to an unacceptable postoperative mortality and necessitated separation of the urinary and fecal streams (32–34). Adequate separation and a corresponding decrease in ascending infection were observed with ureteral anastomosis into isolated rectosigmoid bladders. However, the unacceptable incidence of urinary incontinence and continued biochemical alterations from absorption of retained urine led to the discontinuation of this technique (35). Therefore, the enterocutaneous conduit, with ureteral anastomoses to an isolated segment of ileum or colon, continues to serve as the most satisfactory method of urinary diversion. The complete separation of the upper urinary tract and contaminated bowel has minimized the incidence of retrograde pyelonephritis, while the dynamic intestinal segment, functioning as a conduit rather than a reservoir, decreases absorption of urinary products and minimizes metabolic derangements.

Ileal Conduits

Although Seiffert (36) initially described ureteroileocutaneous diversion, Bricker (27) reported in 1950 on the first clinical application of isolated ileal segments as conduits for urinary diversion. Since that time, the ileal conduit has contributed significantly to the increased success in the management of advanced primary and recurrent pelvic malignancies and has gained acceptance as the most versatile form of urinary diversion. Its application and long-term follow-up in radical pelvic extirpative procedures were recently addressed by numerous authors (37–40).

The method we prefer for creation of an ileal conduit is a modification of the technique described for ileal substitution, as illustrated in Figure 16. A generous segment of ileum is isolated, and after bilateral ureteroileostomy and immobilization of the closed proximal end to the left perilumbar fascia, the distal portion of the segment is tailored to limit ileal redundancy. The ideal conduit length is the shortest intestinal segment remaining free from tension, both at the anastomotic and stomal sites. After removal of a circular cutaneous wedge (approximate diameter, 3 cm) in the right lower quadrant, the distal segment of ileum is delivered through the abdominal wall and matured with the resultant 2- to 3-cm stomal bud. Preoperative selection of the stomal site is desirable to assure proper application of the external appliance. Generally, ureteral stenting is not necessary unless anastomotic compromise is anticipated secondary to excessive pelvic irradiation.

During the past 25 years, 144 ileal conduits were created at the Mayo Clinic during the course of pelvic surgery for benign and malignant gynecologic processes. The charts of these patients were critically reviewed with specific emphasis on the acute and long-term results, as determined by clinical, biochemical, and urographic assessments (N.S. Angerman, M.D., and R.E. Symmonds,

M.D., unpublished data). There were five deaths within 60 days of surgery, resulting in an overall operative mortality of 3.5% (Table 1). Of interest is the observation that all patients who died in the postoperative period had previously been subjected to pelvic irradiation. The major complications directly associated with a urinary conduit included (1) fistula formation (ureteral or conduit) in four patients (one healed spontaneously, two required surgical repair, and one persisted until the patient's death), (2) ureteral obstruction from recurrent cancer in six patients and from mechanical dysfunction in two, (3) stomal necrosis, stenosis, or retraction requiring revision in three patients, and (4) small bowel obstruction or fistula formation necessitating reoperation in five cases (Table 1). In a recently published series from the M. D. Anderson Hospital, similar urologic complications were observed, with 18.6% of the conduit diversions (213 ileal, 33 sigmoid) requiring revision for fistulization, necrosis, or obstruction of either the conduit or the ureter (41). As expected, the major factor adversely affecting successful supravesical urinary diversion was preconduit high-dose pelvic irradiation.

The postoperative morbidity that was associated with the surgical procedures necessitating urinary diversion but that was not directly related to ileal conduit dysfunction is tabulated in Table 2. Chronic pyelonephritis and nephrolithiasis (calculi) occurred in 19 and 12 patients, respectively, and was invariably associated with preoperative upper urinary tract sepsis, a result suggesting the continuation of a preexisting disease process. Furthermore, 16 patients had transient hyperchloremic acidosis, but only 7 required sepecific treatment. These electrolyte imbalances likewise occurred in patients with significant presurgical impairment of renal function. In addition, the incidences of prolonged ileus, pelvic abscess, and wound infection were not unexpected, because of the extent of gastrointestinal and urinary tract manipulation in a frequently irradiated field. As expected, mild pyeloureterectasis, presumably secondary to transient edema at the anastomosis site, was usually demonstrable in the

Table 1. Postoperative Complications Related to the Conduit After Supravesical Urinary Diversion

Type of Complication	Ileal Conduit (144 Patients)		Sigmoid Conduit (54 Patients)	
	Number	%	Number	%
Fistula (ureteral or conduit)	4	2.8	0	—
Ureteral obstruction	8	5.6	2	3.7
Stomal necrosis, stenosis, or retraction	3[a]	2.1	7[b]	13.0
Small bowel obstruction or fistula	5[c]	3.5	3[c]	5.6
Death	5	3.5	2	3.7

[a] Necessitated surgical correction; in another two patients (1.4%), was resolved spontaneously.
[b] Necessitated surgical correction.
[c] Necessitated surgical correction; in another patient (0.7%), was resolved spontaneously.

Table 2. Postoperative Morbidity After Urinary Diversion by Ileal or Sigmoid Conduit

Type of Complication	Ileal Conduit (144 Patients)		Sigmoid Conduit (54 Patients)	
	Number	%	Number	%
Chronic pyelonephritis	19	13.2	14	25.9
Calculi	12	8.3	4	7.4
Ileus (>10 days)	10	6.9	3	5.6
Wound infection	19	13.2	19	35.2
Wound dehiscence	3	2.1	6	11.1
Pelvic abscess	11	7.6	7	13.0
Transient acidosis	16	11.1	10	18.5
Phlebitis	5	3.5	0	—
Pulmonary embolism	2	1.4	1	1.9
Psychoneurologic behavior	3	2.1	5	9.3

immediate postoperative convalescent period, with resolution occurring within 6–12 months.

Of interest was the improvement noted in both the anatomic and functional appearances of the ureterorenal unit after urinary diversion. Preoperative moderately severe pyeloureterectasis, bilateral in 20 patients and unilateral in 13, was resolved in 17 and 11 patients, respectively, after creation of an ileal conduit. In addition, of nine patients with unilateral nonvisualization by exeretory urography, three had return or renal function and six did not; only one required subsequent nephrectomy.

Sigmoid Conduit

Although the ileal conduit provides the most satisfactory method of permanent supravesical diversion with anterior exenteration, the use of the sigmoid colon as a diverting conduit is often an effective alternative when total exenteration is required. With the latter procedure, the use of segment of mobilized sigmoid diminishes operative time by obviating ileoileostomy and minimizes the potential for enteric fistula formation. Like its ileal counterpart, the adequately constructed sigmoid conduit, by actively transporting urine, reduces transit time and exposure of intestinal mucosa to excretory products and reduces reabsorption. Kaplan and associates (42) evaluated conduit dynamics and found that frequent mass contractions of moderate intensity and duration resulted in effective urinary evacuation. In addition, comparative evaluation of the functional status of the two primary conduit systems showed no significant differences, as judged by biochemical and urographic assessments (43, 44). Therefore, the preoperative and intraoperative processes of conduit selection should be determined and, if necessary, modified by the type of exenterative procedure, previous pelvic irradiation, colonic disorders (diverticulosis, colitis), and type of vaginoplasty (sigmoid vagina).

The operative technique for creation of a sigmoid conduit is a modification of the Bricker ileal conduit, as illustrated in Figure 17. After complete pelvic exenteration, the distal 15–0 cm of mobilized sigmoid is isolated (the sigmoidal tributaries of the interior mesenteric vessels are preserved). The proximal end of the segment is closed in two layers, including an initial continuous through-and-through inverted catgut suture and a second reinforcing layer of interrupted 3-0 silk sutures. The ureters are anastomosed to the antimesenteric surface by use of interrupted, full-thickness, mucosa-to-mucosa 3-0 or 4-0 catgut sutures, as described previously. A tension-free union is secured by attaching the ureteral-associated peritoneal flap to the serosa of the bowel beyond the ureterosigmoidostomy, and the closed end of the segment is transfixed to the fascia immediately above the pelvic brim. Stenting of the anastomosis is usually not necessary unless high-dose pelvic irradiation was previously administered. The distal portion of the conduit is exteriorized through a 3- to 4-cm excised cutaneous wedge in the right lower abdominal quadrant.

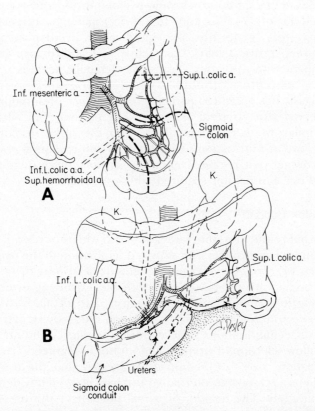

Figure 17. The technique of sigmoid conduit diversion. (*a*). A segment of sigmoid colon is selected and isolated, with preservation of the sigmoidal branches of the inferior mesenteric artery. (*b*). Bilateral ureterosigmoidal anastomoses. The proximal conduit end is transfixed to the perilumbar fascia. The distal end is exteriorized and matured in the right lower quadrant. K = kidney.

The Mayo Clinic series of sigmoid conduit diversions, recently updated, includes 54 cases accompanying exenterative procedures (Angerman and Symmonds, unpublished data). The associated postoperative mortality was 3.7 %, two patients dying within 60 days of surgery. The most frequent complication directly related to conduit construction was unsatisfactory stomal function, including necrosis, stenosis, and retracton (Table 1). Compromise serious enough to warrant stomal reconstruction developed in seven patients (13%); obesity and preconduit irradiation were the dominant contributing factors. In addition, one patient (1.9%) required nephrectomy for ureteral obstruction about 1 month after the operation, and another had progessive bilateral obstruction without recurrent neoplasia and continues to have adequate function with intermittent home dialysis.

The postoperative morbidity not directly influencing conduit function is detailed in Table 2. Wound infections (35.2%), wound dehiscence (11.%), and pelvic abscesses (13%) occurred with frequencies considerably higher than expected and presumably were related to the increased manipulations (transection, closure, and anastomosis) of the contaminated large bowel. In support of this presumption, the corresponding complications with the ileal conduit were significantly fewer. In addition, chronic pyelonephritis and transient acidosis were observed in 14 (25.9%) and 10 (18.5%) patients, respectively. These complications were generally associated with predisposing pathologic conditions—preoperative urinary tract sepsis with the former and functional renal impairment with the latter. Transient metabolic acidosis required treatment in five patients. Although a moderate degree of preoperative pyeloureterectasis was noted (20 patients), no evidence of additional deterioration was observed after ureteral diversion. The frequency of bilateral involvement was similar to that of unilateral, with complete resolution in 65%. Furthermore, two of four patients with prediversion unilateral nonvisualization of the ureterorenal unit regained normal excretory urographic function; the other two did not, but neither required additional therapy.

Transverse Colon Conduit

The high morbidity and mortality rates associated with the creation of either ileal or sigmoid conduits in patients with previous irradiation to the pelvis prompted pelvic surgeons to search for alternative methods of urinary diversion. Conduit necrosis and breakdown of anastomoses with accompanying urine or intestinal leakage leading to metabolic imbalances, sepsis, and fistula formation are not infrequently encountered secondary to radiation-induced vascular compromise. In order for such complications to be avoided, the classic conduit technique was modified to allow selection of ureteral and intestinal segments from outside the field of irradiation. Nelson (45) initially suggested that the transverse colon conduit would be a reasonable alternative and has subsequently demonstrated its effective application. The healthy proximal portion of the ureter (above the pelvic brim) optimizes anastomotic healing, and the transverse colonic mesentery generally imparts an excellent vascular supply and adequate mobility for versatile conduit construction. The indications for the transverse colon conduit continue to expand and currently include anterior and total exenterations after supervoltage irradiation, operation on the fibrotic or scarified pelvis more than once, previous failure of urinary diversions, concomitant sigmoidoanal anastomosis with exenteration, the need for high urinary diversion, and diverticulosis or sigmoidovaginoplasty preventing use of a segment of sigmoid.

The technique requires initial incision and mobilization of the omentum from the transverse colon and its mesentery. The latter is transilluminated for localization of the middle colic and marginal arteries. The appropriate conduit length is estimated, the mesentery is incised, and the colon is transsected (Fig. 18a). A colocolostomy is performed to reestablish bowel continuity, and the mesenteric defect is closed transversely to minimize pedicle compression. The distal end of the conduit is closed in two layers with continuous 2-0 chromic sutures and reinforcing interrupted 3-0 silk sutures. The proximal portions of the ureters are identified, bluntly mobilized, delivered through the retroperitoneum below the level of the ligament of Treitz, and anastomosed to the transverse colonic segment, as previously described (Fig. 18b). The distal end of the conduit is anchored to the retroperitoneum to minimize anastomotic tension, and the stoma is matured in either upper quadrant. Whether the diversion is fashioned in an isoperistaltic or antiperistaltic manner has no apparent effect on

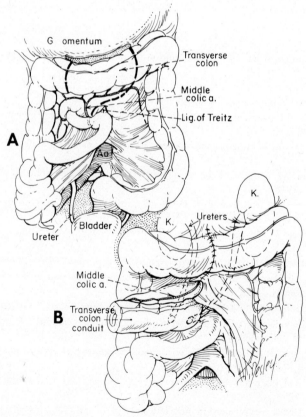

Figure 18. The technique of transverse colon conduit diversion. (a). The middle colic artery is identified, and the transverse colonic segment is isolated. Ao = aorta. (b). The ureter or ureters are mobilized and delivered through the retroperitoneum and are anastomosed to the isolated segment of transverse colon. The conduit is transfixed to the retroperitoneum, and the stoma is matured in either upper quadrant. K = kidney.

conduit function. In addition, antireflux techniques and anastomotic stents are generally not required.

The transverse colon conduit provides a satisfactory alternative to the more traditional methods of urinary diversion in the treatment of benign and malignant pelvic disease. Several authors recently addressed the use of proximal colonic urinary diversion (46–49) and suggested that this technique is superior in instances of preconduit high-dose pelvic irradiation. As the indications for the transverse colon conduit have grown, its use together with that of its sigmoid counterpart permits the surgeon to choose either a high- or a low-colonic diversionary method during the treatment of both benign and malignant disease processes. The associated morbidity and mortality rates are similar to those observed with ileal conduits. Acute pyelonephritis, complications of the conduit stoma, and dysfunction of the ureterocolic anastomosis are conditions most often contributing to postsurgical morbidity. Although now predominantly a secondary technique after initial conduit failure, the transverse colon conduit procedure will undoubtedly gain support as a primary diversionary method as additional results of continuing series become available.

REFERENCES

1. Benson RC, Hinman F Jr: Urinary tract injuries in obstetrics and gynecology. *Trans Am Assoc Genitourin Surg* 47:220, 1955.

2. Rusche C, Morrow JW: Injury to the ureter, in Campbell MF, Harrison JH (eds): *Urology*, ed 3. Philadelphia, WB Saunders Co, 1970, vol 1, p 811.

3. Symmonds RE: Ureteral injuries associated with gynecologic surgery: Prevention and management. *Clin Obstet Gynecol* 19:623, 1976.

4. Mayer HGK: Abflusstörungen der oberen Harnwege nach vaginaler Radikaloperation. *Geburtshilfe Frauenheilkd* 28:338, 1968.

5. Park RC, Patow WE, Rogers RE, et al: Treatment of stage I carcinoma of the cervix. *Obstet Gynecol* 41:117, 1973.

6. Kaskarelis D, Sakkas J, Aravantinos D, et al: Urinary tract injuries in gynecological and obstetrical procedures. *Int Surg* 60:40, 1975.

7. Rampone JF, Klem V, Kolstad P: Combined treatment of stage IB carcinoma of the cervix. *Obstet Gynecol* 41:163, 1973.

8. Webb MJ, Symmonds RE: Wertheim hysterectomy: A reappraisal. *Obstet Gynecol* 54:140, 1979.

9. Brunschwig A, Barber HRK, Roberts S: Return of renal function after varying periods of ureteral occlusion: A clinical study. *JAMA* 188:5, 1964.

10. Hamm FC, Weinberg SR: Management of the severed ureter. *J Urol* 77:407, 1957.

11. Harada N, Tanimura M, Fukuyama K, et al: Surgical management of a long ureteral defect: Advancement of the ureter by descent of the kidney. *J Urol* 92:192, 1964.

12. Carlton CE Jr, Scott R Jr, Guthrie AG: The initial management of ureteral injuries: A report of 78 cases. *J Urol* 105:335, 1971.

13. Politano VA, Leadbetter WF: An operative technique for the correction of vesicoureteral reflux. *J Urol* 79:932, 1958.

14. Paquin AJ Jr: Ureterovesical anastomosis: The description and evaluation of a technique. *J Urol* 82:573, 1959.

15. Landau SJ: Ureteroneocystostomy: A review of 72 cases with a comparison of two techniques. *J Urol* 87:343, 1962.

16. Lee RA, Symmonds RE: Ureterovaginal fistula. *Am J Obstet Gynecol* 109:1032, 1971.

17. Hodges CV, Moore RJ, Lehman TH, et al: Clinical experiences with transuretero-ureterostomy. *J Urol* 90:552, 1963.

18. Smith IB, Smith JC: Trans-uretero-ureterostomy: British experience. *Br J Urol* 47:519, 1975.

19. Udall DA, Hodges CV, Pearse HM, et al: Transureteroureterostomy: A neglected procedure. *J Urol* 109:817, 1973.

20. Sandoz IL, Paull DP, Macfarlane CA: Complications with transureteroureterostomy. *J Urol* 117:39, 1977.

21. Ehrlich RM, Skinner DG: Complications of transureteroureterostomy. *J Urol* 113:467, 1975.

22. Ockerblad NF: Reimplantation of the ureter into the bladder by a flap method. *J Urol* 57:845, 1947.

23. Casati E, Boari A: Contributo sperimentale alla plastica dell' uretere. *Atti Acad Sci Med Nat Ferrara* 68:149, 1894.

24. Demel R: Ersatz des Ureters durch eine Plastik aus der Harnblase (Vorläufige Mitteilung). *Zentralbl Chir* 51:2008, 1924.

25. Thompson IM: Bladder flap repair of ureteral injuries. *Urol Clin North Am* 4:51, 1977.

26. Schoemaker J: Discussion: Intra-abdominale plastieken. *Ned Tijdschr Geneeskd* 47 (Ser 2, Pt A, Sect 1):836, 1911.

27. Bricker EM: Bladder substitution after pelvic evisceration. *Surg Clin North Am*, October 1950, p 1511.

28. Boxer RJ, Johnson SF, Ehrlich RM: Ureteral substitution. *Urology* 12:269, 1978.

29. Fritzsche P, Skinner DG, Craven JD, et al: Long-term radiographic changes of the kidney following the ileal ureter operation. *J Urol* 114:843, 1975.

30. Krupp P, Hoffman M, Roeling W: Terminal ileum as a ureteral substitute. *Obstet Gynecol* 35:416, 1970.

31. Küss R, Bitker M, Camey M, et al: Indications and early and late results of intestino-cystoplasty: A review of 185 cases. *J Urol* 103:53, 1970.

32. Barber HRK, Brunschwig A: Urinary tract fistulas following pelvic exenteration. *Obstet Gynecol* 28:754, 1966.

33. Symmonds RE: Use of the colon for urinary diversion. *Clin Obstet Gynecol* 10:217, 1967.

34. Zincke H, Segura JW: Ureterosigmoidostomy: Critical review of 173 cases. *J Urol* 113:324, 1975.

35. Jensen PA, Symmonds RE: The rectosigmoid urinary reservoir with anterior pelvic exenterations: An evaluation. *Obstet Gynecol* 26:786, 1965.

36. Seiffert L: Die "Darm-Siphonblase." *Arch Klin Chir* 183:569, 1935.

37. Cohen SM, Persky L: A ten-year experience with ureteroileostomy. *Arch Surg* 95:278, 1967.

38. Remigailo RV, Lewis EL, Woodard JR, et al: Ileal conduit urinary diversion: Ten-year review. *Urology* 7:343, 1976.

39. Abrams HJ, Buchbinder MI: Experience with ileal ureters. *Bull NY Acad Med* 53:329, 1977.

40. Pitts WR Jr, Muecke EC: A 20-year experience with ileal conduits: The fate of the kidneys. *J Urol* 122:154, 1979.

41. Swan RW, Rutledge FN: Urinary conduit in pelvic cancer patients: A report of 16 years' experience. *Am J Obstet Gynecol* 119:6, 1974.

42. Kaplan AL, Hulme GW, Laskowski T, et al: The sigmoid conduit as a means of urinary diversion. *South Med J* 60:688, 1967.

43. Symmonds RE, Gibbs CP: Urinary diversion by way of sigmoid conduit. *Surg Gynecol Obstet* 131:687, 1970.

44. Symmonds RE, Jones IV: Sigmoid conduit urinary diversion after exenteration. *Prog Gynecol* 6:729, 1975.

45. Nelson JH Jr: *Atlas of Radical Pelvic Surgery.* New York, Appleton-Century-Crofts, 1969, p 181.

46. Morales P, Golimbu M: Colonic urinary diversion: 10 years of experience. *J Urol* 113:302, 1975.

47. Schmidt JD, Hawtrey CE, Buchsbaum HJ: Transverse colon conduit: A preferred method of urinary diversion for radiation-treated pelvic malignancies. *J Urol* 113:308, 1975.

48. Schmidt JD, Buchsbaum HJ, Jacobo EC: Transverse colon conduit for supravesical urinary tract diversion. *Urology* 8:542, 1976.

49. Schlesinger RE, Berman ML, Ballon SC, et al: The choice of an inestinal segment for a urinary conduit. *Surg Gynecol Obstet* 148:45, 1979.

7
Complications
of Bladder Surgery
and Cystoscopy

William Maxted

BLADDER SURGERY
Suprapubic Incision—Cystotomy

The alternative incisions available to approach the lower abdomen and pelvis and the details of technique for each are well known to the gynecologic surgeon. Therefore, the focus of this section will be those anatomic and technical points relevant to facilitating the suprapubic approach to the urinary bladder and minimizing the risk of complications (1). The urinary bladder is an extraperitoneal pelvic structure, access to the anterior surface of which is gained by opening the transversalis fascia at its attachment to the periosteum of the pubic bone to enter the prevesical space.

Having developed the prevesical space to the extent necessary, avoiding going too inferiorly or posteriorly, in order to minimize risk of venous injury and bleeding and to expose the anterior wall of the urinary bladder, the surgeon then bluntly reflects the inferior peritoneal edge cephalad, to expose an additional area of the anterior bladder wall adequate for the cystotomy incision required. The peritoneum must be reflected from the anterior bladder wall so that injury to the intestine is avoided while the cystotomy incision is made. A cystotomy tube is easily and most desirably placed at the most superior aspect of the anterior wall of the urinary bladder (1). The cystotomy incision is made by a stab into the lumen of the urinary bladder with a 10 blade, the sharp edge being directed caudally, through the anterior bladder wall, which has been previously grasped between two Allis clamps and tented anteriorly. This fixation of the anterior wall averts the risk of injury to the posterior bladder wall or even of perforation through the posterior wall. The incision is then extended sharply to the degree required. Any of the readily available drainage tubes may be used, but a mushroom catheter seems to be less irritating to the bladder wall and thus less of a problem with postoperative bladder muscle spasms. However, if

151

significant hematuria with clots is anticipated, a Malecot catheter gives more effective drainage and is preferable. If urinary drainage is the only requirement and is anticipated to be of relatively short duration, a 24 F caliber tube is adequate. If bleeding or long-term use is anticipated, a larger tube of 30–32 F is desirable to prevent obstruction by clots or early occlusion by deposition of urinary salts. The cystotomy incision is closed with a running suture of 0 chromic gut that incorporates the full thickness of the bladder wall. The tube is transfixed by the suture being tied around it. The apex of the bladder is fixed to the fascia of the anterior abdominal wall to facilitate access to the cystotomy, should replacement be necessary. It is advisable to transfix the tube to the skin with a heavy nonabsorbable suture, to further ensure against the tube's being accidentally dislodged.

Cystotomy in the Radiated Bladder

In the radiated bladder, suprapubic cystotomy should be avoided unless a significant indication exists for electing this mode of bladder drainage. The radiation effects on the anterior abdominal wall and the wall of the urinary bladder preclude the likelihood of spontaneous closure with removal of the suprapubic tube, leading to the need for secondary surgical closure of the cystotomy tract. There is also a tendency for the cystotomy tract to increase in width, leading to urinary leakage around the cystotomy tube and to resultant skin and nursing care problems.

Bladder Injury

Injury to the urinary bladder of the patient with a gynecologic malignancy might occur as a result of the malignancy itself or as a result of the treatment of the malignancy. Injury to the urinary bladder of the patient undergoing treatment for gynecologic malignancy might occur from radiation or during the course of surgical treatment. The surgical injury might be recognized immediately or escape detection, to become manifest during the postoperative course.

When an injury to the urinary bladder is recognized at the time of surgery, its extent and location, especially as related to the terminal course of the ureters, must be accurately defined. The bladder is then mobilized as necessary in order to ensure obtaining closure without any tension (1). It might well be desirable to place catheters in the ureters, to facilitate definition of their relation to the bladder injury and its repair, in order to avoid the risk of ureteral injury. After this procedure has been accomplished, the edges of the injury should be prepared by excising traumatized, shredded, or devascularized bladder wall to obtain healthy edges and hemostasis. The defect is then closed with a continuous running 0 chromic suture, full-thickness bites of bladder wall being taken and care taken not to strangulate tissue along the line of closure. A second imbricated layer incorporating perivesical fascia or peritoneum and burying the initial layer is highly desirable. Involvement of the area of ureteral entry in the injury may require disconnection of the ureter and ureteral implantation for optimum repair with minimal risk of ureteral injury. This is a safer approach than attempting primary repair without implantation when the injury closely approaches the area of ureteral entry. Bladder decompression can be accomplished equally well with indwelling urethral catheter or suprapubic tube drainage. This drainage should be maintained for 10–14 days or longer, depending upon the quality of tissues and closure and the patient's postoperative course.

The urinary bladder afflicted with radiation changes and compromise in the quality of blood supply, together with increased interstitial fibrosis, demands special consideration. These effects seriously compromise the normal process of healing, causing marked delay into complete failure of the healing process. Consequently, the risk of injury to the previously radiated urinary bladder must be minimized. When injury does occur, repair must be meticulous, the maximum number of layers of closure used, and particular attention paid to avoiding compromise of perfusion of the wound edges. When the risk of fistula formation exists or there are posterior injuries in the vaginal cuff or anterior injuries in the anterior abdominal wall, interposition of an omental flap might be helpful in avoiding such a complication (2). Bladder decompression must be maintained for a significantly longer time than in the nonradiated bladder. The duration must be determined by the severity of radiation change in the urinary bladder and the sense of security with respect to the quality of repair of the injury. Several weeks or longer would not be unusual.

The bladder must be left open to drain at all times. Continuous drainage will prevent an increase in intravesical pressure and the resultant risk of disruption of the bladder closure and urinary extravasation. Urinary bladder distention or premature discontinuation of bladder drainage might well be complicated by urinary extravasation; all that this complication portends will be discussed in the next paragraph. The possibility exists that this complication can occur even when decompression has been maintained for what should have been an adequate period of time. The impact of this complication can be minimized by placing, at the time of repair, a small Penrose drain to the area of injury, to permit the escape of any extravasated urine and nonoperative treatment of any urinary extravasation by simple replacement of the indwelling catheter. However, should urinary extravasation occur in the absence of provision for drainage, prompt surgical intervention for drainage is mandatory. The other bladder injury complication of concern is breakdown of a repair of an injury in that area of the urinary bladder related to the anterior vagina, with the breakdown causing the development of a vesicovaginal fistula.

Should a bladder injury go unrecognized at the time of surgery and thus fail to be repaired, the inevitable urinary extravasation might manifest itself through one or more of the following spectra: There might be immediate urinary drainage through either the abdominal incision or vagina. There might be a somewhat persistent ileus or the development of systemic sepsis. In the rare instance of intraperitoneal extravasation without external drainage, the patient might experience anuria. Thus, a patient manifesting any of the preceding complications might be considered for urinary extravasation, the source then to be localized to either the ureter or the urinary bladder.

While the patient's renal function and metabolic status are being assessed, any defect defined is being treated, and antibiotic levels are being obtained for treatment of any sepsis, intravenous pyelography to evaluate the upper urinary tracts should be performed as soon as appropriate in the patient's clinical course. If this study is normal, retrograde gravity-filled cystography should be performed under the strictest aseptic technique. Both oblique views and a postemptying view are needed to detect any posterior extravasation that can be obscured by an anterior view with a full bladder (1). If the intravenous pyelogram is consistent with ureteral obstruction, with or without demonstrated extravasation of the contrast medium, and there is no extravasation of the contrast medium from the urinary bladder on cystography, the site of urinary extravasation must be placed in the ureter. Should the cystographic studies reveal extravasation of the contrast medium, which then indicates a bladder injury, immediate surgical drainage of the anatomic areas affected by the urinary extravasation, repair of the bladder defect, and provision for urinary bladder drainage as in the situation of injury recognized at surgery must be undertaken. On occasion, a small bladder defect can be healed nonsurgically by placement of an indwelling urethral catheter and use of broad antibiotics to treat any possible infection. Inadequate drainage of extravasated urine or extravasation and diffusion of infected urine carries the risk of delayed abscess formation.

Radiation Cystitis

Radiation cystitis is a term employed to describe a number of lesions in the urinary bladder with a spectrum of signs and symptoms. The types of reaction to radiation in the urinary bladder can be divided, based on onset of symptomatology, into acute, subacute, and chronic (3).

The most important variable in determining urinary bladder reaction to intense radiation is the presence of preexisting disease. Destruction of tumor that has invaded the bladder wall may result in a persistent defect and fistula formation. Infection adds to the reactivity of the bladder. Prior treatment, whether it be surgery or radiation, usually reduces the tolerance for further radiation.

The changes of acute radiation cystitis usually begin 4–6 weeks after a course of treatment is begun (3). These changes will be manifest as symptoms of bladder irritation: urgency, frequency, and dysuria. They will be accompanied by a reduction in functional bladder capacity. Pathologically (3), the early response to radiation includes varying degrees of injury to the basal epithelial cells, a hyperemic phase, injury to the fine vasculature and connective tissue, interstitial edema, and desquamation of epithelial cells. The endothelial cells of fine blood vessels show degenerative and necrotic changes, the swollen cells occluding the lumen to varying degrees. Varying degrees of ulceration of the bladder mucosa may occur. Susceptibility to infection increases as a result of radiation damage to the tissue. A spectrum of changes occurs in the blood vessels: the walls thicken and the lumens narrow as a result of endothelial proliferation, subendothelial and medial fibrosis occurs, the number of fine vessels gradually decreases, and telangiectatic vessels are gradually produced. The connective tissue undergoes hyalization. The progressive reduction in the fine vasculature and the increase in the connective tissue lead to gradual atrophy or breakdown of epithelium in regions seriously affected, leading to delayed ulceration. Endoscopic evaluation at this acute stage reveals diffuse, intense hyperemia of the bladder mucosa. Lysis of a tumor that has fully invaded the bladder wall can lead to bladder perforation and the development of a vesicovaginal fistula. Treatment at this stage consists of symptomatic relief in the form of Pyridium and nonnarcotic analgesics. Parasympathetic blocking drugs may decrease the irritability, with a resultant decrease in frequency and urgency. The average case will subside rapidly after the course of therapy is completed.

Painless hematuria is the usual presenting manifestation of subacute radiation cystitis. It will usually occur suddenly 6 months to 2 years after the completion of therapy (3). There may be associated bladder irritative symptoms when mucosal ulceration occurs. Pathologically, there is a progressive reduction in the fine vasculature and an increase in the amount and density of the connective tissue (3). In general, the bladder becomes increasingly susceptible to infection and ulceration. The mucosal ulcerative lesions may heal slowly with reepithelialization or scarring or result in fistula formation, depending upon the degree of devitalization of vasculature and associated secondary infection.

Endoscopically one will observe an overall pale mucosa with telangiectatic lesions. It is the rupture of one of these vessels that is the source of hematuria. There might be sharply demarcated mucosal ulcerative lesions resulting from obliterative ischemia from involvement of smaller arterioles. This ulcerative lesion must be differentiated from recurrent tumor. The ulcer of radiation cystitis will usually occur on the posterior wall of the urinary bladder and be sharply demarcated from adjacent normal mucosa. Induration at the base of the lesion or heaped-up mucosa about the margin of the lesion suggests tumor invasion as the etiology of the lesion. Deep coagulation of bleeding areas carries a risk of fistula formation. Transfusion may be necessary because of the magnitude of blood loss secondary to bleeding. The majority of the ulcers will heal with conversative management including irrigation with a three-way Foley catheter. Secondary bacterial infection is controlled by appropriate drug therapy. Control of infection is important because persistent infection will increase the risk of fistula formation.

Intense radiation can lead to extensive scarring and fibrosis of the bladder wall manifest from 1 to 5 years after completion of therapy as a contracted urinary bladder. The patient will experience profound diurnal and nocturnal urinary frequency, bladder pain and dysuria, and in some cases, continuous urinary dribbling. Hematuria is less common at this stage.

Pathologically, the fine vessels progressively deteriorate slowly through obliterating endarteritis and fibrosis and sclerosis of the vessels, and the amounts of connective tissue in the bladder wall increase (3). These changes lead to increased ischemia and progressive atrophy and necrosis of the epithelium. The fibrosis and induration of the bladder wall lead to considerable contraction of the bladder and reduction in functional bladder capacity. The dilated telangiectatic vessels are dilated and fragile and may become the source of repeated and serious hemorrhage. Scarring of the intravesical portions of the ureters can lead to a complicating obstruction that may be associated with upper urinary tract dilatation, pyelonephritis, and impaired renal function (3). Intravenous pyelography is necessary to assess the effects on the upper urinary tract. A cystogram will define an irregular contracted urinary bladder. Cystoscopy will reveal a very pale urinary bladder mucosa with a telangiectatic vascular pattern. Once a contracted urinary bladder occurs, the resultant symptoms are irreversible and a diversionary procedure must be employed if it is appropriate with respect to the status of the patient's malignancy.

Bladder Bleeding

Gross hematuria in the patient who has or has been treated for a gynecologic malignancy often presents one of the more challenging therapeutic problems encountered in the total management of this category of patients. Hematuria might be the manifestation of a bacterial infection of the urinary bladder. This condition will promptly clear with appropriate drug treatment of the infection. Unfortunately, more often hematuria is a sign of a more serious problem involving the urinary bladder, with respect to either its prognostic significance or the therapeutic challenge presented. The bleeding might be from neoplastic tissue that has invaded the full-thickness bladder wall or from radiation or chemotherapeutic drug effects on the bladder wall and bladder mucosa. The precise etiology must be defined through cystoscopy; sometimes a biopsy is required to differentiate between radiation cystitis with ulcer formation and direct tumor invasion with tumor necrosis.

When cystoscopy defines the source of bleeding as tumor, careful trans-urethral resection of necrotic tumor with exposure of viable tumor and tumor vessels will often permit effective control of the bleeding through transurethral electrocoagulation (4). Caution must be exercised to prevent perforation or fistula formation from too aggressive resection. Whether it has been feasible to resect the tumor or not, a period of bladder rest with an indwelling three-way catheter is carried out with sterile water to dilute any further bleeding, thus preventing clot formation and catheter obstruction with its attendant potential for reactivating major bleeding.

When the cause of bleeding is found to be radiation cystitis, management will depend upon the stage. Rarely will the bleeding be the result of diffuse changes in the mucosa in the acute stage of radiation cystitis, but when this is the situation, bladder rest with three-way catheter irrigation as previously described will be indicated and most likely will be successful. Hematuria is more likely to be a problem in subacute and chronic radiation cystitis. In this condition hematuria results from either rupture of a telangiectatic vessel or mucosal ulceration. In either case electrocoagulation of the bleeding vessels or tissue will usually be successful in controlling the bleeding. Also, in both cases a period of bladder rest with a three-way catheter and continuous irrigation is necessary for definitive management.

The major challenge is the patient who is not amenable to the measures just described because of the nature of the problem in the urinary bladder or who fails to respond to these measures (5). For this patient we would employ intravesical formalin instillation or, in a rare situation, urinary diversion with or without cystectomy.

Anesthesia, general or spinal, is required for the instillation of formalin because of the associated discomfort. Preliminary cystoscopy is first performed, all clots are removed, and to the extent possible, necrotic tissue is removed. An effort is made to control any major bleeding points with light fulguration. Cystography must be performed to demonstrate the competency of the ureterovesical junction, to exclude the presence of vesicoureteral reflux, for reflux of formalin can lead to ureteral and renal parenchymal coagulation necrosis. When reflux is demonstrated, measures to prevent backward flow of the formalin solution into the ureters must be taken: The patient is placed in a reversed Trendelenburg's position and occlusion of the ureters with Fogarty catheters is considered (6). Additionally, the solution should be instilled by gravity flow only at low pressures.

Formalin solutions ranging in strength from 1% to 10% have been employed. It seems most prudent to begin with a 1% solution and progress to increasing concentrations, as necessary. In the preparation of the solution careful attention must be paid to the details of formulation of its strength. Formalin, which is a 37% solution of formaldehyde, must be diluted with sufficient sterile distilled water to make a 1% formalin solution, that is, 0.37% formaldehyde. Fair recommends passive irrigation of the bladder with from 500 to 1,000 ml of a 1% formalin solution over a 10-minute period followed by irrigation with 1,000 ml of distilled water. Catheter drainage for a minimum of 24 hours is then maintained.

If the initial effort is unsuccessful in controlling bleeding or if bleeding recurs, the procedure can be repeated with increased strengths of formalin.

The intravesical use of formalin is not without potential for significant complications (7). Fistula formation, upper urinary tract dilatation secondary to ureterovesical obstruction, and marked bladder fibrosis with loss of bladder capacity have been reported.

In that rare patient in whom all the previously described measures have been employed and failed, one must consider, depending upon the patient's overall status and stage of disease, upper urinary tract diversion. Often, urinary diversion alone will be effective in bringing about control of the bladder bleeding.

Neurogenic Bladder

A comprehensive treatise on neurogenic bladder is beyond the scope of this section. Discussion will be confined to that aspect of neurogenic bladder dysfunction encountered after extensive pelvic surgery. The motor innervation responsible for the contraction of the smooth muscle of the urinary bladder and for effective emptying of the urinary bladder is autonomic parasympathetic. The motor cells in the sacral cord discharge impulses that are conducted by the pelvic nerve (nervi erigentes) to synapse in ganglia at the urinary bladder, to then innervate the smooth muscle of the urinary bladder (8, 9). Thus any injury to the pelvic nerves such as surgical trauma, recurrent pelvic tumor, or pharmacologic compromise of parasympathetic function through the use of drugs with parasympathetic blocking (parasympatholytic) effects will compromise the con-tractile function of the bladder muscle (10). This effect will be manifest in the patient as difficulty in initiating urinary flow, as a weak, dribbling stream with the need to strain or with significant residual urine, after voiding or as the inability to void, that is, urinary retention (11). This spectrum of neurogenic dysfunction will be accentuated by any preexisting lower urinary tract obstructive dysfunction.

General principles of management of neurogenic bladder are as follows: Nearly all neurogenic bladder patients will eventually recover adequate bladder function; in some patients, however, this recovery can take months. Until recovery occurs, one must protect the bladder from the effects of chronic overdistention and the total urinary tract from infection. There is little benefit in performing urodynamic studies at this time. For the patient unable to void or carrying a significant residual urine (greater than 100–150 ml), use of an indwelling urethral catheter with constant drainage is mandatory until function improves to an acceptable level of residual urine. Recovery can often be expedited by making bladder emptying easier by decreasing outflow resistance through empiric urethral–bladder neck dilation and pharmacologic augmentation of parasympathetic activity with parasympathomimetic drugs, for example, Betenchol in a minimum dose of 25–50 mg by mouth every 6 hours as tolerated and begun the day before catheter removal. Periodic urine cultures should be obtained to monitor bacteria in the urine. Specific therapy should be directed by culture and sensitivity studies begun 24 hours before catheter removal. Adherence to these principles should protect the urinary tract. The serial upper tract evaluation through intravenous pyelography is not necessary.

CYSTOSCOPY
Purposes of Cystoscopy

Cystoscopy and urethroscopy, by offering direct visual inspection of the interior of the urinary bladder and urethra, afford an opportunity for more accurate clinical staging of neoplasms of the female genital tract and for the evaluation of primary lower urinary tract signs and symptoms (1). When upper urinary tract abnormalities have been defined on an excretory pyelogram during the initial staging, evaluating the patient by means of gynecologic malignancy cystoscopy provides a more precise definition of the pyelographic findings through ureteral catheterization and retrograde pyelography. Signs and symptoms of intrinsic lower urinary tract disease, whether in the early postoperative course or at some time remote from treatment, might well be elucidated through cystoscopy.

Gynecologic malignancies that have spread beyond the organ of origin may involve the urinary tract either through direct extension with invasion or through the effects of dissemination to the regional lymph nodes with secondary ureteral obstruction. Thus cystourethrography, by permitting careful visual inspection of the mucosa of the urethra and the urinary bladder, will define evidence of direct invasion of the urethra or urinary bladder, providing a more accurate definition of extension and clinical staging. Early invasion of the outer wall of the urinary bladder by extending neoplasms might be manifest by bullous edematous changes in the mucosa of the urinary bladder superficial to the area of extrinsic invasion. These changes will consist of large, variably sized, clear bullous blebs completely involving the mucosa over the area of invasion; the area of mucosal involvement will usually be rather sharply demarcated from the adjacent normal mucosa. More advanced invasion through the wall of the urinary bladder will be manifest by frank tumor replacing the bladder mucosa. These mucosal changes will consist of variably sized solid tumor nodules projecting into the lumen of the urinary bladder, often with a zone of bullous edema interposed between the tumor nodules and adjacent normal mucosa. These changes may involve an area of bladder wall deformed and invaginated by the extrinsic tumor mass. A variable extent of tumor replacing bladder mucosa may undergo necrosis and present the endoscopic picture of hemorrhagic necrosis with, at times, no apparent viable tumor to be observed. On occasion, areas of necrotic tumor can be covered by a shaggy film of opaque white-gray exudate. At other times the necrotic tumor or exudate can be the site of patchy superficial calcification, particularly when complicated by urinary infection.

When the endoscopic picture of necrotic invasive tumor is encountered and transurethral biopsy is entertained, there are two important points to be considered. First, in order for the possibility to be maximized of obtaining viable tissue from which the surgical pathologist can confidently make a diagnosis, sampling should be done at the periphery of the tumor at its junction with normal-appearing bladder mucosa. Second, biopsy of necrotic tumor, particularly in an area related to the anterior vaginal wall, carries the grave risk of perforation and fistula formation. Should evidence consistent with neoplastic invasion of the urinary bladder be discovered on cystoscopy, it then becomes most important to accurately define the precise location and extent of the observed changes within the urinary bladder. It is especially important to note the relation of any evidence of tumor invasion to the bladder neck and trigone and vesical ureters. The accuracy of these observations is important, not only in enhancing the accuracy of clinical staging but also in planning therapy and in anticipating the potential for the development of complications such as vesicovaginal fistula or ureteral obstruction.

Early in the postoperative course of treatment of the patient who has undergone extensive pelvic surgery and in whom urinary diversion has not been performed, one might encounter a number of lower urinary tract complaints. Some of the more common are disturbances in the mechanics of voiding ranging from marked difficulty to inability to void to varying patterns of urinary incontinence. Urinary tract infection might also be a problem. Cystoscopy, by defining an obstructive entity in an anatomic outlet in the patient with bladder muscle hypotonia and ineffective voiding or urinary tract infection, might enable us to benefit the patient by relieving that obstruction through dilation. The question of the etiology of incontinence, overflow, or incontinence resulting from a urinary-vaginal fistula can be resolved through the definition and localization of any fistula proximal to the urethra, urinary bladder, or ureter. Insights into the factors responsible for urinary tract infection or its refractoriness to treatment can often be gained that lend themselves to treatment resulting in control of the urinary infection. Cystoscopy can play a valuable role, both diagnostically and therapeutically, in the postoperative anuric patient or the patient with acute renal failure in whom the question of ureteral obstruction exists. Cystoscopy allows evaluation of the trigone and intravesical ureters and access to the ureteral orifices for diagnostic ureteral catheterization and retrograde pyelograms as well as for placement of ureteral catheters to establish upper urinary tract drainage and to provide temporary relief of obstruction in the management of the metabolic complications of obstruction.

Tumor recurrence or late complications from the specific therapy for a given tumor might be manifest as signs or symptoms of urinary tract disease. Cystoscopy, through visual inspection of the interior of the urinary bladder, can be most valuable and informative in elucidating the etiology of a problem and thus defining its prognostic significance. The spectrum of endoscopic manifestations of the presence of tumor invasion in the urinary bladder has been previously discussed. Hematuria, in the patient who has received radiation therapy, is often a sign of radiation cystitis, the sum of those changes in the wall of the urinary bladder resulting from radiation.

The location of a urinary-vaginal fistula can be accurately defined only through cystourethroscopy. The location of the fistula within the urinary bladder and its extent and relation to the bladder neck and ureteral orifices must be known in planning repair; this information can be obtained only through cystoscopy. The patient in whom dysfunction of voiding or urinary infection develops long after initial treatment can often be successfully managed through information gained from cystoscopy.

On occasion, an intravenous pyelogram performed at a time remote to the primary treatment of a tumor will be abnormal in a way that may suggest recurrence of tumor or late complications of treatment.

Not infrequently, the intravenous pyelogram will not enable one to localize the point or extent of pathology. Again, cystoscopy, by providing access to the ureteral orifice for ureteral catheterization and retrograde pyelography, will give us that desired information.

Cystoscopic Procedures

The anesthesia necessary for cystoscopy must be individualized for the patient and the anticipated procedure to be performed. The emotionally stable patient in whom minimal manipulation is anticipated can comfortably tolerate the procedure with topical urethral anesthesia or, at most, intravenous Valium occasionally supplemented with Demerol, provided no medical contraindications exist. If transurethral biopsy might be necessary, provision should be made for anesthesia standby so that the patient is totally prepared for the anesthetic procedure that might be necessary in order for the surgical procedure to be performed. Cystoscopy is performed with the patient in the dorsal lithotomy position, either on a conventional cystoscopy table, where water flow is easily managed, or on a conventional operating room table. Initial calibration of the urethra with a Bougie-a-bole will aid in the selection of the cystoscope of appropriate size; generally, a cystoscope in the range of 17−21 F caliber is adequate for diagnostic evaluation of the urinary bladder. Sterile water for irrigation is employed for distention of the urinary bladder. The instrument is introduced through the urethra to the lumen of the urinary bladder with the obturator in place.

The cystoscope must be introduced with great care in order to avoid bladder trauma or perforation in the patient with known extensive pelvic tumor, gross hematuria, or suspected radiation cystitis. The patient with a markedly contracted bladder, the wall of which is relatively unyielding, is at risk for perforation through too vigorous introduction of the cystoscope. With removal of the obturator, any urine remaining in the urinary bladder will flow forth. An aliquot should be taken for culture and the total residual volume measured, because if the patient was instructed to void immediately before this examination, this measurement will serve as an assessment of the effectiveness of bladder emptying through residual urine determination. All urine must be evacuated before the examination begins; any remaining urine will interfere with the clarity of the visual image. If there is active bleeding, the bladder lumen must be evacuated of any clots and gently and thoroughly irrigated, to optimize visualization. Systematic and thorough examination of the urinary bladder using the right-angle lens is then undertaken. The endoscopic findings relevant to the evaluation in the patient with neoplasms of the female genital tract have been reviewed earlier in this section. Care should be taken to avoid excessive distention of the urinary bladder, for this might precipitate troublesome bleeding in the presence of certain pathologic conditions.

Should findings consistent with neoplastic invasion of the urinary bladder be noted, biopsy confirmation is generally desirable. Classic tumor nodularity lends itself to biopsy by the cold cup technique, but a cystoscope of wider caliber will be necessary to accommodate the biopsy forceps. The ACMI 25 F easily accommodates the forceps, but a 24 F sheath can also be used by advancing the biopsy cup distal to the end of the examining telescope before introducing the forceps through the cystoscope sheath. The biopsy specimen should be examined to ensure that adequate tissue was obtained for pathologic study. The biopsy site should be examined for bleeding, which is readily controlled by spot electrocoagulation with the Bugbee electrode. An indwelling catheter is generally not necessary unless bleeding was troublesome to control. With bullous edema or extensive tumor necrosis, generally a deeper biopsy of the bladder wall will be required to ensure an adequate sampling. Electrocautery using the resectoscope loop will be necessary. One must bear in mind the cellular and architectural distortion of the biopsy speciman resulting from this form of biopsy; cytologic changes can present a difficult problem of interpretation for the pathologist. This distortion can be minimized by taking a generous biopsy with pure cutting current without using any coagulation current. It would be prudent not to take a biopsy specimen from an area related to the vagina because of the risk of causing fistula formation. Any bleeding is then controlled by spot electrocoagulation with the resectoscope loop. One must be most careful, in using electrocautery in areas of deep tumor, not to cause tumor necrosis and bladder perforation with urine extravasation or fistula formation. Generally, because of the depth of the biopsy and the greater potential for delayed bleeding, an indwelling catheter is used to prevent this complication. Not infrequently, when one is faced with recurrent pelvic tumor that is manifesting itself by urinary bladder signs or symptoms, significant tumor bulk will be palpable vaginally, lending itself to safer biopsy, with less potential for morbidity through transvaginal needle biopsy.

Ureteral Catheterization

A section on cystoscopy in a treatise on complications of gynecologic oncology must address itself to the subject of ureteral catheterization. Previously, the potential for ureteral involvement through both local extension and lymphatic involvement was mentioned. Early postoperative ureteral obstructive problems appearing as anuria or acute renal insufficiency and delayed ureteral obstruction through tumor recurrence or complications of therapy lend themselves to diagnostic evaluation and palliative management through ureteral catheterization and retrograde pyelography and through the placement of ureteral catheters. Neoplasms of the proximal vagina, uterine cervix, and uterine corpus, by virtue of their anatomic relation to the bladder base and trigonal area, often obliterate the intravesical ureters when they invade the urinary bladder, making ureteral catheterization technically impossible because of loss of normal landmarks. When the ureteral orifices are visible and the catheterization is for diagnostic retrograde pyelographic studies, a 5 F olive-tipped catheter is best employed and advanced with the aid of the catheterizing element to a distance of approximately 25 cm, provided no resistance is encountered. Efforts at advancement must be terminated when any resistance is encountered, to avoid the risk of ureteral perforation.

After a preliminary film is taken and inspected, approximately 4 ml of contrast medium is slowly and gently injected; then a second film is taken. The findings in that initial film will dictate subsequent films. If ureteral catheterization is being done because of acute renal failure in which the possibility exists of the need for leaving that catheter indwelling for palliative drainage, a 6 F whistle-tip ureteral catheter is employed. The ureteral catheter is fixed in place by being fixation-tied to an indwelling urethral Foley catheter, each catheter then being attached to appropriate drainage devices for accurate monitoring of urinary output.

REFERENCES

1. Harrison JH, Gittes RF, Perlmutter AD, Stamey TA, Walsh PC: *Campbell's Urology,* ed. 4. Philadelphia, WB Saunders Co, 1978, pp 22, 241, and 364.

2. Kiricuta I, Goldstein AMB: The repair of extensive vesicovaginal fistulas with pedicled omentum: A review of 27 cases. *J Urol* 108:724–727, 1972.

3. Rubin P, Casarett GW: *Clinical Radiation Pathology.* Philadelphia, WB Saunders Co, 1968, Vol 1, pp 58–59, 337–344, 350–351, 353, and 355.

4. Brown RB: A method of management of inoperable carcinoma of the bladder. *Med J Aust* 1:23, 1969.

5. Kumar S, Rosen P, Grabstald H: Intravesicle formation for the control of intractable bladder hemorrhage secondary to cystitis or cancer. *J Urol* 114:540, 1975.

6. Bright JF, Tosi, SE, Crichlow, RW, Selikowitz SM: Prevention of vesicoureteral reflux with fogarty catheters during formalin therapy. *J Urol* 118:950, 1977.

7. Fair WR: Formalin in the treatment of massive bladder hemorrhage: Techniques, results and complications. *Urology* 2:669, 1973.

8. Fletcher TF, Bradley WE: Neuroanatomy of the Bladder and urethra. *J Urol* 119:153, 1978.

9. Lec JF, Maurer VM, Block GE: Anatomic relations of pelvic autonomic nerves to pelvic operations. *Arch Surg* 107:324–328, 1973.

10. Watson PC, Williams DI: The urological complications of excision of the rectum. *Br J Surg* 40:19–28, 1952.

11. Fowler JW, Bremner DN, Moffat LEF: The incidence and consequences of damage to the parasympathetic nerve supply to the bladder after adbominoperineal resection of the rectum for carcinoma. *Br J Urol* 50:95–98, 1978.

8

Urologic Complications Secondary to Radiation Alone or Radiation and Surgery

Richard C. Boronow

The spectrum of urologic surgery in the nonradiated patient is discussed in some detail in the preceding chapter. Anatomy and physiology are reviewed, and the specific techniques used in a variety of urologic procedures are described.

The primary purpose of this chapter is to consider the problem of urologic complications occurring in an irradiated field. These complications will be discussed individually (in a general sense), as well as those factors that in my experience predispose to complications. Prevention considerations and management alternatives will also be detailed. To be sure, the management of these complications is often quite complicated, challenging the surgeon both in terms of technical skill and surgical judgment.

GENERAL CONSIDERATIONS

Before each of the various complications is considered, it seems appropriate to review a number of general factors that must be carefully assessed before reaching a therapeutic decision: (*1*) the nature of the radiation, (*2*) the nature of any prior surgery, (*3*) the status of the patient, and (*4*) technical considerations and cautions.

The nature of the radiation is of paramount concern. When possible, it is desirable to review in detail the written treatment records, dosimetry and other physicist's calculations, portal films, and brachytherapy films. The endarteritis induced by radiation injury (which may predispose to fibrosis or, in more severe cases, to necrosis and slough and occasionally to fistula) has quantitative features

163

that must be considered. For example, let us contrast two situations: The first is a patient who had had a preoperative radium implant (that delivered 3,000 or 4,000 rads to point A) and in whom a ureterovaginal fistula then developed after a radical hysterectomy. The second is a patient who had received external beam therapy *and* intracavitary therapy (in relatively standard contemporary doses) and in whom a small central recurrence then developed that was treated by a radical hysterectomy. The same injury—a ureterovaginal fistula—then developed in the patient. The clinician cannot simply consider this occurrence a case of ureterovaginal fistula but must consider all the conditions under which the fistula arose.

When we refer to the radiated patient, we are generally thinking about the patient receiving both external beam therapy and radium (or other brachytherapy). Most reports of radiation-induced complications concern patients treated by radiation alone. Yet, most of the complications occur when surgery is combined with intracavitary and/or external beam therapy.

The nature of any prior surgery is also important. Primarily, the degree of radicality and the attendant devascularization of the central (visceral) pelvis must be considered. In addition to the radicality, information about any other prior surgery and any postoperative morbidity (febrile or otherwise) may indicate the likelihood of difficult pelvic adhesions.

The status of the patient must be assessed. Quite obviously, the aggressiveness of the approach depends on such factors as the degree of disability caused by the complication, the patient's cancer status, and other medical considerations that reflect the patient's general health and prognosis, as well as technical factors such as significant obesity.

Technical considerations are all influenced by the foregoing. There is little, if any, margin for technical error when operating in an irradiated field. Often the pelvis is filled with radiated loops of small bowel adherent from prior surgery, and this condition introduces the potential for G.I. complications as well. Retroperitoneal spaces frequently lose some of their identity, and safe, clean dissection planes are often significantly altered secondary to prior surgery and/or prior radiation. Major vascular injury can ensue.

Although only scant data are available to permit quantifying the risk of operating in an irradiated field, some data will be included where appropriate in this chapter. It is of interest at the outset to cite the report of Swan and Rutledge (1) on 256 cases of conduit diversion at the M. D. Anderson Hospital and Tumor Institute. Thirty-five patients had conduit diversion as part of their primary (no prior radiation) exenterative procedure for cancer, and there was a 10% operative mortality. Of the 24 patients having conduit diversion for urologic injury without cancer (but secondary to surgery and irradiation), these authors quoted a 25% mortality. They commented on this "surprising and inexplicable finding" and suggested that it "most likely reflects the hazards of dissection in patients with previous radical surgery and irradiation."

One other point: Through this entire section, the variable of age (relevant to the dose of radiation energy) must be kept in mind. As noted, endarteritis and sclerosis are common denominators of radiation injury. The degree of endarteritis, with subsequent devascularized tissues, may be viewed as a constant once the radiation therapy has been delivered. The progressive small vessel compromise associated with aging and/or progressive arteriosclerotic changes may be viewed as a variable, a progressive and additive phenomenon. Although the initial injury might not be significant enough to cause serious structural change, when the progressive aging and/or arteriosclerotic changes ensue, they may (in an additive fashion) be sufficient to create late complications. This is probably "the straw that breaks the camel's back" and explains vesical and rectal fistulas, for example, that develop 10 and 15 years after the radiation therapy.

SPECIFIC COMPLICATIONS

Ureteral Injury

Ureteral Stricture

Moss and colleagues have observed, "In its course through the parametrium, the ureter lies a scant 1.5 cm from the lateral vaginal fornix. High doses exceeding the usual cancericidal levels are routinely delivered to this portion of the ureter. The tolerance of the ureter (to radiation energies) is emphasized by the rarity of late ureteral complication" (2) page 426. Clearly, dose is a factor. Closely akin to dose is the type of uterine-vaginal applicator that is used. Systems such as the Ernst applicator, with its short source-applicator surface distance, will produce very high surface doses; with sidearms fully extended into the vaginal fornix, the applicator may produce especially intense ureteral doses.

Ureteral stricture with secondary hydronephrosis of varying degrees and severity will occasionally occur incident to radiation therapy alone but is much more likely to follow radical pelvic surgery preceded by radiation therapy. Ureteral stricture with secondary hydronephrosis has been considered a relatively uncommon observation (3), but that impression has been challenged by two more contemporary reports from Buchler and associates (4) and from Underwood and associates (5). These are recorded in Table 1.

Kottmeier (3) reported an incidence of 0.83%, and when nine cases in which there was operative intervention and six cases in which radioactive colloidal gold was injected into the parametrium were deleted, the incidence was 0.4%. The report of Graham and Abad (6) stresses the role of reactive salpingitis in aggravating radiation injury, which was noted in five of their nine cases. Interestingly, in three instances there was ureterovaginal fistula as well. Shingleton and associates (7) found an instance of 0.42% and stressed that stricture is delayed 1, 2, or even more years in this "radiation only" group, as contrasted with the more prompt development of stricture seen in patients treated with combined radiation and radical surgery. Buchler and associates (4) reported a 4% incidence. Five of the cases were associated with symptomatic radiation cystitis, whereas 17 cases were found in asymptomatic patients. Slater and Fletcher (8) found a 1.67% incidence of ureteral stricture in the absence of recurrent cancer. Sixteen of their 26 patients had some type of surgical procedure after the radiation therapy, for a variety of reasons (including pelvic abscess and radiation complications), leaving 10 (0.65%) in whom stricture developed secondary to radiation therapy only. Underwood and associates (5) found an incidence of 0.33% in symptomatic stricture and, in an effort to determine the frequency of silent injury, reviewed 100 cases 5 or more years

Table 1. Ureteral Stricture Secondary to Radiation Therapy for Cancer of the Cervix

Author	Number of Cases	Number of Strictures	Percent Stricture
Kottmeier[3]	3,484	29 (total)	0.83
Kottmeier[3]	3,469	14 (deleting patients operated on or treated with gold)	0.4
Graham, Abad[6]	1,100	9	0.8
Shingleton, Fowler Pepper, Palumbo[7]	715	3	0.42
Buchler, Kline, Peckham, Boone, Carr[4]	515	22	4.0
Slater, Fletcher[8]	1,555	26	1.67
Slater, Fletcher[8]	1,539	10 (deleting patients having surgery)	0.65
Underwood, Lutz, Smoak[5]	2,393	8 (symptomatic)	0.33
Underwood, Lutz, Smoak[5]	100	4 (asymptomatic)	4.0

after treatment. They found pyelographic evidence of stricture in 4% of cases, an incidence that is identical with that reported by Buchler et al.

When radical hysterectomy is carried out after radiation therapy, the stricture rate is higher and the development more prompt. In the Shingleton et al. report (7), the rate was at least 10 times higher than with radiation therapy alone. One hundred thirty-two patients had combined therapy, and in seven (5.3%) stricture developed. All seven patients had preoperative radium, and four of the seven had external beam therapy as well. Burch and Chalfant (9) reported hydronephrosis in 9 of 200 patients (4.5%) when radical hysterectomy was preceded by a radium insertion that usually delivered 5,000 rads to point A. Churches and associates (10) reported four cases of hydronephrosis and four cases of complete obstructive uropathy among 274 operations (2.9%) when radical hysterectomy was preceded by a radium system that delivered approximately 6,000 rads to point A. Temporary hydronephrosis was observed in 27 of the 274 patients (9.9%). Rampone, Klem, and Kolstad (11) reported on 537 Stage IB patients treated with preoperative radium applications followed by radical hysterectomy. Significant, nonfistulizing ureteral injury occurred in seven patients (1.3%), but persistent injury was noted in only two (0.3%). It should be noted that the surgery as described is clearly a more conservative modification of the radical hysterectomy. The radium dose used in this experience was in the range of 5,000–6,000 rads to point A.

Management of Ureteral Stricture
The first consideration, in the patient in whom nonfistulizing ureteral stricture is identified, is the total clinical picture. In the occasional patient in whom ureteral stricture is found in conjunction with pelvic abscess secondary to active salpingitis or to postoperative hematoma, attention should be directed primarily to the

inflammatory process, either by excision and drainage or by drainage alone, as the case dictates. The ureter should be left undisturbed (awaiting quiescence of the pelvic inflammation) for at least 6 months, yet with continued observation of the renal units by serial pyelograms. If progressive obstruction portends loss of the kidney before surgery in the pelvis can safely be undertaken, percutaneous nephrostomy is the preferred diversion.

Sometimes the stricture may be associated with radiation-induced vesical fistula. Surgical correction of these defects must be delayed and is discussed in another section.

Since most developing obstructive uropathy occurs secondary to recurrent cancer, one must suspect this problem initially. A swollen leg is commonly associated with recurrent disease and, unilaterally, is highly suspicious. Leg edema secondary to high-dose pelvic radiotherapy does occur, but it is very uncommon (and is usually only mild) and is normally bilateral. Sciatic-distribution leg pain is a most ominous symptom of malignant involvement.

If other findings such as central recurrence, parametrial recurrence (bulky and often unilateral), and palpable groin or neck nodes are discovered, the diagnosis may be confirmed by biopsy. Weight loss is suspicious for recurrence, but can and does occur with profound radiation injury. A metastatic work-up is always indicated when obstructive uropathy is found.

The especially difficult patients to manage are those with obstructive uropathy and no other findings or symptoms. In these cases, one must formulate a plan of follow-up. If the pyelogram confirms that the obstruction is very low in the pelvis, near the bladder, and yet there are no palpable findings to suggest recurrent cancer, radiation injury is most probable. A more distal (from the bladder) point of obstruction may more likely be reactive cancer in the nodes. Retrograde ureteral catheterization is to be avoided, if at all possible, because of the risk of introducing infection. If necessary, catheterization should be done by the bulb retrograde technique.

We no longer explore all these patients promptly. Postradiation progression of disease is rarely dealt with satisfactorily by surgical intervention, and chemotherapy should be reserved for the emergence of symptoms to palliate. The routine aggressive treatment of recurrent nodal disease in the asymptomatic patient produces toxicity and morbidity that, in my view, are not justified by the results. There are anecdotal exceptions, so exception is sometimes made for the young or especially healthy, good-risk patient.

Intervention should be reserved, in most instances, for urologic considerations and preservation of renal function. In this context, depending on the severity of the obstructive uropathy, serial intravenous pyelograms (IVPs) are obtained at 4–6-week intervals and then at less frequent intervals if the change is not significantly progressive. On the other hand, if reasonably significant obstruction develops, intervention is indicated. Often, one must consider both the degree of obstruction and the time during which it develops and/or changes. The following two cases illustrate this point.

Case 1: TB. This 240-lb, 38-year-old patient with Stage IB adenosquamous carcinoma of the cervix was treated with full radiotherapy in April 1975. In March 1977, a radical hysterectomy and pelvic lymphadenectomy was carried out for a small central recurrence and an omental pedicle was swung into the retroperitoneal space for neovascularization. There was a normal preoperative IVP. Figure 1 is the postoperative IVP showing mild hydronephrosis on the tenth postoperative day, just before discharge. It is not an unusual picture. Figure 2 was obtained May 11, 1977 (approximately 1 month later) and reflects significant increasing hydronephrosis despite the effort at neovascularization. Urologic consultation was obtained, and reimplantation of the left ureter into the bladder was carried out; it strictured. A bladder flap was then done and it, too, strictured. Finally, an isolated ileal segment was interposed with success and, most recently, the 2-year follow-up IVP continues to be normal.

This case demonstrates the more rapid onset of ureteral stricture when radical surgery is combined with full radiotherapy. Radical surgery in the radiated field is complicated by increased paraureteral fibrosis. The use of conventional urologic procedures in this field may have been doomed to fail from the outset. Indeed, they were unsuccessful until fresh, nonradiated tissue was brought in to bridge the gap.

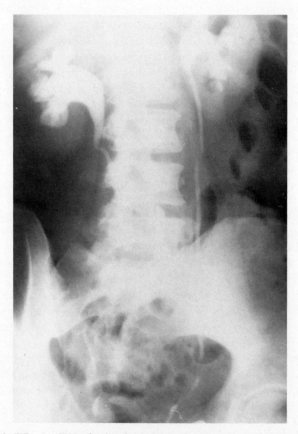

Figure 1. Case 1, TB: An IVP obtained 10 days after surgery. This pyelogram does not reflect an unanticipated degree of hydronephrosis after radical hysterectomy and pelvic lymphadenectomy.

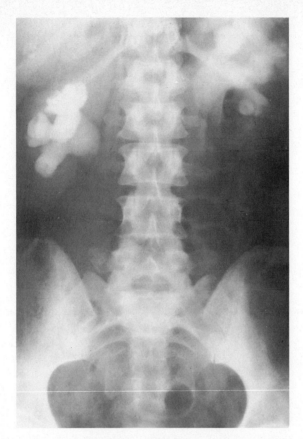

Figure 2. Case 1, TB: An IVP taken approximately 6 weeks after surgery. This pyelogram demonstrates the rapid deterioration that characterizes injury from a combination of surgery and full-pelvis radiotherapy.

Case 2: BM. This 45-year-old woman had Stage IB carcinoma of the cervix and was treated with rotational cobalt, 6,000 rads, but no radium was used. Then, on August 30, 1968, she had a radical hysterectomy and node dissection; there was no evidence of metastatic spread. Her preoperative IVP was normal. Figure 3 is an IVP taken on September 16, 1968; significant hydronephrosis is evident. A repeat IVP 2 weeks later showed a stable condition. This gross distortion persisted for over 4 months before it was resolved. Figure 4 is an IVP obtained in late January 1969; the IVP is finally back to normal. The last IVP recorded was obtained in April 1975; it was normal.

This case represents radical surgery in a heavily irradiated field but without the intensive central boost of radium implantation. Significant hydronephrosis was present. This case reflects the critical decision the clinician must make, along with careful follow-up. A stable situation, rather than progression, was observed. The temptation to intervene was with us continually during our period of observation, but we were willing to temporize because the condition was stable and not complicated by any secondary pyelonephritis. IVPs were obtained every 10 days initially, then every 2 weeks until we were certain the situation was stable.

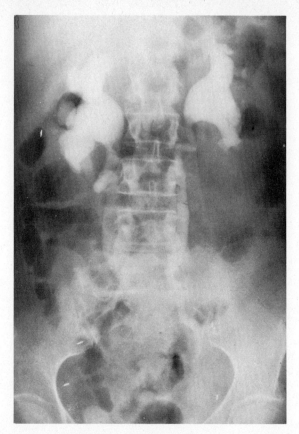

Figure 3. Case 2, BM: An IVP taken 16 days after radical hysterectomy and pelvic lymphadenectomy preceded by 6,000 rads of whole-pelvis radiation and no radium implant.

The conservative approach was justified by the ultimate return to normal of both renal units.

If the point of significant injury is in the parametrium, we have had, selectively, success with ureteroneocystostomy. The ureter is mobilized only enough for reimplantation; it is kept attached to most of the parametrium. Primary mobilization is done with the bladder (bringing the bladder to the ureter rather than the ureter to the bladder). The ureter is reimplanted into the lateral dome, away from the most intense radiation effect. We use a full-thickness, through-and-through, mucosa-to-mucosa technique, usually with six 4-0 chromic catgut sutures. Four or five 4-0 silk sutures are then placed very superficially in the ureter and more snugly in the bladder for a second external layer. If the length of ureter that must be sacrificed is sufficient to place any degree of tension on the suture line, the tension may be relieved by one or several sutures from the adjacent bladder to the pelvic side wall, peritoneum, or muscle (the so-called psoashitch).

Some surgeons have simply incised the encasing fibrotic tissue, without reimplantation, with reported success. We fear that cicatrix is likely to be replaced by more cicatrix and favor reimplantation. Others (12,13) have

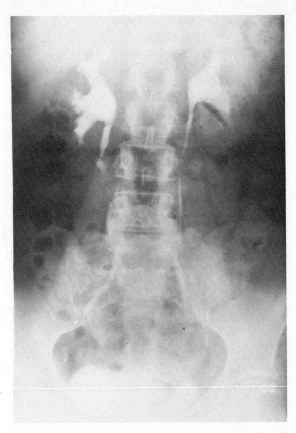

Figure 4. Case 2, BM: The gross distortion in Figure 3 remained unchanged for over 4 months and there was no intervention. This IVP was obtained 5 months after the study in Figure 3.

reported success with placement of an intervening segment of ileum when the length of ureter sacrificed is too great for bladder implantation. This is a very suitable technique that should be in the clinician's armamentarium. If the stricture is unilateral, a more direct approach (in experienced hands) is the ureteral-ureteral anastomosis above the radiated field.

Case 3: EJ. This 48-year-old patient was first seen in March 1972 with a bulky Stage III cancer of the cervix and was treated with 5,000 rads of whole-pelvis radiation, plus a chimney port; the periaortic nodes received 5,000 rads. She had two radium applications as well. In September 1974, the right kidney could not be visualized and the left was hydronephrotic. The patient was believed to have metastatic cancer although this was not confirmed histologically, and she was treated with combined chemotherapy. The last normal IVP was obtained in October 1973. Recently, progressive obstructive uropathy was documented on the left kidney but it did not suggest reactive cancer. A computerized tomographic scan revealed hydronephrosis of the left kidney and a small contracted kidney on the right. A renal scan revealed negligible activity in the right system.

At surgery (April 1980), with a creatinine level of 1.5 and a creatinine clearance of 43 ml/min, the patient's pelvis was explored and an extensive radiation reaction found so that all planes were obliterated. The same intense changes were noted in the periaortic chain. The right kidney was small and contracted. No periaortic nodes were palpated. Peritoneal washings were obtained and were subsequently reported as negative. The radiation reaction in the pelvis was as intense as I have seen. The left ureter was divided well above the pelvic brim, above the level of the common iliac vessels, and seemed reasonably healthy. A 6-inch intestinal segment was taken from the upper ileum with fairly good vascularity, and an end-to-side uretero-ileal anastomosis was carried out using six through-and-through, full-thickness 4-0 catgut sutures for the primary anastomosis and four 4-0 silk sutures to reinforce the anastomosis. The distal segment was anastomosed side-to-side to the bladder with a mucosa-to-mucosa, full-thickness closure using the same material. The side-to-side technique was used because the natural curve in the intestinal segment lent itself to easy approximation to the dome of the bladder as shown in Figure 5.

Initial pyelograms revealed essentially no change. Six weeks later, there was still essentially no improvement and, curiously, the right system (untouched during the surgery) showed some concentration from the small contracted kidney. A further follow-up pyelogram, taken approximately 3½ months postoperatively, revealed definite improvement on the left. The BUN level was 12, the creatinine, 1.2. Clearance studies were not determined at this examination.

It should be apparent that a variety of management techniques can be applied. Individualization requires experience and critical judgment on the part of the clinician, often with intraoperative assessment of the relative health, and/or damage, and vascularity of the tissues involved.

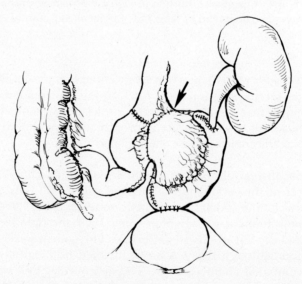

Figure 5. Use of a segment of fairly healthy proximal ileum to bypass a lengthy segment of severely damaged ureter. Note (arrow) that the incision in the mesentery of small bowel was deliberately short, just long enough to allow mobilization but short and broad enough to prevent vascular compromise.

Ureteral Fistulas

Ureteral fistulas secondary to radiation therapy alone is virtually nonexistent. But ureteral fistulas secondary to surgery and radiation therapy are vastly more frequent than with comparable surgery alone. Data are quite elusive. It would appear that a fivefold to tenfold increase in fistulization may be anticipated in the best of hands (14).

Ureteral Fistula Prophylaxis

There has been a clear trend in the last decade or two to modify the radicality of the radical hysterectomy and pelvic lymphadenectomy when radiotherapy, especially full radiotherapy, has been applied; but modification is usually introduced if radiotherapy is delivered by radium application only. The ureter must be handled especially carefully as it is cleared from the parametrium; longitudinal vascularity must be preserved; the ureterovesical junction should not be completely skeletonized; some degree of lateral soft tissue and blood supply should be preserved.

A variety of techniques have been recommended for handling the ureter after dissection. The two most frequently mentioned are (*1*) the technique of Green (15): carefully suturing, with very fine catgut, the ureter to the superior vesical artery (Fig. 6); and (*2*) the technique of Novak (16): using a sling of peritoneum from round ligament to lateral sigmoid cul-de-sac peritoneum, elevating the ureter anteriorly without sutures (Fig. 7). Both lift the ureter anteriorly into a more intraperitoneal position, out of the serum, blood, and potentially infected pelvic pool that may contribute to ureteral injury. I have routinely used the latter technique.

Closure of the vaginal cuff and use of Hemovac suction catheters are championed by some as a preferred method of keeping the collection in the pelvis to a minimum. I have continued to leave the cuff open with iodoform gauze and/or a Penrose drain. We have swung omentum or omental pedicles (with vascularity intact) into the bladder base area, usually suturing the omentum to the anterior vaginal cuff, and occasionally wrapping the distal ureter. This was not helpful in Case 1 but was in Case 5.

In the rare case of central recurrence after radiation therapy (Case 1), suitable for radical hysterectomy and pelvic lymphadenectomy, some have felt that the complication rate is too high to justify this approach and have tended to recommend exenteration procedures. The argument is made that the risk of postoperative fistula is so high that visceral diversion will most likely be required to manage complications and preferably should be used in the context of primary management. No ironclad rules are permissible (the patient in Case 1 is disease-free and viscerally intact); they are always subject to change. Distinguished surgeons who felt strongly about this matter 20 years ago have more recently championed "modified" exenterative procedures. This approach was stressed by Moore and co-workers (17) (Fig. 8) and should be considered in the category of prophylaxis against ureteral fistula and vesical fistula.

Case 4: AE. This 39-year-old patient had received radiation therapy for Stage I carcinoma of the cervix, and (after primary healing) an increasing firmness was felt in the cervix. Primary treatment was carried out in June and July of 1965. All fornices were reached, and it was an early Stage IIA lesion. Radiation therapy

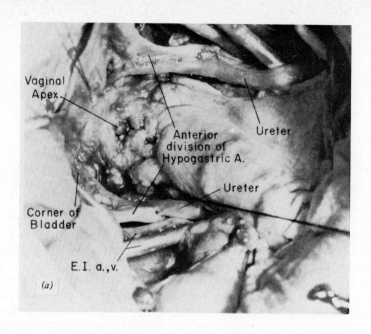

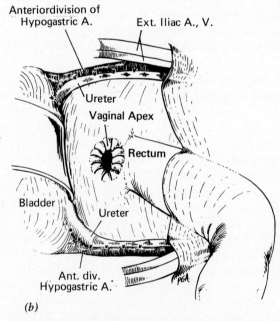

Figure 6. (*a*) The surgical field after bilateral ureteral suspension to the anterior division of the hypogastric artery. The fine chromic catgut sutures are visible, with this technique serving to replace and stabilize the ureters in a gently curving course along the side walls of the pelvis and well up out of the pelvic hollow. The external iliac artery and vein are designated E.I. a. and v. (*b*) Diagramatic representation of the ureteral suspension technique photographed in Figure 6*a*. Note that a few sutures are also employed to anchor the lowermost portion of the ureters to the corners of the bladder just proximal to the ureterovesical junction. (Green, Ref. 15.)

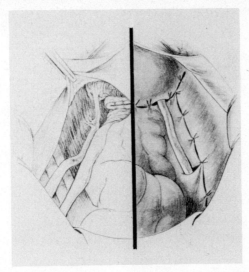

Figure 7. The technique of Novak demonstrating intraperitoneal placement of the right ureter (right half of illustration) and the classic retroperitoneal replacement of the ureter (left half of illustration). (Novak, Ref. 16.)

details included use of two Ernst applicators, each with 100 mg of radium, for 45 hours on July 9, 1965, and for 35 hours on July 15, 1965, for a total of 8,000 mg hours. This procedure delivered a calculated 14,500 rads at the cervical os, 6,300 rads at point A, and 2,200 rads at point B. External therapy was given in 31 days through two anterior pelvic portals and two posterior pelvic portals for a midplane dose of 4,278 rads. By March 1966, biopsies revealed viable cancer. There was no gross cancer, and the disease was believed to be confined to the cervix although the anterior fornix was suspiciously thickened.

Pelvic exenteration was discussed with the patient and her husband; they vehemently refused consideration of this procedure. Accordingly, a modified anterior pelvic exenteration was carried out after the technique of Moore and colleagues (radical hysterectomy and pelvic lymphadenectomy with incontinuity resection of the base of the bladder and terminal ureters and bilateral ureteroneocystostomy with suprapubic cystostomy). Residual cancer was found in the cervix but did not extend beyond it. Twenty nodes were microscopically negative. The patient's convalescence was smooth. Her voiding function returned to normal with acceptable residual volumes and reasonably normal bladder sensation. The IVP also returned to normal. She continues well to date.

Modifying the bladder-base resection technique just described is performing radical hysterectomy in the usual fashion but transsecting the ureters as they enter the parametrial tunnel and at the ureterovesical junction and then reimplanting them in the bladder dome. This procedure may be applicable when central recurrence is small and no extension is suspected, either preoperatively or intraoperatively. This procedure greatly simplifies the dissection in the parametria, allows a better *en bloc* parametrial dissection, sacrifices the most heavily irradiated 2 or 3 cm of distal ureter, and allows reimplantation in the

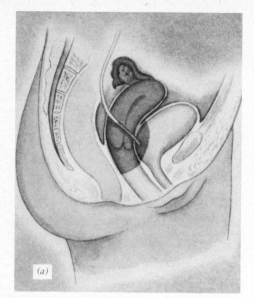

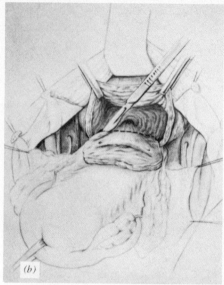

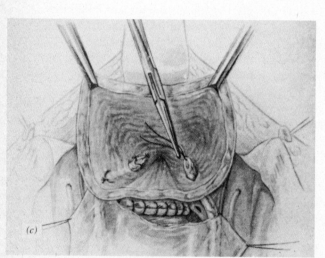

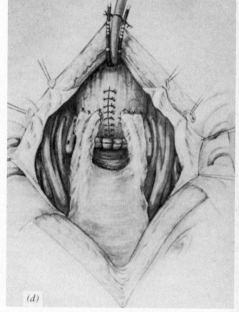

Figure 8. (*a*) Diagram indicating the approximate area of the ureters and bladder excised in the operation of modified pelvic exenteration. (*b*) The ureters have been transected as they enter the parametrial tunnel, facilitating resection of the parametria as a whole and, in this figure, a segment of the base of the bladder is being excised, remaining firmly in continuity with the anterior cervix and vaginal wall. (*c*) Ureteroneocystostomy is now carried out. (*d*) Reconstruction is now completed and attention is directed to the vertical bladder closure. Several sutures from the peritoneal flap and periureteral tissues to the outer bladder wall are used to take tension off the mucosal sutures. (Moore et al., Ref. 17.)

176

least radiated area of the bladder. We have used this technique on several occasions without postoperative problems.

Management of Ureteral Fistulas

The principles of management of ureteral fistulas are very similar to those discussed in more detail in the section called "Management of Ureteral Stricture." Again, one must have a number of techniques in mind and be able to individualize and apply them as the occasion arises, carefully analyzing the clinical presentation of disease, the radiation damage, and such features as obesity, medical considerations, and psychological factors.

Two management points seem especially worthy of stressing: (1) although prompt intervention may be appropriate in the nonirradiated field and is championed by some, I believe that the wise approach is to delay repair at least 3–4 months. (2) One must use tissue with good vascularity, and this often requires a departure from techniques that may be employed with good success in nonirradiated tissues; insistence on the rote employment of these techniques is doomed to result in a high failure rate.

The unusual instance of unrecognized transsection with prompt leakage would be the only situation in which one might consider immediate reoperation. However, most fistulas will develop later than is commonly seen in nonirradiated patients, with the endarteritis of irradiation therapy apparently being "the straw that breaks the camel's back," the feature that simply won't allow an injury to heal. With most of these patients, it is far safer to await quiescence of the inflammatory response in the surgical field rather than risk reoperation on already partially devitalized tissues. To ignore this rule, gained through bitter experience by many pelvic surgeons, is to risk major problems with poor wound healing, as well as a variety of other visceral and vascular complications that are occasionally lethal.

Bladder Injury

Bladder Fistulas

One of the most troublesome complications in obstetrics and in gynecologic surgery is the vesicovaginal fistula. Most of these fistulas can be corrected, however, with well-defined surgical techniques. Especially vexing, however, is the vesicovaginal fistula arising in an irradiated field. It usually defies the standard techniques for vesicovaginal fistula closure.

The incidence of radiation-induced vesicovaginal fistulas varies from series to series, depending to some extent on dose, radium geometry, and the experience of the clinicians or institutions reporting. Most important seem to be specific features of the uterovaginal radium therapy. It is recognized that with most systems currently used, the posterior bladder wall receives 6–8 times more radiation than the anterior bladder wall. Severe acute reactions in the bladder are common, although not commonly crippling, when so-called cancericidal doses of radiation are employed in contemporary therapy.

With such contemporary systems and doses, the vesical fistula rate is usually well less than the 3%–5% not infrequently reported in the literature 10–20 years ago. As higher doses of radiation are employed in an effort to eradicate larger volumes of disease, the fistula rate tends to rise. This fact is reflected in the general trend toward a difference in rate with each progressive stage of disease, as shown in Table 2 (18). In this study, the corrected vesicovaginal fistula incidence (with radiotherapy only) for all stages was 1.2%.

As Fletcher states "At least 90% of the vesico- or rectovaginal fistulae have developed when there was massive central disease or extensive vaginal involvement. In both instances therapy had to be extra-radical, at times with additional interstitial gamma ray treatment in the form of sources in the vagina or interstitial implant. In a few patients, a fistula developed when a compact radium system consisting only of an afterloading tandem with a protruding source was used with heavy radium loading" (19).

Every essayist reviewing hysterectomy experience, radical or conservative, acknowledges the increased risk of fistula when one combines surgery and radiation therapy. In an earlier review of 79 patients with vesicovaginal fistulas associated with cancer seen on the Gynecologic Service at the M. D. Anderson Hospital and Tumor Institute from 1944 to 1965, we observed that the addition of a hysterectomy in an irradiated field introduced a near fourfold increase in fistula formation (18). This fact is reflected in the righthand column of Table 2. Most of these hysterectomies were of the conservative type.

Although a vesicovaginal fistula caused by hysterectomy will usually develop within the first 2 or 3 postoperative weeks, in our series of combined therapy the interval from operation to fistula was 12.6 weeks (if two late fistulas occurring at 2 years and 5 years after operation were excluded, the interval was 7.7 weeks) (18).

Some increased risk is to be expected with the additional compromise of the central pelvic blood supply that hysterectomy produces. Although all surgeons

Table 2. Vesicovaginal Fistulas in Cervical Cancer Cases Treated Entirely at M. D. Anderson, 1948–1964[a]

Stage	Number of Cases Treated with Radiation Only	Number of Fistulas	Fistulas (%)	Number of Cases Treated with Radiation and Surgery	Number of Fistulas	Fistulas (%)
IA	157	0	0	13	1	7.1
IB	405	6	1.5	47	2	4.2
IIA	570	2	0.35	50	1	2.0
IIB	510	4	0.78	77	4	5.2
IIIA	507	8[b]	1.6	32	2	6.2
IIIB	464	17[b]	3.7	18	0	—
IV	116	2[c]	1.2	4	0	—
Total	2,729	39[d]		241	10	
Average			1.4[d]			4.1

SOURCE: Boronow and Rutledge[18]. Used by permission.

[a]The data in this table are at variance with the data in the text because the table lists the number of fistulass through the year 1964 in those patients treated solely at M.D. Anderson Hospital.

[b]Includes four recurrent (malignant) fistulas: one State IIIA at 11 months and three Stage IIIB at 5, 11, and 16 months.

[c]One patient received palliative transvaginal therapy only.

[d]There were 34 fistulas apparently from radiation, exclusive of recurrence, for a rate of 1.2%

recognize some risk, it is difficult to quantify and no doubt varies with radiation doses, the nature of the operation, and the technical skill of the surgeon. Nevertheless, the margin of safety is reduced. As emphasized in Table 3, a technical error or deviation in procedure—even a small one—may be poorly tolerated. Similarly, we documented that in the follow-up of the radiated patients, gentle handling of tissues is essential when one examines, takes a biopsy of, or packs clinical vaginal and/or cervical radiation necrosis.

In a recent report of radiation combined with extrafascial hysterectomy in the treatment of the so-called barrel-shaped lesion of the cervix, O'Quinn and M. D. Anderson co-workers reflected on the hazards of combined therapy and stressed features to reduce the fistula risk. The vesicovaginal fistula rate was approximately 6% in the 1954–1969 group of cases compared with a rate of 1.3% in the 1970–1976 experience (20). Thus, with meticulous precision both in radiation planning and in surgical technique, the risk in combined therapy can be significantly minimized.

In the classic report of Kottmeier (3), the incidence of vesicovaginal fistula was approximately 0.8% in patients treated with radiation only at the Radiumhemmet in Stockholm, and when radical hysterectomy of the Meigs variety was added after full radiotherapy, either for a persistent disease or later for recurrent disease, the vesicovaginal fistula incidence was about 15%.

In the more contemporary report of Webb and Symmonds (14), radical hysterectomy and pelvic lymphadenectomyy was associated with a vesical fistula rate of 0.7% among 423 patients not given radiotherapy; and among the 141 patients with a history of prior radiotherapy, the vesicovaginal fistula rate was 7.1%.

Management of Bladder Fistulas
The radiation or radiation surgery–induced vaginal fistula is difficult, sometimes impossible, to correct surgically. The pathologic changes of severe radiation injury—endarteritis, necrosis, slough, and fistula formation—create an anatomic field most unfavorable for conventional techniques. To try them is to invite chaos.

Table 3. Additional Factors Predisposing to Vesical Fistulas

Factors	Number of Cases
Cancer	
Fresh, untreated cases	3
Recurrence	10
Bladder entered	
Hysterectomy	5
Radium insertion	1
Radiation necrosis biopsy and/or fulguration	
Bladder base	4
Vaginal apex	9
Vaginal packing for bleeding	3
Instrumentation of pelvic abscess	3

SOURCE: Boronow and Rutledge[18]. Used by permission.

The defect is usually large, there is poor mobility of tissues due to fibrosis, and there is compromised blood supply in the region of the fistula. As noted, standard surgical techniques rarely yield satisfactory results unless the defect is extremely small. When these standard approaches fail, as they usually do, diversionary procedures have been commonly employed in the past. During the past several decades, a reasonable amount of experience has accumulated with a variety of additional techniques so that virtually no patient is doomed to continual wetness, and many can be managed without diversionary procedures.

Colpocleisis

Colpocleisis, either partial or complete vaginal closure, is a technique that has achieved some degree of popularity in this country, and the experience at the M. D. Anderson Hospital with colpocleisis was quite sizable (Table 4) (18). Marshall has recently updated the Marshall and Twombly experiences of an earlier decade (21,22).

Continence is usually, but not always, achieved, and frequently several procedures are required. Loss of coital function may be a major consideration in the sexually active patient when complete colpocleisis is carried out. Stone formation has been reported but is not common. Pyelonephritis can be a chronic problem, especially among patients with some element of obstructive uropathy before closure, but it is rare with normal upper urinary systems. As would be expected, chronic pyelonephritis can lead to progressive renal deterioration in already compromised renal units. We looked at that problem in comparison with the use of urinary diversion in the M. D. Anderson experience and documented the fact that colpocleisis does not improve upper renal systems and, in many instances, cause their deterioration. Although deterioration can occur with conduit diversion, this is generally a technical error, and one should generally anticipate improvement in compromised renal units (Tables 5 and 6) (18). The technique of colpocleisis of Twombly and Marshall (21,22) is demonsttrated in

Table 4. Primary Management of Vesicovaginal Fistula

Method	Number of Cases
Partial colpocleisis	20
Complete colpocleisis	7
Ileal conduit[a]	22
No closure	18
Spontaneous closure	5
Conventional closure	1
Latzko closure	2
Ureterosigmoidostomy	2
Anterior exenteration	1
Method unknown, closed elsewhere	1
Total	79

SOURCE: Boronow and Rutledge[18]. Used by permission.

[a]Includes two cases of isolated sigmoid conduit.

Table 5. Effect on Intravenous Pyelography of Fistula Management Methods

Method	Number of Renal Units Available for Study[a]	Postoperative Evaluation		
		Number of Renal Units Unchanged	Number of Renal Units Improved	Number of Renal Units Deteriorated
Partial colpocleisis	16	11	0	5
Complete colpocleisis[b]	10	7	0	3
Ileal conduit[c]	32	14	11	7

SOURCE: Boronow and Rutledge[18]. Used by permission.

[a]With pretreatment and posttreatment studies. (A renal unit is an individual renal collecting unit.)

[b]Includes two cases initially treated by partial colpocleisis.

[c]Includes two cases initially treated by partial colpocleisis.

Table 6. Comparison of Preoperative and Postoperative Intravenous Pyelography in Ileal Conduit Cases

Preoperative Grade	Number of Renal Units[a]	Postoperative Grade	
		0–I	II–IV
0–I	21	18 (86)[b]	3 (14)
II–IV	11	9 (82)	2 (18)
Total	32	27	5

SOURCE: Boronow and Rutledge[18]. Used by permission.

[a]A renal unit is an individual renal collecting system.

[b]Figures in parentheses are percentages.

Figure 9, and the technique of Blaikley (23), the basic technique used in the M. D. Anderson experience, is demonstrated schematically in Figure 10.

Neovascularization

Because of the problem of compromised vascularity in the operative field, a number of techniques have been described to bring in an improved blood supply. In these neovascular procedures a pedicle of fresh tissue is usually brought in between layered suture lines, for additional support as well as for a new blood supply. We have stressed the necessity of extremely wide mobilization of the fistula margins so as to approximate the initially fixed and rigid tissues *without* tension. Recurrent cancer must, of course, be excluded by appropriate biopsies, clinical means, and a metastatic work-up. Enough time should be allowed to elapse between fistula formation and attempted closure to permit full quiescence of the acute radiation injury and maturation of the fistula margins. We have used 12 months as our guide (24).

Gracilis Muscle

Kottmeier (3) makes reference to success in closing vesical fistulas in the irradiated field by using the interposed gracilis muscle. He mentions that "in post-radiation cases, the operation as a rule has to be repeated one or two times." He describes the wide mobilization of the margin (see preceding text) as

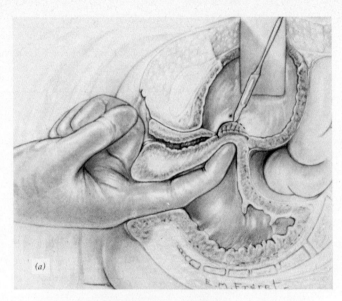

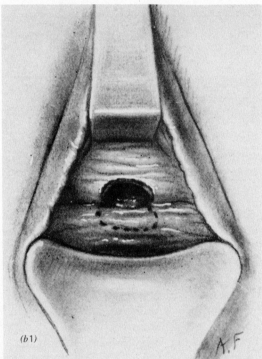

Figure 9. (*a*) With the finger in the rectum, the proposed patch of posterior vaginal wall is outlined via suprapubic cystostomy. This procedure delineates the area of posterior vaginal wall that will fit the fistula. (Marshall V, Twombly G: Further experiences with an operation for the repair of vesicovaginal fistula caused by radiation. *Cancer* 5: p 429, 1952.) The delineated vaginal patch defined from above is evident (*b*1). Liberal removal of vaginal mucosa is then begun, the delineated patch left intact (*b*2). Then transverse closure approximates the external margins of excision (*b*3). (Twombly G et al., Ref. 22.)

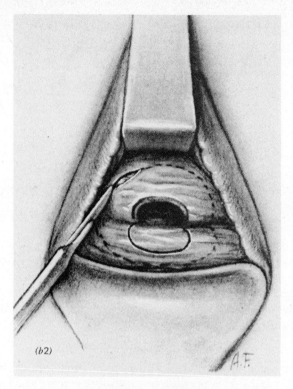

(b2)

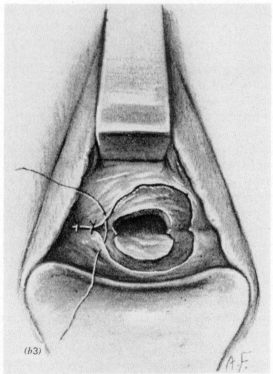

(b3)

Figure 9. (Continued)

183

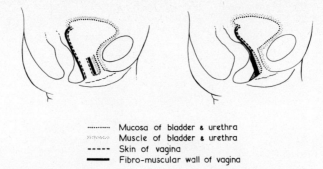

    ········· Mucosa of bladder & urethra
    ░░░░░░░░ Muscle of bladder & urethra
    - - - - - Skin of vagina
    ━━━━━ Fibro-muscular wall of vagina

Figure 10. Diagram before (left) and after (right) use of the colpocleisis technique for closing a large vesicovaginal fistula. The upper part of the posterior vaginal wall has been used to fill the defect and the lower vaginal skin has been excised. (Blaikley, Ref. 23.)

"scrupulous dissection of the fistula and the surrounding tissues." Credit is generally given to Ingelman-Sundberg (25), but the procedure appears to have been described in 1928 by Garlock (26) of New York. The late John Graham (27) probably had the most extensive personal experience with this technique of anyone in this country.

Omentum

Bastiaanse (28) is generally credited with popularizing the use of omentum in these difficult problems. It is possible to carefully preserve the vascular arcades and mobilize generous portions of omentum for use in the pelvis. As mentioned, we have used omentum to cover the pelvic floor when ureters and bladder base have been denuded in the course of extended surgery after radiation.

Case 5: LH. This 30-year-old patient had been treated for Stage IB cervical cancer elsewhere and had a large vesicovaginal fistula encroaching on one ureteral orifice, and her defunctionalized bladder was extremely small from disuse for many years (Fig. 11*a*). An abdominoperineal approach was used with two surgeons, the fistula was widely mobilized and closed, the compromised ureter was reimplanted (Fig. 11*b*), and the bladder was closed. The bladder was so contracted from its defunctionalized state that it had to be carefully closed over a Foley catheter inflated only 5 cc (Fig. 11*c*). This was inserted before closure to avoid the potential trauma of blind insertion at the completion of the case. This tiny bladder, completely mobilized, was then "wrapped" with a network mesh of mobilized omentum (Fig. 11*d*). The patient has been continent for 6 years after the surgery, has a normal IVP, and has gradually reexpanded her bladder capacity up to voided volumes of 3 and 4 oz and negligible residual volume.

Bulbocavernosis-Labial Fat Pad

Martius's description (29) of the labial musculo-fatty pad technique and his reported success suggested to us that, since this tissue is the most proximally available source of neovascularization, this technique is worthy of further use. It also seemed the least complicated approach, so we adopted this technique for radiation-induced vaginal fistula repair and have reported our earlier experi-

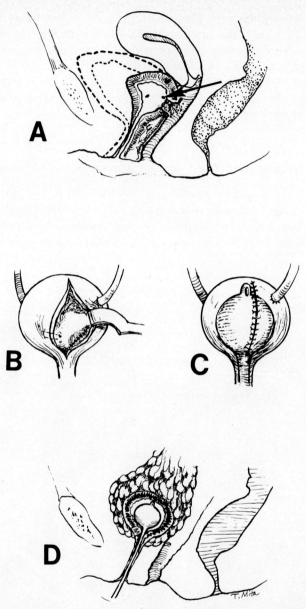

Figure 11. The small, defunctionalized bladder (*a*) is noted as having a large vesicovaginal fistula, and the left ureteral orifice is in the fistula margin. The compromised ureteral orifice was reimplanted (*b*) and the fistula margins thus safely and widely mobilized and approximated. The contracted bladder was then closed over a 5-cc Foley catheter bulb (*c*), and the small, contracted bladder was wrapped with an omental pedicle (*d*) and functions normally 6 years later.

ence (24,30). The technique is illustrated in Figure 12. Most of the cases were rectovaginal fistulas, and the success rate was 82% with the first operation (30). However, we were not nearly so successful with the vesicovaginal fistulas, and despite technical closure in one remarkable case (Fig. 13), the bladder was not truly functional and continual dribbling persisted. We have recently incorporated the labial fat pad technique with conduit diversion, and this will be described in the next section.

Undiversion
Through serendipity, we devised another approach that we recently reported (31).

Case 6: LB. A large radiation vesical fistula had developed in this 53-year-old patient, who was managed by primary ileal conduit. She prevailed in her insistence on being "put back to normal." Our initial experience with the labial

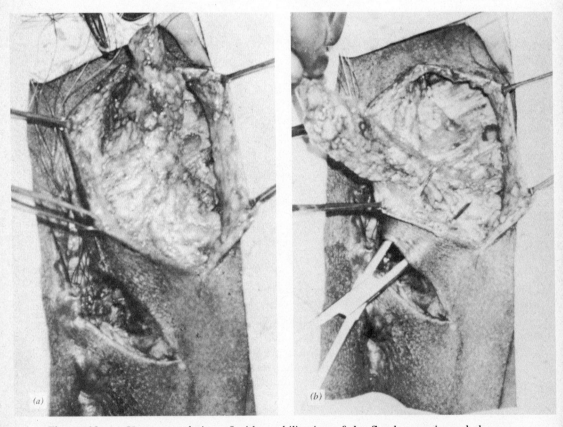

(a)   (b)

Figure 12. (a) Upon completion of wide mobilization of the fistula margin and closure without tension, the musculofatty contents of the labia are developed with thin skin flaps. (b) A nonconstricting tunnel is made under the vulvar skin once the pedicle has been developed. (c) The pedicle is brought in without twisting the base, and if it is too long, it

fat pad technique had been frustrating, but because she was a patient whose urinary stream had already been diverted, we considered reevaluating the approach. It seemed somewhat analogous to fecal stream diversion for rectal fistula correction, our routine procedure in for all radiated patients. We waited 12 months. After closure using the Martius technique, the bladder was watertight. Five months later the ileal conduit was taken down and the distal stomal end freshened and simply anastomosed end-to-side to the dome of the bladder with satisfactory results (Fig. 14). The patient now voids and empties her bladder, waits a short time for the conduit to empty residual urine into the bladder, and then voids again. This "double voiding" technique maintains a very acceptably low residual urine volume, and the patient's IVPs have been stable for 4 years.

This fortunate outcome encouraged the planned use of this staged diversion, bladder closure, undiversion approach on a second suitable patient. This fistula, too, healed without incident and the patient remains well.

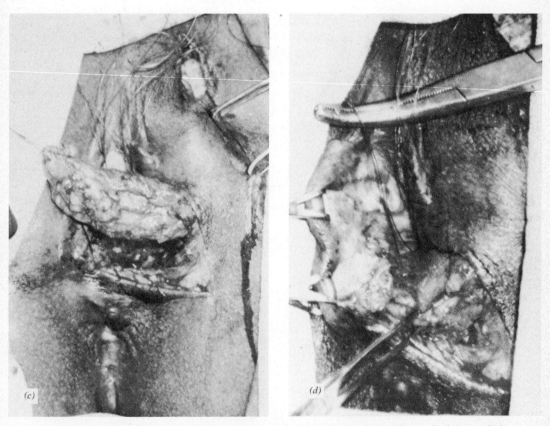

(c)

(d)

can be trimmed. It is encouraging to have to tie a bleeding point at the end of the pedicle. (d) The pedicle has been secured to the contralateral angle and interposed across the suture line before closure of the vaginal mucosa. The Allis clamp reflects the pedicle downward. (Boronow, Ref. 24.)

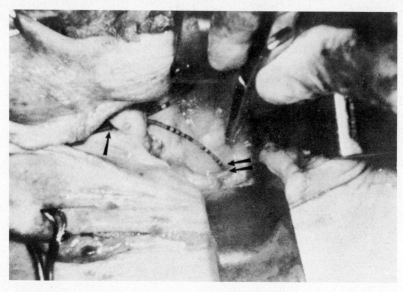

Figure 13. A large urethrovesicovaginal fistula noted on viewing the interior of the bladder. The urethral meatus is marked with one arrow, and the right ureteral orifice (right at the margin of the fistula) is marked with two arrows. This case was successfully closed with the first operation. (Boronow, Ref. 24.)

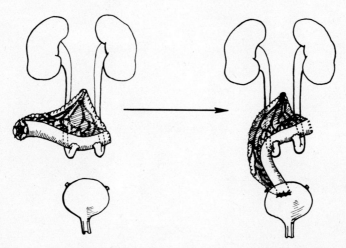

Figure 14. A schematic drawing of undiversion. The ileal conduit, previously constructed and functional, illustrated on the left, is taken down and ileocystostomy performed. (Kwon and Boronow, Ref. 31.)

Myocutaneous Pedicles
The use of gracilis myocutaneous pedicles is applicable to this clinical setting, and the preliminary experience, although anecdotal, has been encouraging.

Conduit Diversion
Conduit diversion was used in 22 cases in the M. D. Anderson experience (18). Twenty cases were ileal conduit, and two were isolated sigmoid conduit. Conduit

diversion was used in two additional cases in which colpocleisis failed and in three additional cases referred after primary vaginal closure attempts were unsuccessful elsewhere. While not without potential significant as well as lesser complications (see following text), conduit diversion is the most expedient method of dealing with radiation-induced vesicovaginal fistula. In general, there seems to be a trend away from primary conduit diversion toward some of the techniques just described wherein normal, or essentially normal, bladder function may be maintained. In cases in which radiation-induced ureteral stricture has produced obstructive uropathy, it is obvious that this condition may well progress and will certainly not be improved by transvaginal technique. Conduit diversion does offer the potential of correcting obstructive uropathy. Reference again is made to Tables 5 and 6. In this particular experience, when deterioration does occur (7 of 32 renal units), one must accept technical factors. However, two of the seven deteriorations were only minor. Table 6 reflects a closer look at the degree of preoperative and postoperative change with the use of Bricker's classification of obstructive uropathy (0—none, I—mild, II—moderate, III— severe, IV—nonvisualization). Among patients with moderate or more severe hydronephrosis, 82% showed significant improvement postoperatively, whereas 18% remained in essentially the same category. Although all the numbers in this series were small, the percent of changes for better and for worse were comparable to those reported from the institution of Bricker (32).

Hemorrhagic Cystitis

The mechanism of hemorrhagic cystitis is the same as that of fistula, but the injury is less profound. It is often an indolent problem taking many months to resolve. Occasionally, it will progress to fistula formation. Problems include anemia from chronic blood loss, pain from bladder spasm if the bleeding is heavy, and chronic infection.

In mild cases, vigorous oral hydration must be maintained and urinary tract antisepsis, as indicated, will usually suffice.

In more severe cases, three-way catheter drainage in the hospital may be periodically required. We have found endoscopic inspection, often repeated with judicious cautery of particularly active bleeding points, very valuable and adequate for the majority of cases.

We have used instillation of formalin (33) with uniformly good results in the few patients treated.

Case 7: SJ. This 29-year-old para IV had a bulky Stage IB carcinoma of the cervix and was treated by radiation therapy consisting of 4,000 rads of whole-pelvis radiation in 4 weeks and 6,500 mg hours of radium with the Fletcher tandem and ovoids in two applications. Therapy was complete in August 1976, and from December 1977 through January 1978, the patient was hospitalized on several occasions because of profuse hematuria. Bladder irrigation, urinary antiseptics, cystoscopy, and fulguration of bleeding points failed to control the problem. A 5% formalin solution was instilled in the bladder under general anesthesia, but all the solution was immediately expelled owing to immediate and severe bladder spasms. A second attempt was made under spinal anesthesia, and about 80 cc of formalin solution was retained in the bladder for 3−5 minutes. Subsequently, the patient has had no further gross hematuria over almost 2 years of follow-up.

Defunctionalizing the bladder with conduit diversion occasionally works in refractory cases. Cystectomy should be reserved for that rare case in which all other measures fail and in which hemorrhage becomes life-threatening.

Conduit Complications

The mortality associated with urinary conduit surgery seems to average 10%–15%, with ranges reported of from 5% to 20%. Subgroups of patients who have more radical surgery (such as exenteration and/or cystectomy, and/or surgery in an irradiated field) skew the mortality and morbidity rates of the total group upward (although a recent challenge to this view has been reported and will subsequently be cited) (34). There is also general agreement that technical problems associated with the urinary diversional part of the operation account for about one-third of the morbidity and mortality.

Complications due generally to technical errors include hydronephrosis (by far the most common complication), gangrene of the intestinal segment, retraction and/or stenosis of the stoma, and leaking of the ureteral and/or intestinal anastomosis.

Parkhurst has stressed, "By adhering strictly to Halsted's principles of hemostasis, asepsis, atraumatic handling of tissue and reapproximation of divided tissue without tension or dead space, the procedure is not difficult but does require attention to detail, intelligent assistance, and frequent performance for familiarity and speed" (35). Bricker's group similarly stresses "meticulous attention to technical detail" (32). Conduit diversion in radiated tissue demands special responsiveness to these admonitions. The reader is referred to Butcher et al.'s detailed discussion of complications (32) and Parkhurst's succinct discussion of diagnosis and management of complications (35) based on an analysis of both series, which total close to 900 cases. Butcher's paper (the Bricker group) introduced the system of classification of assessing individual renal units that is used in follow-up assessment by most essayists. This system is recorded in Table 7.

Swan and Rutledge (1) studied 189 patients with urinary conduit diversion associated with exenterative surgery (Group I) and an additional 57 patients who had diversion for urologic complications of therapy (Group II). Two hundred thirteen patients had ileal conduits and 13 had sigmoid conduits. These patients, the vast majority of whom had undergone radiation therapy, had a higher conduit fistula rate than is generally reported. In this series, revision of the conduit was carried out on 46 occasions (18.6%) for early and late complications. Conduit fistula accounted for 17 of the 26 early revisions, whereas progressive obstructive uropathy, either stomal or ureteral, accounted for 15 of the 20 long-term follow-up revisions. Table 8 depicts the relation of preoperative factors to postoperative urinary tract follow-up. Surgery in the irradiated field, complicated by the technical problems inherent in developing a training program, enhanced the potential for problems. This fact underscores the necessity of careful judgment as well as technical skill in the conduit construction.

Critical judgment begins with selection of the intestinal segment. The sigmoid with larger vessels is often suitable, all other factors being equal, but when especially high doses of external beam therapy have been employed, the radiation effect may be too profound. Nelson was among the first gynecologists

Table 7. Classification of Renal Status After Ureteroileal Urinary Diversion

By Individual Renal Collecting System — Intravenous Pyelography	Grade
Normal intravenous pyelogram	0
Minimal or questionable hydronephrosis	I
Definite hydronephrosis	II
Massive hydronephrosis	III
Kidney not visualized by intravenous pyelograms	IV

By individual patient

Satisfactory: Those patients having never had clinical evidence of pyelonephritis, whose pyelograms show no hydronephrosis on either side (Grade 0–I) or whose pyelograms are improved postoperatively.

Unsatisfactory: All patients having recurrent bouts of pyelonephritis or patients whose pyelograms show no improvement in preoperative hydronephrosis or the occurrence of a higher grade of hydronephrosis postoperatively than preoperatively.

SOURCE: Butcher et al.[32]. Used by permission.

Table 8. Relation of Preoperative Factors to Postoperative Urinary Tract Follow-up

					Renal Function					
	Fistula		Stomal Stenosis/ Dehiscence		Normal, Improved, or Stabilized Renal Disease		Progressive Renal Disease		Nonfunction	
Preoperative Factors	%	Number[a]	%	Number[a]	%	Number[a]	%	Number[a]	%	Number[a]
Age (60 yr or over)	17	9/54	2	1/54	84	36/42	14	6/42	0	
Weight (over 200 lb)	13	1/8	0		57	4/7	29	2/7	14	1/7
5,000 r — ± radium, ± surgery	19	11/57	5.2	3/57	47	24/51	31	16/51	22	11/51
Urologic studies Normal	12	18/147	5	8/147	80	104/129	13	16/129	7	9/129
Abnormal	11	1/85	2.4	2/85	74	63/85	12	10/85	14	12/85

SOURCE: Swan and Rutledge[1]. Used by permission.

[a]Number of patients in each category available for analysis. The patient differentials under the heading "Renal Function" signify patients with unknown renal follow-up.

to use an isolated segment of transverse colon for conduit diversion (36) (Fig. 15). Our preference has been sigmoid colon when total exenteration is performed and, if not, ileum. By running the small bowel from the cecum beyond the terminal ileum, which ordinarily contains the most intense radiation changes, when the more proximal ileum is reached, acceptable vascularity is usually found. Only occasionally have we had to go to the junctional area of ileum and jejunum. The high jejunum is to be avoided because one may encounter significant electrolyte abnormalities such as hyperkalemia, hyponatremia, hypochloremia, and alkalosis. Another point concerning the development of the conduit seems worthy of reemphasis, and that is Bricker's admonition to avoid

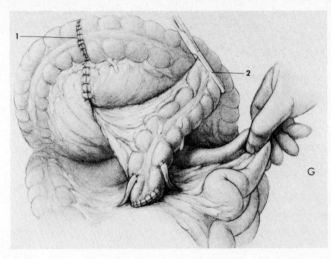

Figure 15. End-to-end anastomosis of the transverse colon and its mesentery has been completed, and the ureterointestinal anastomosis has been completed in the isolated segment. (Nelson, Ref. 36.)

excessively long incisions into the mesentery isolating the segment. Such an incision compromises already somewhat compromised vascularity, and torsion can more easily occur.

The second area of technical concern involves, of course, the ureters. When they are markedly scarred and unsuitable for use, there is no point (and not inconsiderable risk) in trying to free them from their encasement in dense pelvic fibrosis that may also involve pelvic vasculature. They should be mobilized from the pelvis at a point where they seem reasonably healthy and free and then, if necessary, cut back successively in small increments until bleeding from the fresh end is evident. We employ the anastomotic technique of Bricker. This is an end-to-end anastomosis of the ureters to the intestinal segment, without tunneling. The ureters are cut square, not beveled, and are anastomosed near the proximal end of the segment. We do not use catheter splints or stents. Nor have we found it necessary to spatulate and conjoin the ureters although this technique appears to be gaining favor and has certainly been reported with good results (34). Usually, six through-and-through sutures of 4-0 catgut are placed in all layers of the ureter and intestine, the so-called mucosa-to-mucosa technique, for the first layer of the anastomosis. Four to six similarly fine silk sutures are placed to the adventitia of the ureter, the ureteral musculature being carefully avoided, and to the serosa of the bowel, to complete the second layer. In my own experience, adherence to these principles (in an obviously modest-sized personal series) has resulted in no conduit revisions, either early because of leaks or late because of deteriorating obstructive uropathy. We have however, had one significant stoma-skin stricture.

The fact that the carefully selected ileal segment can be used with good success and a reasonably low complication rate expected has further been recently documented by Malgieri and Persky (34). Between 1970 and 1975, 136 adults underwent ureteroileal bypass. Of these patients, 36 had preoperative radiation for various pelvic malignancies, 44 had malignancies with no irradiation, and 56 were operated on for neurogenic bladders. Major morbidity in the irradiated group included wound infections (33%), ureteroileal leaks (19.4%), and paralytic ileus (13.9%). The average postoperative stay was 8–11 days longer than for the other two groups (Table 9). In contrast, however, the overall incidence of reoperation for various complications in the irradiated group was only 11%, compared with 25% for the group not given preoperative radiation and 30.4% for those operated on for neurogenic bladders. Most significantly, none of the patients in the irradiated group required reexploration and surgical correction of ureteroileal urinary fistulas (Table 10). These essayists conclude with this observation: "Current methods of urinary diversion are by no means totally satisfactory, regardless of the pathological indication. Although this study makes no attempt to prove the superiority of ileal segments over other types, it does suggest that the ileal loop is still a viable operative technique to divert the urine in patients who have had prior irradiation for pelvic malignancies" (34). This certainly is this author's view as well. A current view with immense personal perspective is recorded by Bricker (37).

Long-term follow-up of conduit-diverted patients is important; obstruction, calculus, and progressive deterioration without obstruction all pose fairly significant risks (38).

Case 8: EL. In 1971, this patient was a 42-year-old para V who was free from disease 6 years after total pelvic exenteration was performed for recurrent carcinoma of the cervix. Conduit stomal stenosis was evident, and a filiform probe was required to start dilation of the conduit. The patient had young children in school, so we fashioned a series of polyethylene dilators that she could clean and use at home until she was able to return for conduit revision. An

Table 9. Complications After Ureteroileal Diversion

	Group I (%) (Number of Patients)	Group II (%) (Number of Patients)	Group III (%) (Number of Patients)
Death	2.8 (1)	6.8 (3)	1.8 (1)
Sepsis	2.8 (1)	0	1.8 (1)
Ureteroileal leak	19.4 (7)	4.5 (2)	3.6 (2)
Ureteroileal obstruction	2.8 (1)	9.1 (4)	5.4 (3)
Paralytic ileus	13.9 (5)	4.5 (2)	7.1 (4)
Bowel obstruction	5.6 (2)	4.5 (2)	3.6 (2)
Stomal stenosis	5.6 (2)	2.3 (1)	17.9 (10)
Wound infection	33 (12)	22.7 (10)	12.5 (7)
Wound dehiscence	2.8 (1)	2.3 (1)	1.8 (1)
Pyocystis	2.8 (1)	2.3 (1)	3.6 (2)
Pulmonary problems	0	2.3 (1)	0
Cardiac problems	0	4.5 (2)	0
Electrolyte abnormality	0	0	0
Renal failure	5.6 (2)	2.3 (1)	10.7 (6)
None	30.6 (11)	54.5 (24)	44.6 (25)

SOURCE: Malgieri and Persky[34]. Used by permission.

Table 10. Incidence of Secondary Operations

	Group I (Number of Patients)	Group II (Number of Patients)	Group III (Number of Patients)
Dehiscence	1	3	1
Stomal revision	2	1	11
Loop obstruction	1	2	3
Bowel obstruction	0	1	1
Recurrent cancer	0	3	0
Loop-enteric fistula	0	0	1
Total	4 (11%)	10 (25%)	17 (30.4%)

SOURCE: Malgieri and Persky[34]. Used by permission.

impressively sizable conduit calculus was documented after pyelography was performed. Subsequently, the stoma was revised and stone removed. It was possible to accomplish removal by mobilizing the entire conduit into the intraperitoneal portion, and there was enough mobility to allow drawing it upward and excising the distal stenotic 2 cm. The patient has remained well (Fig. 16).

Case 9: ES. In October 1967, this 44-year-old patient was admitted in uremia through the University of Mississippi Medical Center Emergency Room to the internal medicine service. She was transferred when a review of her old record revealed that she had had a radical hysterectomy and pelvic lymphadenectomy in 1961, which was followed about 8 months later by central recurrence, then by vigorous radiotherapy. Subsequently both a rectovaginal and a vesicovaginal fistula developed; she had the fecal stream diverted by a transverse colostomy in 1964 and the urinary stream diverted by ileal conduit in 1965. The patient was stuporous and in uremia, and the initial impulse was not to intervene. The status of the disease, of course, was unknown and only presumed to be progressive and the cause of the problem. The alert gynecologic resident, who had arranged for the transfer, had removed the conduit appliance and observed the stenosis. Dilation was accomplished to effect good drainage, and once the uremia was resolved, metastatic work-up failed to reveal any evidence of cancer. The stoma was revised, and at the same time the rectovaginal fistula was closed by Martius technique (this is among the cases included in Ref. 18). The colostomy was subsequently closed. The bladder damage was too extensive to be amenable to local correction, but the patient continues free from disease.

It is appropriate to conclude this segment with the recommendation of Parkhurst: "The necessity for lifetime supervision is important. Periodic inspection of the stoma and collecting device, together with radiographic study of the diverted urinary tract, is mandatory to prevent the development of stomal problems and nephrolithiasis which are significant complications. A carefully programmed review study is urged for all institutions where this procedure is performed frequently."

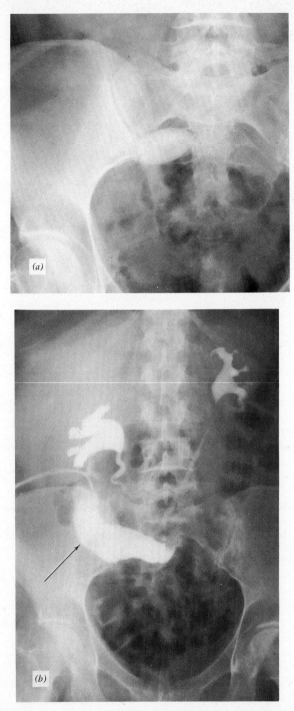

Figure 16. Case 8: EL: (*a*) A Closeup view of the abdominal flat film revealing a large calculus in the right lower quadrant. (*b*) Retrograde filling of the ileal conduit confirmed the calculus within the distal segment of the conduit.

REFERENCES

1. Swan RW, Rutledge FN: Urinary conduit in pelvic cancer patients. *Am J Obstet Gynecol* 119:6, 1974.

2. Moss WT, Brand WN, Battifora H: *Radiation Oncology Rationale, Technique, Results.* St. Louis, The CV Mosby Co, 1973.

3. Kottmeier HL: Complications following radiation therapy in carcinoma of the cervix and their treatment. *Am J Obstet Gynecol* 88:854, 1964.

4. Buchler DA, Kline JC, Peckham BM, Boone MLM, Carr WF: Radiation reactions in cervical cancer therapy. *Am J Obstet Gynecol* 111:745, 1971.

5. Underwood PB, Lutz MH, Smoak DL: Ureteral injury following irradiation therapy for carcinoma of the cervix. *Obstet Gynecol* 49:663, 1977.

6. Graham JB, Abad RS: Ureteral obstruction due to radiation. *Am J Obstet Gynecol* 99:409, 1967.

7. Shingleton HM, Fowler WC, Pepper FD, Palumbo L: Ureteral strictures following therapy for carcinoma of the cervix. *Cancer* 24:77, 1969.

8. Slater JM, Fletcher GH: Ureteral strictures after radiation therapy for carcinoma of the uterine cervix. *Am J Roentgenol* 111:269, 1971.

9. Burch JC, Chalfant RL: Preoperative radium irradiation and radical hysterectomy in the treatment of cancer of the cervix. *Am J Obstet Gynecol* 106:1054, 1970.

10. Churches CK, Kurrle GR, Johnson B: Treatment of carcinoma of the cervix by combination of irradiation and operation. *Am J Obstet Gynecol* 118:1033, 1974.

11. Rampone JF, Klem V, Kolstad P: Combined treatment of Stage IB carcinoma of the cervix. *Obstet Gynecol* 41:163, 1973.

12. Krupp P, Hoffman M, Roeling W: Terminal ileum as ureteral substitute. *Obstet Gynecol* 35:416, 1970.

13. Perry CP, Massey FM, Moore TN, Erickson CA: Treatment of irradiation injury to the ureter by ileal substitution. *Obstet Gynecol* 46:517, 1975.

14. Webb MJ, Symmonds RE: Wertheim hysterectomy: A reappraisal. *Obstet Gynecol* 54:140, 1979.

15. Green TH Jr: Ureteral suspension for prevention of ureteral complications following radical Wertheim hysterectomy. *Obstet Gynecol* 28:1, 1966.

16. Novak F: *Surgical Gynecologic Technique.* Padova, Italy, Piccin Editore, New York, John Wiley & Sons, 1978.

17. Moore C, Atherton D, Haynes DM: Modified pelvic exenteration. *Surg Gynecol Obstet* 118:59, 1964.

18. Boronow RC, Rutledge F: Vesicovaginal fistula, radiation, in gynecologic cancer. *Am J Obstet Gynecol* 111:85, 1971.

19. Stockbine MF, Hancock JE, Fletcher GH: Complication in eight hundred thirty-one patients with squamous cell carcinoma in the intact uterine cervix treated with three thousand rads or more whole pelvis radiation. *Am J Roentgenol* 108:293, 1970.

20. O'Quinn AG, Fletcher GH, Wharton JT: Guidelines for conservative hysterectomy after irradiation. *Gynecol Oncol* 9:68, 1980.

21. Marshall VF: Vesicovaginal fistulas on one urological service. 4J Urol 121:25, 1979.

22. Twombly GH, Marshall VF: Repair of vesicovaginal fistula caused by radiation. *Surg Gynecol Obstet* 83:348, 1946.

23. Blaikley JB: Colpocleisis for difficult vesicovaginal and rectovaginal fistulas. *Am J Obstet Gynecol* 91:589, 1965.

24. Boronow RC: Management of radiation-induced vaginal fistulas. *Am J Obstet Gynecol* 110:1, 1971.

25. Ingelman-Sundberg A: Pathogenesis and operative treatment of urinary fistulae in irradiated tissue, in Youssef AF (ed); *Gynecologic Urology.* Springfield, Ill., Charles C Thomas Publisher, 1960.

26. Garlock JH: The cure of an intractable vesicovaginal fistula by the use of a pedicled muscle flap. *Surg Gynecol Obstet* 47:225, 1928.

27. Graham JB: Vaginal fistulas following radiotherapy. *Surg Gynecol Obstet* 120:1019, 1965.

28. Bastiaanse MAVB: Bastiaanse's method for surgical closure of very large radiation fistulae of the bladder and rectum, in Youssef AF (ed): *Gynecologic Oncology.* Springfield, Ill., Charles C Thomas Publisher, 1960.

29. Martius H: In McCall ML and Bolten KA (eds): *Operative Gynecology.* Boston, Little Brown & Co, 1956.

30. Boronow RC: The complicated vaginal fistula. *J Med Assoc Ga,* January 1, 1973.

31. Kwon TH, Boronow RC: Urinary undiversion: Use in management of radiation induced bladder fistula. *Gynecol Oncol* 8:164, 1979.

32. Butcher HR Jr, Sugg WL, McAfee CA, Bricker EM: Ileal conduit method of ureteral urinary diversion. *Ann Surg* 156:682, 1962.

33. Strom SH, Donaldson MH, Duckett JW, Weim AJ: Formalin treatment for intractable hemorrhagic cystitis: A review of the literature with sixteen additional cases. *Cancer* 38:1785, 1976.

34. Malgieri JJ and Persky L: Ileal loop in the treatment of radiation-treated pelvic malignancies: A comparative review. *J Urol* 120:32, 1978.

35. Parkhurst EC: Experience with more than five hundred ileal conduit diversions in a 12 year period. *J Urol* 99:434, 1968.

36. Nelson JH Jr: *Atlas of Radical Pelvic Surgery,* ed 2. New York, Appleton-Century-Crofts, 1977.

37. Bricker EM: Current status of urinary diversion. *Cancer* 45:2986, 1980.

38. Pitts WR Jr, Muecke EC: A twenty-year experience with ileal conduit: The fate of the kidneys. *J Urol* 122:154, 1979.

9

Complications of Pelvic and Aortic Lymphadenectomy

M. Steven Piver

Shashikant B. Lele

Pelvic lymphadenectomy is normally performed as a therapeutic procedure at the time of radical hysterectomy and vaginectomy for (*1*) diethylstilbestrol-related clear-cell adenocarcinoma of the vagina or cervix; (*2*) infants with embryonal rhabdomyosarcoma limited to the vagina or cervix; (*3*) early-stage carcinoma of the uterine cervix (Stage IB or IiA); and (*4*) recurrent postirradiation cervical carcinoma limited to the cervix or vagina. However, para-aortic lymphadenectomy is primarily used as a staging procedure in women with gynecologic malignancies. This is in contrast to the more extensive therapeutic aortic lymphadenectomy in patients with testicular malignancies. Women with locally advanced cervical carcinoma (Stages IIB–IV) have approximately a 30% incidence of aortic node metastases, all of which would be out of the standard field of pelvic irradiation (Table 1) (1). Similarly, women with Stage I endometrial carcinoma who have Grade III poorly differentiated carcinomas or deep invasion of the myometrium have a high incidence of aortic node metastases (Table 2). Also, if the cervix is involved, there is a high incidence of aortic node metastases. Patients with ovarian carcinoma clinically limited to the ovary (Stage I) have approximately a 10% incidence of subclinical aortic node metastases (Table 3).

Therefore, patients with locally advanced cervical carcinoma, with endometrial carcinoma that is poorly differentiated and involves the cervix or invades deeply into the myometrium, or with early ovarian carcinoma should have preadjuvant therapy–staging para-aortic lymphadenectomy. The chapter will review the intraoperative and postoperative complications related to para-aortic and pelvic lymphadenectomy (Fig. 1). Knowledge of the tributaries to the aorta,

Table 1. Incidence of Para-Aortic Node Metastases in Locally Advanced Cervical Carcinoma

	Stage II		Stage III		Stage IV	
	Patients		Patients		Patients	
Author	Number	%	Number	%	Number	%
Sudarsanam et al.[a]	7/43	16.2	3/19	15.7	0/3	0.0
Buchsbaum[a]	1/12	8.3	7/20	35.0	1/2	50.0
Nelson et al.[a]	9/63	14.2	15/39	38.4	0/2	0.0
Rutledge[a]	7/50	14.0	14/41	34.1	0/1	0.0
Piver[a]	6/44	13.6	18/49	36.7	4/7	57.1
Total	30/212	14.1	57/168	33.9	5/15	33.3
			92/395=23.5%			

[a]Cited in Ref. 1.

Table 2. Aortic and Pelvic Node Metastases in Stage I Endometrial Carcinoma[a]

	Number of Patients	Pelvic Node Metastases (%)	Aortic Node Metastases (%)
Grade:			
I	65	3.1	1.5
II	50	10.0	4.0
III	25	36.0	28.0
Myometrial invasion:			
Endometrium	55	3.6	1.8
Superficial invasion	61	11.5	9.8
Intermediate invasion	10	10.0	0.0
Deep invasion	14	43.0	21.0

[a]Cited in Ref. 1.

Table 3. Ovarian Cancer Stage I and II Aortic Lymph Node Metastases

Author[a]	Number of Patients	Percent
Knapp	24	12.5
Musumeci	28	7.0
Delgado	10	20.0
Piver	5	0.0
Total	68	10.3%

[a]Cited in Ref. 1.

inferior vena cava, and major pelvic vessels as well as the relationship of the pelvic side wall structures to the endopelvic fascial planes and the avascular paravesical and pararectal spaces should lessen such complications.

PARA-AORTIC LYMPHADENECTOMY: ANATOMIC CONSIDERATIONS

Inferior Vena Cava

The visceral venous tributary encountered includes the right ovarian vein, which enters the inferior vena cava at the level of the second lumbar vertebra. The left ovarian vein drains into the left renal vein and is normally not encountered during staging para-aortic lymphadenectomy. The inferior vena cava is in intimate contact with the right side of the abdominal aorta. Below the renal veins, the surgeon must be aware of the lumbar veins that have connecting posterior branches with the vertebral veins. In the performance of a staging para-aortic lymphadenectomy, however, these veins are not normally encountered.

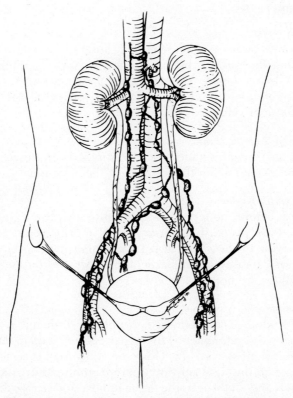

Figure 1. The pelvic and para-aortic lymph nodes.

Abdominal Aorta

Lumbar Arteries

Like the lumbar veins, the four paired lumbar arteries that are related to the upper four lumbar vertebra are not normally encountered at the time of staging para-aortic lymphadenectomy.

The Celiac Artery (Axis), Superior Mesenteric Artery, and Renal Arteries

The celiac artery, superior mesentery artery, and renal arteries are not normally encountered at the time of staging para-aortic lymphadenectomy.

Inferior Mesenteric Artery

The inferior mesenteric artery arises at the level of the third lumbar vertebra, giving off the left colic artery to the descending colon and two to three sigmoid arteries to the sigmoid colon and continuing as the superior hemorrhoidal artery to the rectum.

Right and Left Ovarian Arteries

The right and left ovarian arteries arise from the anterior abdominal aorta at approximately the level of the second lumbar vertebra.

Para-Aortic Lymph Nodes

Preaortic Lymph Nodes

The preaortic lymph nodes are situated on the anterior surface of the abdominal aorta surrounding the inferior mesenteric artery, superior mesenteric artery, and celiac axis. When a staging para-aortic lymphadenectomy is performed, the lymph nodes surrounding the inferior mesenteric artery are removed but the superior mesenteric or celiac axis nodes are not.

Left Lumbar Aortic Lymph Nodes

The left lumbar aortic lymph nodes are in continuity with the left common iliac lymph nodes and extend along the left side of the abdominal aorta.

Right Lumbar Lymph Nodes

The right lumbar lymph nodes are in continuity with the right common iliac lymph nodes and are primarily anterior to the inferior vena cava but may be lateral and posterior to the vena cava. In a staging para-aortic lymphadenectomy, the anterior lateral right lumbar lymph nodes are routinely removed but the retrocaval nodes are not.

Lymphatic Drainage

In cervical and endometrial carcinoma, lymphatic drainage is initially to the pelvic lymph nodes and subsequently to the para-aortic chain in the region of the second to the fifth lumbar vertebra. However, in ovarian carcinoma there may be direct drainage on the right side anywhere from the bifurcation of the aorta to the renal vessels and on the left side to the lumbar and preaortic lymph nodes, usually below the level of the renal vessels.

Duodenum

The third, or horizontal, portion of the duodenum crosses perpendicular to the inferior vena cava and the abdominal aorta and lies in intimate relationship to the anterior surface of the aorta and the vena cava.

Nerves

The lumbar plexus is related intimately to the laterally situated psoas muscle and is, therefore, not normally encountered at the time of staging para-aortic lymphadenectomy. The superior and inferior hypogastric plexus are in close proximity to the abdominal aorta. The sympathetics on the left are just lateral to the abdominal aorta and can be encountered, whereas the sympathetics on the right in the retrocaval area are not encountered.

Ureters

The left ureter is not normally encountered at the time of staging para-aortic lymphadenectomy. However, the abdominal portion of the right ureter lies just lateral to the right lumbar chain of lymph nodes and may be encountered on the lateral border of the inferior vena cava.

COMPLICATIONS OF PARA-AORTIC LYMPHADENECTOMY

Incision-Related Complications

Many of the complications of staging para-aortic lymphadenectomy in women with carcinoma of the uterine cervix are related to the type of incision and the use of subsequent external radiation therapy. Transperitoneal staging para-aortic lymphadenectomy frequently results in segments of the ileum or jejunum adhering to the undersurface of the incision and thus restricting the normal mobility of the intestine. This process results in a higher radiation dose to the adherent segment of small intestine, leading to possible obstruction and/or fistula. However, the use of a retroperitoneal J-shaped incision (Fig. 2) for staging para-aortic lymphadenectomy before external irradiation therapy has significantly decreased these complications (2). Patients undergoing staging para-aortic lymphadenectomy at the time of primary surgery for endometrial or ovarian carcinoma require a transperitoneal approach.

Venous Complications

Because of their thin walls, veins are not uncommonly injured. Small lacerations of the vena cava can be controlled by using one hand to apply sponge stick pressure over the defect and the other hand to repair the lacerations with fine cardiovascular sutures as the defect is slowly uncovered from beneath the sponge stick (Fig. 3). A larger injury to the vena cava or other large veins should be initially controlled by laparotomy packs. A vena caval defect is slowly exposed by

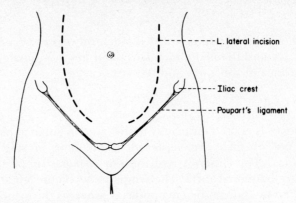

Figure 2. J-shaped retroperitoneal incisions for para-aortic lymph node biopsy.

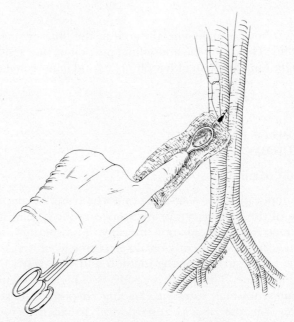

Figure 3. Control of bleeding and repair of an inferior vena cava injury.

progressively retracting the pack off the injured area until the edge of the defect is in view. If bleeding still obscures the field, gentle occlusion of the area above and below the defect with sponge sticks will allow for repair of the defect. Interrupted mattress sutures are then placed so as to evert the walls of the vein. Vascular clamps on the vena cava or major vein should be avoided, if possible, since they tend to worsen the injury.

Extensive injury to the vena cava below the renal veins is best managed by ligating the vena cava below and above the damaged area and not by attempting to repair an extensive defect. Remediation can be accomplished using heavy nonabsorbable suture on a swedged-on needle and passing around the vena cava. This procedure will prevent excessive acute blood loss and reduce the risk of pulmonary embolism from the resultant clot formation that occurs at the site of extensive vena caval repair. Morbidity from ligation of the infrarenal portion of the vena cava is minimal.

Although there have been survivors after ligation of the suprarenal portion of the vena cava, most patients will not survive such a procedure. The reported survivors are those in whom the right kidney was also removed at the time of ligation or resection of the suprarenal portion of the inferior vena cava. Therefore, injury to the inferior vena cava above the renal veins must be repaired (3).

Severe damage or inadvertent ligation of the left renal vein proximal to its tributaries will not result in death of the left kidney because of the multiple communicating veins in this area. However, this is not true of the right renal vein, which must be repaired if damaged or inadvertently ligated.

Arterial Complications

Thick-walled arteries can withstand much trauma, and major injuries to the aorta are infrequent. Most arterial injuries require clamping above and below the injured area with aortic vascular clamps and repair of the defect by closely approximated interrupted cardiovascular sutures to achieve close intimal approximation. Larger defects in the arterial wall that cannot be repaired by simple everting of sutures should be repaired by saphenous vein tissue patching. This vein is easily removed from the inguinal area and will withstand arterial pressures, whereas abdominal veins such as the ovarian vein will not (4).

Inferior Mesenteric Artery
Ligation of the inferior mesenteric artery is not advocated at the time of staging para-aortic lymphadenectomy. If the inferior mesenteric artery is inadvertently injured, it is important to ascertain whether there is arterial backflow indicating anastomosis between the middle and left colic artery. If there is no arterial backflow, reimplantation of the inferior mesenteric artery into the aorta should be considered to prevent postoperative ischemia to the descending colon and rectosigmoid. The resultant diarrhea is easily managed, but the adverse effects of ligation of the inferior mesenteric artery and subsequent irradiation to this area are not known.

Nerve Complications

Because of the superior and lateral location of the branches of the lumbar plexus, these nerves are rarely encountered or injured at the time of staging para-aortic lymphadenectomy. However, segments of the left sympathetic plexus are frequently resected, causing postoperative concern because the contralateral leg feels cool to the examiner in contrast to the warm, vasodilated ipsilateral leg.

Duodenal Complications

Care must be taken in mobilizing and subsequently retracting the horizontal portion of the duodenum at the time of exposing the superior portion of the aortic nodal specimen.

Postoperative Complications

Of the first 56 women in our study who underwent staging para-aortic lymphadenectomy for locally advanced cervical carcinoma, 34 sustained no major postoperative complications (5). Complications were related primarily to the lungs, the wound, and the intestine (Table 4). Prolonged ileus is a frequent complication of staging para-aortic lymphadenectomy. Ileus is not, however, secondary to resection of the nerve supply to this area but most likely results from excessive packing of the intestines to expose the retroperitoneal lymph nodes.

PELVIC LYMPHADENECTOMY: ANATOMIC CONSIDERATIONS

Avascular Spaces: Paravesical and Pararectal

The development of the avascular spaces allows visualization of the major vessels of the retroperitoneal pelvic area, helping to prevent injury to unsuspected branches, and allows for control of bleeding without injury to important structures. Dissecting the fibrofatty tissue along the anterior surface of the internal iliac artery and superior vesical artery to the bladder allows one to create the paravesical space by blunt dissection lateral to the superior vesical artery. By staying lateral to the superior vesical artery, one will not encounter significant bleeding before reaching the inferior portion of the obturator fossa. The pararectal space is developed by blunt dissection along the medial portion of the internal iliac artery and the lateral border of the rectum. Blunt dissection close to the rectum prevents inadvertent injury to the branches of the internal iliac vein along the pelvic side wall.

Lymphatics

The pelvic lymph nodes should be removed as a whole and consist of those surrounding the (1) external iliac artery and vein to the inguinal ligament, (2) the

Table 4. Postoperative Complications of Para-Aortic Lymphadenectomy[a]

Complication	Number of Patients
Pneumonitis	6
Wound infection	5
Prolonged Ileus	5
Fever of undetermined origin	2
Partial intestinal obstruction	1
Pyelonephritis	2
Thrombophlebitis	1
Total	22
No complications	34

[a]Cited in Ref. 5.

internal iliac artery with its continuation, the superior vesical artery, to the bladder, (3) the obturator fossa around the obturator artery, vein, and nerve, (4) the common iliac artery and vein, and (5) the sacral nodes that lie medial and inferior to the common iliac vessels. The sacral nodes are rarely encountered and normally do not contain metastatic deposits.

Pelvic Nerves

Except for the obturator nerve, all other sacral plexus somatic motor branches lie deep to the endopelvic fascia and exit from the pelvis by the greater sciatic foramen and are, therefore, not encountered during pelvic lymphadenectomy. Along the psoas muscle one must recognize the genitofemoral nerve.

Ureters

The ureters cross the common iliac vessels medially and lie on the medial portion of the peritoneum. Retraction medially of the ureters prevents injury during pelvic lymphadenectomy.

Common Iliac Artery and Vein

The right common iliac vein lies lateral to the right common iliac artery, whereas the left common iliac vein is medial to the left common iliac artery.

Internal Iliac Artery

The posterior division of the internal iliac artery gives off three parietal branches—iliolumbar, lateral sacral, and superior gluteal—which are not normally encountered during pelvic lymphadenectomy. The anterior division gives off the uterine, superior vesical, middle hemorrhoidal, obturator, internal pudendal, and inferior gluteal.

Internal Iliac Vein

The branches of the internal iliac vein are formed in part by veins draining the pelvic viscera and are similar to the internal iliac artery branches with the exception that a superior vesical vein is not normally present.

COMPLICATIONS OF PELVIC LYMPHADENECTOMY

Arterial Complications

Complete occlusion of the common iliac artery will result in loss of the corresponding limb in approximately 100% of patients, whereas complete occlusion of the external iliac artery will result in loss of the extremity in 13% of patients. Laceration of or a small injury to the common or external iliac arteries is repaired by everting interrupted cardiovascular mattress sutures; if the injury is more extensive, a saphenous vein patch is used. A completely transected iliac artery is repaired by everting mattress cardiovascular sutures. Occasionally, an oblique fish mouth anastomosis is required because of the small caliber of the vessels (Fig. 4). More extensive arterial defects that cannot be easily repaired by (*1*) suture or (*2*) saphenous vein patching will require arterial graft replacement.

Venous Complications

Excessive traction and stripping of the major veins will lead to an increased incidence of pelvic thrombophlebitis and subsequent pulmonary embolism. The use of preoperative and postoperative heparin and gentle dissection of the pelvic veins may reduce this complication. Small bleeding from the external iliac vein may be controlled by gentle pressure. If it is not controlled, suture ligation should be carried out. The principles outlined for control of bleeding from the inferior vena cava apply to major injuries of the iliac veins. Most iliac vein defects are repaired by fine everting interrupted cardiovascular mattress sutures. When injury is extensive, the external iliac vein must occasionally be ligated with the realization that there will be postoperative swelling of the extremity. Because of venous thrombosis, graft replacement is usually not successful except on rare occasions (6).

Nerve Complications

Inadvertent transection of the obturator nerve should be repaired, if possible, to prevent postoperative difficulties with adduction of the leg. However, if the nerve is not repaired, most patients will have complete recovery of function if they undergo postoperative physiotherapy. Injury to the genitofemoral nerve does not require repair.

Lymphatic Complications

Lymphocyst

The transected lymph vessels continue to deposit lymph, so extraperitoneal drainage is required to prevent the accumulation of fluid. In some instances the fluid becomes encapsulated and a lymphocyst forms. In a series of 610 radical hysterectomies and pelvic lymphadenectomies, this complication occurred in 3% of the cases (18) (7). Careful pelvic examination postoperatively is important to ensure early recognition of this complication. Certain lymphocysts are also

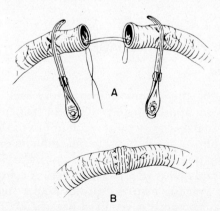

Figure 4. The repair of arterial injury by oblique everting anastomosis.

diagnosed by ultrasonography or lymphangiography. Lymphocysts can cause pressure on the pelvic portion of the ureter, leading to hydroureter, hydronephrosis, pyelonephritis and, occasionally, complete loss of renal function. The formation of lymphocysts may be decreased by (1) ligating all lymphatics leading into this area and (2) draining the pelvic side wall by continuous negative catheter pressure. The catheter not only removes the fluid but collapses the potential space by approximating the pelvic peritoneum to the pelvic side wall. Small lymphocysts that do not cause pain, that are not confused with possible recurrent or persistent cancer, and that do not cause ureteral obstruction normally require no treatment and regress spontaneously. Lymphocysts causing hydroureter should be drained retroperitoneally by excision of a portion of the cyst wall. Also, catheter drainage with negative pressure should be used to cause complete collapse of the walls of the cyst, thus preventing reaccumulation of lymph fluid. The hydroureter will normally then be resolved.

Peripheral Lymphedema

Significant lymphedema occurred in 10% of 610 patients undergoing radical hysterectomy and pelvic lymphadenectomy but was not related to whether or not the patients had prior pelvic irradiation (7). However, lymphedema has been related to the extent of the pelvic lymphadenectomy. Lymphedema occurred in 11%–30% of the patients, with the higher incidence associated with those surgeons doing the more extensive pelvic lymphadenectomy (8). Normal lymphatic drainage cannot be restored, but in severe cases symptomatic control of lymphedema has been achieved by staged subcutaneous excisions (9).

Ureteral Injuries

Inadvertent ligation of the ureter can be treated by simple deligation if the ureter appears viable after removal of the ligature. Inadvertent transection or laceration of the ureter requires division of the ureter at the point of injury. The upper or middle portion of the ureter requires repair by means of a spatulated watertight anastomosis to prevent subsequent stricture formation. An oblique or spatulated suture line will allow for a wider anastomosis (Fig. 5). In end-to-end ureteroureterostomy, (1) the anastomosis should be made tension-free by caudad mobilization of the kidney if necessary; (2) the ends of the ureter should be debrided to excise the damaged area; (3) care must be taken in handling the ureter so as not to disturb the longitudinal blood supply within the periureteral sheeth; and (4) an oblique or spatulated anastomosis should be performed to prevent stricture. Ureteral stents placed cystoscopically at the time of ureteral injury allow for more accurate placement of the sutures with less handling and damage to the ureter. In a clean ureteral injury, however, stents may not be necessary. Ureteral stents should be used if there is any tension on the anastomosis or if there has been previous radiation to that portion of the ureter. Injury to the lower portion of the ureter within several centimeters of the bladder cannot be repaired by ureteroureterostomy and is best repaired by an antireflux submucosal ureteroneocystotomy. A cystotomy is performed and the ureter is brought through the full thickness of the bladder just superior to the previous ureteral orifice. A submucosal tunnel is created and the ureter anastomosed to the bladder mucosa (Fig. 6).

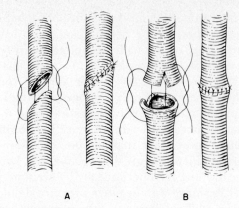

A   B

Figure 5. The repair of middle and upper third ureteral injury by (a) oblique or (b) spatulated anastomosis.

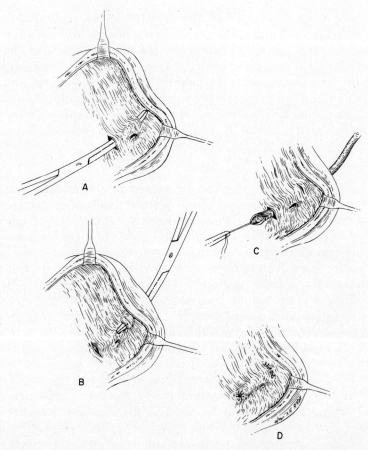

Figure 6. The repair of lower third ureteral injury by antireflux submucosal ureteroneocystotomy: (*a*) Creation of submucosal tunnel; (*b*) Ureter brought through full thickness of bladder; (*c*) Ureter brought through submucosal tunnel; (*d*) Mucosal to mucosal anastamosis between ureter and bladder.

210

REFERENCES

1. Piver MS: Para-aortic node biopsy in staging women with cervical, ovarian and endometrial carcinoma: A review. *J Surg Oncol* 12:365–370, 1979.

2. Berman ML, Lagasse LD, Watson W, et al.: The operative evaluation of patients with cervical carcinoma by an extraperitoneal approach. *Obstet Gynecol* 50:658–664, 1977.

3. Duckett JW, Lifland JH, Peters PC: Resection of the inferior vena cava for adjacent malignant diseases. *Surg Gynecol Obstet* 136:711–716, 1973.

4. Bergan JJ, Dean RH, Yao JST: Vascular injury in pelvic cancer surgery. *Am J Obstet Gynecol* 124:562–566, 1976.

5. Piver MS, Barlow JJ: Para-aortic lymphadenectomy in staging patients with advanced local cervical cancer. *Obstet Gynecol* 43:544–548, 1974.

6. Romanucci D: External iliac vein segment replacement by Teflon graft. *JAMA* 216:231, 1971.

7. Webb MJ, Symmonds RE: Wertheim hysterectomy: A reappraisal. *Obstet Gynecol* 54:140–145, 1979.

8. Martinbeau PW, Kjorstad KE, Kolstad: Stage IB carcinoma of the cervix, the Norwegian Radium Hospital 1968–1970: Results of treatment and major complications: I. Lymphedema. *Am J Obstet Gynecol* 131:389–394, 1978.

9. Miller TA, Harper J, Longmire WP: The management of lymphedema by staged subcutaneous excisions. *Surg Gynecol Obstet* 136:586–592, 1973.

10
Complications of Vulvar and Vaginal Surgery

Maurice J. Webb

Malignant diseases of the vulva and vagina account for about 1% of all gynecologic cancers each, and squamous cell carcinoma is the most prominent type (1,2). The fact that both sites are richly supplied with lymphatics and are in close proximity to the bladder and rectum can make the treatment of malignancy in this region a considerable challenge. Likewise, when one considers that complications of treatment can be severe and that the diseases are rare, it is not surprising that most patients with malignancies of these organs are referred to major centers for management.

Management of complications due to treatment of vulvar and vaginal malignancies will be dealt with in this chapter; the emphasis will be on prevention.

VULVA

There is general agreement that surgery is the primary treatment for cancer of the vulva (3,4). Irradiation, cryosurgery, laser surgery, and chemotherapy are all used for specific indications but, with the exception of intraepithelial cancer, only as secondary treatment for recurrent disease (5). Although local excision, skinning vulvectomy, and simple vulvectomy are surgical procedures used in the treatment of intraepithelial disease (6–8), we will concentrate mainly on complications of radical vulvectomy with inguinal or pelvic lymphadenectomy in the treatment of invasive vulvar cancer. These can be divided into early complications (usually arising in the second or third week postoperatively) and late complications.

Early Complications

Skin Necrosis and Separation
Skin necrosis and separation is by far the most common complication (9–11), for seldom is there not some degree of skin necrosis, especially in groin incisions.

Although in the majority of cases skin loss is minimal, in some cases large areas of the skin flap may necrose. This problem may be minimized in a number of ways. Firstly, the undermined skin flaps should be the full thickness of skin and fat, to prevent interference with the vascular supply. Likewise, undermining of flaps should be carried out only to allow adequate approximation of skin edges and no further. Use of the "butterfly" incision (12), which removes a strip of groin skin together with the underlying nodes, has diminished the frequency of this problem. Others have suggested a vertical midline inverted tennis racquet incision to avoid this complication (13). Particular care should be taken after completion of the groin dissection to trim off any obviously devascularized skin before the incision is closed. Fluorescence with fluorescein and ultraviolet light may be of help in noting devascularized areas. Tension when suturing skin edges should be avoided, for the resulting edema and pressure will invariably lead to sloughing. Likewise, pressure dressings over the flaps only aggravate the problem. Suction wound drainage is essential and will help in avoiding both pressure and sepsis from seromas beneath the flaps.

If skin necrosis occurs, debridement should be carried out once the lines of demarcation between viable and dead tissue have become obvious. The high-pressure pulsating water jet commonly used for dental hygiene is useful in tissue debridement, as is the whirlpool bath. Honey has been used as an aid to wound healing. When the gaping wound is clean and granulating, a decision can be made whether to skin-graft the defect or allow it to granulate and epithelialize slowly. Even large areas epithelialize rapidly.

Sepsis
It is impossible to sterilize the skin of the perineum and inguinal region completely, and for this reason some degree of postoperative sepsis is inevitable. This complication usually involves only some purulent discharge and localized inflammation around the incisions, but it can extend to severe cellulitis, septicemia, and rarely, necrotizing fasciitis (Fig. 1). Because the edema from wound inflammation tends to compromise skin flap viability further, we use prophylactic antibiotics in an attempt to reduce the frequency of this complication. Attention to the usual surgical principles of good skin preparation, hemostasis, aseptic technique, and wound drainage is, however, more important.

Hemorrhage
Although the subcutaneous tissues of the vulva and groin have a rich blood supply, intraoperative blood loss can be kept to a minimum if most of the dissection is done with the cutting cautery. Few bleeding points, apart from the clitoral and pudendal vessels, require suture ligation. Postoperative suction drainage is for collection of serum and lymphatic fluid and should not be used as an alternative to good hemostasis. Pressure dressings are difficult to apply, are not necessary, and may lead to further necrosis of skin flaps.

A major complication after groin dissection is rupture of the femoral artery, which often leads to exsanguination (10,11). This rare complication usually follows necrosis and sepsis in the inguinal incision and occurs 2–3 weeks postoperatively. Transplanting the sartorius muscle over the exposed vessels at the time of surgery guards against this serious complication (Fig. 2). If femoral artery rupture occurs, it may be possible to insert a saphenous vein graft,

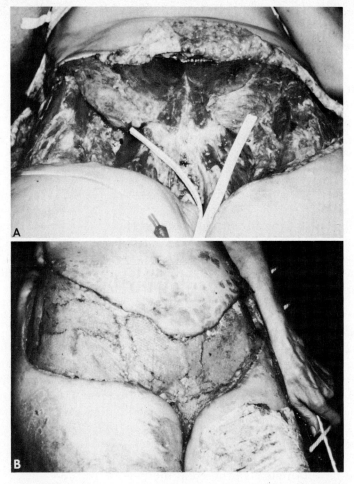

Figure 1. (*a*) Postvulvectomy necrotizing fasciitis after debridement. (*b*) Necrotizing fasciitis after skin grafting.

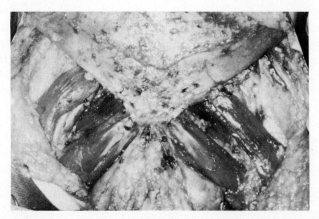

Figure 2. A sartorius muscle transplant to cover the femoral vessels.

depending on the degree of infection in the groin incision. Another alternative is insertion of an extra-anatomic axillofemoral Dacron graft in order to bypass the infected area.

Seroma
Use of the cautery for dissection seals many lymphatic vessels, and some surgeons actually ligate the lymphatics in the femoral canal to prevent lymph from escaping under the flaps postoperatively. However, suction drainage beneath the groin incisions has greatly reduced this complication. Occasionally, after removal of the drains (when the amount draining is less than 50 ml/24 hours), a seroma will re-collect, and it should be repeatedly aspirated with a needle until cured.

Thrombophlebitis
Thrombophlebitis is probably the most common potentially serious complication of vulvectomy and groin dissection. Thigh-high antiembolism stockings or leg wrapping with elastic bandages, early mobilization starting the day after surgery, and use of minidose heparin just before and for a few days after surgery are effective prophylactic measures that are easily instituted.

Femoral artery thrombosis has been reported but is uncommon (11).

Nerve Damage
Some degree of anesthesia or hyperesthesia around the inguinal incisions is not uncommon, and it usually diminishes with the passage of time. Trauma to the femoral nerve, which is fortunately much less common, results usually from an overly enthusiastic dissection. The femoral nerve may easily be avoided by approaching the femoral triangle from the lateral aspect where the nerve lies. The fascia over the sartorius muscle is divided and reflected medially, care being taken to stay close to the undersurface of the fascia and thereby avoid trauma to the nerves. There are no significant lymphatics around the nerve, and so it does not need to be as completely exposed as the femoral vessels.

If the lithotomy position is used for this operation, the usual care must be taken to avoid peroneal nerve palsy from pressure by the stirrups at the knee.

Fecal Fistulas and Incontinence
Radical vulvectomy involves resection of a considerable portion of the perineum and even more if the primary lesion is situated in this region. It is a matter of surgical judgment whether adequate margins can be obtained in a particular case that will still allow preservation of adequate anal sphincteric control. Often one may need to perform posterior exenteration rather than compromise on the radicality of the dissection (14–16). If the anus and rectum are left intact, care must be taken to see that any sphincteric damage is repaired during closure; otherwise, the patient will be incontinent of flatus or feces. Plication of the levators in the midline gives added control, but a common cause of rectovaginal fistula is deeply placed sutures penetrating the rectum. Inserting a finger in the rectum during the placement of these sutures will prevent this problem.

Fluid and Electrolyte Balance
It is important to realize that, although groin dissection is, on the whole, well tolerated, most of these patients are elderly and may not tolerate the consider-

able loss of fluid, protein, and electrolytes from the large skin dissection. Care must be taken, therefore, to replace fluids lost in suction drainage and to monitor the patient's electrolyte status. Superimposed sepsis may further aggravate this process, and considerably more fluid is lost postoperatively if a pelvic lymph node dissection has been performed concurrently.

Late Complications

Lymphedema
Persistent lymphedema of the lower extremities is a very common late complication of groin dissection. In most cases, however, it is relatively insignificant and causes the patient few problems. More than half of the patients in our series were noted to have some degree of leg edema after the initial postoperative course, but in only 8 of 219 patients was it significant enough to be labeled "severe" (K.C. Podratz and R.E. Symmonds, unpublished data). Frequent elevation of the legs, wearing of support stockings, and occasional use of massage and diuretics by the patient will help to reduce the degree of edema. Occasionally, a patient with chronic lymphedema will experience recurrent attacks of lymphangitis, which may make the patient quite toxic. Fortunately, this condition usually responds quickly to antibiotics. Lymphedema is usually more severe if the patient receives postoperative pelvic irradiation.

Hernia
Care must be taken during the groin dissection to close the external inguinal ring and the femoral canal; otherwise, postoperatively, inguinal or femoral hernia may occur (9). If a pelvic lymph node dissection is performed together with the groin dissection, the inguinal ligament should be split along its length so that access to the retroperitoneal area is gained. The inguinal ligament should not be divided for this purpose, for this procedure is associated with an unacceptably high rate of abdominal wall hernia postoperatively.

Prolapse
Vaginal and uterine prolapse is not an uncommon long-term complication of radical vulvectomy. It is due largely to excision of the supporting perineum, but interference with the nerve and vascular supply of the perineal musculature probably also contributes to the problem. Careful plication of the levator muscles at operation, to build up the perineum, is important prophylaxis (17). Management of the complication, once it occurs, is difficult, for pessaries usually are not retained and surgical repair has a high recurrence rate.

Urinary Symptoms
Many patients complain of "spraying" of urine or a misdirected urinary stream after radical vulvectomy. By carefully designing the incisions around the urethra, leaving a small triangle of mucosa intact above the meatus, one will avoid sharp upward angulation of the urethral opening. Likewise, during closure of the vulvar incisions, care must be taken to see that the urethra remains centrally placed.

Often it may be necessary to remove a considerable portion of the urethra in order to excise widely around the malignancy. Approximately two-thirds of the urethra may be resected without the patient being made incontinent. If partial urethral resection is necessary, plication sutures placed at the urethrovesical junction will help ensure continence (18). Urethral mucosal prolapse occasionally occurs and is best treated by excision.

Sexual Dysfunction

Radical vulvectomy often results in considerable sexual dysfunction, yet very little has been written on this subject. Contracture of scar tissue resulting in introital stenosis is a well-recognized problem but one that can usually be satisfactorily resolved surgically. Use of a vertical incision at the fourchette closed transversely or of a Z-plasty will usually enlarge the introitus adequately and often will also take care of introital fissuring on coitus.

Clitoral excision often results in loss of the ability to achieve orgasm, but this is not universal. Particular attention is now being paid to performing less than radical excision of microinvasive or in situ disease. Local excision and skinning vulvectomy will prevent many of these problems (6,19).

VAGINA

Primary vaginal cancer is relatively uncommon, but because of the intimate association of the vagina with the bladder and rectum, it presents particular problems in treatment. Although surgery has a well-defined place in the management of in situ disease and also invasive cancer involving the upper third of the vagina, it is not possible, short of exenteration, to provide adequate surgical treatment of an invasive lesion in the middle or lower third. Radiotherapy may be used whatever the location of the lesion, but again treatment is hampered by the close proximity of the bladder and rectum. Either method of treatment may seriously impede subsequent sexual ability and necessitate consideration of procedures to preserve or reestablish vaginal function. It is for all these reasons that treatment must be carefully individualized.

Complications

Urinary Fistula

Vesicovaginal and ureterovaginal fistulas may develop after surgical treatment of vaginal cancer, usually following radical hysterectomy and partial vaginectomy for cancers in the upper third of the vagina. Attention to the well-known surgical principles of minimal handling of the ureter and preservation of its longitudinal blood supply, pelvic suction drainage, and prolonged catheter drainage of the bladder after radical dissection should keep the rate of urinary fistula below 2% in the nonirradiated patient.

If a fistula develops, investigation requires an intravenous pyelogram, cystoscopy with retrograde studies of the ureters if indicated, and dye studies to define the site of the leak. If ureteric damage has resulted in hydronephrosis, an attempt should be made to pass a ureteric catheter, via cystoscopy, past the obstruction. Spontaneous healing can be expected in a significant number of patients, with or without the presence of a splinting ureteral catheter, provided that the patient has not received previous pelvic irradiation and that there is no significant ureteral obstruction with upper urinary tract infection. When pyeloureterectasis and infection exist above the level of the ureteric fistula, a nephrostomy must be performed on the affected side if kidney function is to be preserved. The leaking ureter may then be surgically repaired in 3–6 months by one of various methods, including ureteroneocystostomy, transureteroureterostomy, bladder extension flaps, or ileal conduit interposition, depending on the individual circumstances. As is the case with all fistulas, it is always important to exclude recurrent malignancy as the cause of the fistula.

If the fistula is vesicovaginal, a large-bore urethral catheter should be inserted and left to drain for 6 weeks. When continued leaking occurs at that stage, the fistula is very unlikely to close spontaneously, and therefore the catheter can be removed. The temptation to attempt surgical repair before 3 months postoperatively should be avoided. Excellent results can be obtained on the first attempt at repair if careful attention is paid to the following principles of fistula repair: excision of the fibrotic fistula tract, wide mobilization of the surrounding tissues, careful approximation of each layer in a watertight fashion without tension, meticulous hemostasis, and adequate, closely supervised postoperative bladder drainage via a wide-bore catheter. With large defects, vulvar fat pad or skin flaps of the Martius type may be preferable to closure of the mucosal defect under tension. Although most gynecologists prefer the vaginal approach for repair of vesicovaginal fistulas, occasionally the abdominal approach is indicated, especially if there is a complex defect involving the vesical neck or ureters (20).

Loss of Urethral Floor

The problem of loss of urethral floor may range from a tiny fistula that virtually causes no incontinence to complete loss of the urethral floor, bladder neck, and trigone. Although many methods of urethral reconstruction have been described, most suffer from the fact that the resultant inert noncontractile tube does not provide continence for the patient. Because most of these patients have less tissue loss than it may appear, use of the anteriorly retracted urethral "roof" to construct a narrow-bore contractile tube, as described by Symmonds (21), is our preferred method of repair. A labial myocutaneous flap is again often used in the repair (Fig. 3). Of 50 patients who underwent reconstruction with the use of this technique, 74% were completely continent and another 14% were significantly improved, but 40% of the patients subsequently required a retropubic suspension of the Marshall-Marchetti-Krantz type to achieve complete continence (22).

Stress Incontinence

Although not always avoidable, stress incontinence may be minimized by not resecting the segment of vaginal mucosa just beneath the urethra and bladder neck at the time of vaginectomy. If the mucosa from this region needs to be excised, careful plication of the pubococcygeus muscle beneath the urethrovesical junction at the time of resection may prevent stress incontinence subsequently.

Rectovaginal Fistula

Rectovaginal fistula after irradiation should always be managed with a defunctioning colostomy before repair is attempted, and this rule often applies also to

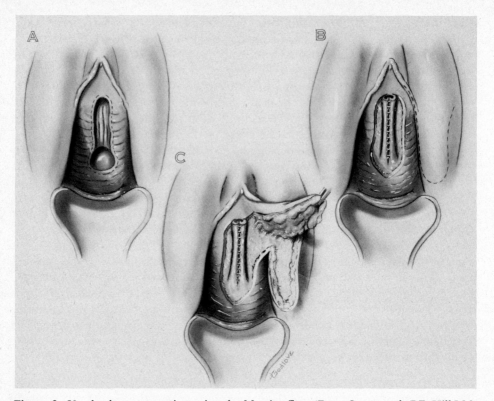

Figure 3. Urethral reconstruction using the Martius flap. (From Symmonds RE, Hill LM: Loss of the urethra: A report on 50 patients. *Am J Obstet Gynecol* 130:130, 1978. By permission of the CV Mosby Co.)

high rectovaginal fistulas without prior irradiation, especially if a previous repair has failed (23). Low rectovaginal fistulas in the nonirradiated patient, even if of large size, can usually be successfully repaired transvaginally without a previous colostomy. Again, wide mobilization, layered closure without tension, and perfect hemostasis are the secrets to success.

It is important in dealing with fistulas due to irradiation to be sure that the radionecrosis is not still progressing before surgical repair is attempted and also that recurrent malignancy has been excluded. Continuing enlargement of a fistula by progressive radionecrosis may occur for many years after the initial radiation treatment. Bricker has developed an extremely innovative technique for closing a large defect: He constructs a loop of rectosigmoid to cover the fistula and reimplants the distal sigmoid into the loop (Fig. 4).

Vaginal Stenosis
The problem of vaginal stenosis can often be avoided during surgical resection of vaginal lesions by the use of plastic surgical procedures such as Z-plasties, skin flaps and grafts, and transverse closure of vertical incisions. However, stenosis is, unfortunately, a common complication of vaginal irradiation (24, 25). Regular coitus after irradiation or the use of dilators or molds, together with the use of vaginal estrogen cream, helps prevent complete obliteration of the vagina after

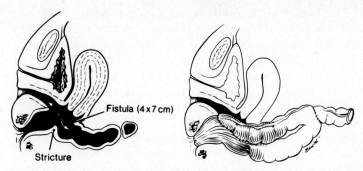

Figure 4. The Bricker technique for repair of a large rectovaginal fistula. (From Bricker EM, Johnston WD: Repair of postirradiation rectovaginal fistula and stricture. *Surg Gynecol Obstet* 148:499, 1979. By permission.)

treatment. Even if the vagina is not required for sexual function, if it is allowed to stenose, adequate follow-up examinations to check for recurrence of the malignancy become impossible.

VAGINAL RECONSTRUCTION

Considerably more attention is now being paid to vaginal reconstructive procedures when treatment of a genital tract malignancy results in loss of vaginal function. This is a direct result of patient demands for sexual rehabilitation, the availability of better surgical techniques for reconstruction, and, with more long-term survivors as a result of improvements in treatment, greater concern for improving the quality of life.

The most commonly used procedure is the McIndoe vaginoplasty, in which split-thickness skin grafts sutured over a foam-rubber mold are inserted into the vaginal cavity. After vaginectomy or exenteration, a pack is left to create a cavity, and after 5–7 days, when the cavity is cleanly granulating, the mold with attached grafts is inserted. The most common complication of this procedure is vaginal stenosis and stricture formation. This operation, therefore, requires that the patient wear a vaginal mold intermittently, to prevent stenosis.

In an attempt to obviate having the patient wear a mold, segments of both small and large bowel have been used to construct a neovagina (26). The most commonly used segment is sigmoid colon, and this tissue has provided a functional vagina in many instances. Intestinal fistulas have been a problem when the patient has had previous pelvic irradiation, mainly when a rectosigmoid anastomosis is performed rather than a sigmoid colostomy. Prolapse of the neovagina, segmental sloughing, and excessive mucus production by the bowel mucosa have also been troublesome. However, stenosis is less common than with skin grafts.

Rotational skin flaps from buttocks and thighs have also been used, with limited success (27, 28). Often, however, vulvectomy is necessary, along with vaginectomy; and here, obtaining adequately sized skin flaps for coverage of the vulvar defect and construction of a vagina may be a problem. A simple vulvoplasty to construct an external vaginal pouch has been described by Williams (29). There are few problems related to performance of the procedure, and it allows for satisfactory vaginal function in many instances. A major drawback is that the angle of the neovagina is practically vertical. In the vaginal agenesis patient who has had the Williams procedure, pressure on the perineum from coitus may eventually produce a vaginal tract, but in the usual oncology patient who has had a vaginectomy, the amount of fibrosis and scarring prevents this. Another difficulty is fissuring of the skin at the newly constructed introitus. This problem occurs when the thin skin and the scar at this location are stretched during coitus.

Recently, interest has focused on the use of myocutaneous flaps, both to reconstruct the vagina and to cover large vulvar and perineal defects (30–32). The gracilis myocutaneous flap has been the most commonly used (Fig. 5). The main advantages of this procedure are that the flaps are available even if large areas of the vulva and perineum have been excised and also that the actual bulk of the newly created vagina helps cover the denuded pelvic floor, a source of much morbidity in the postexenteration patient. Disadvantages are the operating time involved in creation and placement of the flaps and difficulties

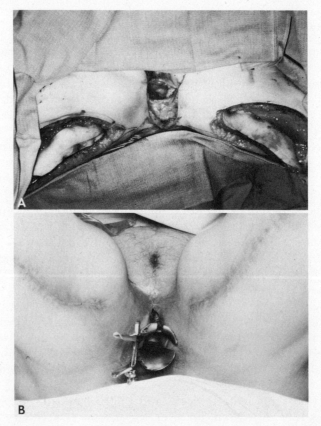

Figure 5. (a) Gracilis myocutaneous flaps before vaginal reconstruction. (b) An adequate vagina 6 weeks postoperatively.

experienced with necrosis of all or portions of the flaps when the dominant vascular pedicle has been compromised. Intravenous fluorescein intraoperatively helps in predicting viability (33).

VULVOPLASTY

Management of large skin defects of the vulva, perineum, and groin is a continuing problem, found most commonly after resection of recurrent vulvar malignancy. Adequate reconstruction requires familiarity with many plastic surgical techniques and considerable ingenuity and adaptability. Free skin grafts to cover skin defects are useful, but they present the problem of morbidity associated with the donor site. Fortunately, there is usually ample redundant skin around the thighs and buttocks that may be used for local skin flaps (Fig. 6). The general rule here is that in the design of a skin flap, the length of the flaps should not exceed the width of the pedicle; otherwise, viability will be compromised. Hematoma and seroma formation under the flaps can be problem, and therefore suction drainage is mandatory.

Gracilis myocutaneous flaps are now often used to cover vulvar and perineal defects. In many instances reported in the recent literature, however, myocutaneous flaps have been used when a simple local skin flap obviously would have sufficed and would have resulted in considerably less morbidity. When vaginal reconstruction is also required, the gracilis flap is invaluable.

Groin defects are particularly suited for coverage by means of tensor fascia lata flaps (Fig. 7); gluteal flaps are less satisfactory. Again, however, these procedures should be reserved for large defects. They should not be used indiscriminately to cover the raw area after a routine vulvectomy and groin node dissection, with the supposed justification that a small area of skin loss commonly occurs after this procedure.

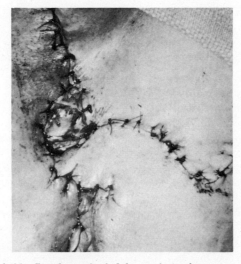

Figure 6. A rotational skin flap from the left buttock used to cover a perineal defect after resection of recurrent vulvar cancer.

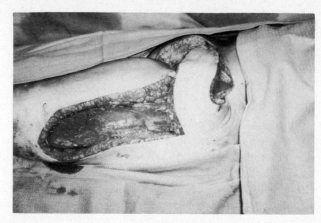

Figure 7. A tensor fascia lata flap to cover a large left groin defect.

CONCLUSION

Although the treatment of vaginal and vulvar cancer involves mainly external procedures, the problems presented in management can tax even the most experienced oncologist. As better preoperative, intraoperative, and postoperative management allows more radical procedures to be performed, and as these better treatment modalities improve patient survival, the oncologist will be called on to provide reconstruction for and rehabilitation of these patients. To this end, he will draw not only on his understanding of the disease as a gynecologist but also on a broad familiarity with developing techniques within other disciplines, such as plastic surgery, gastrointestinal surgery, and urology.

REFERENCES

1. Cutler SJ, Young JL Jr (eds): Third National Cancer Survey: Incidence data. *Natl Cancer Inst Monogr* No. 41, 1975.
2. Rutledge F: Cancer of the vagina. *Am J Obstet Gynecol* 97:635, 1967.
3. Way S: Carcinoma of the vulva. *Am J Obstet Gynecol* 79:692, 1960.
4. Kuipers T: Carcinoma of the vulva. *Radiol Clin (Basel)* 44:475, 1975.
5. Townsend DE: Cryosurgery. *Obstet Gynecol Annu* 4:331, 1975.
6. Rutledge F, Sinclair M: Treatment of intraepithelial carcinoma of the vulva by skin excision and graft. *Am J Obstet Gynecol* 102:806, 1968.
7. Woodruff JD, Julian C, Puray T, et al: The contemporary challenge of carcinoma in situ of the vulva. *Am J Obstet Gynecol* 115:677, 1973.
8. Boutselis JG: Intraepithelial carcinoma of the vulva. *Am J Obstet Gynecol* 113:733, 1972.
9. Boutselis JG: Radical vulvectomy for invasive squamous cell carcinoma of the vulva. *Obstet Gynecol* 39:827, 1972.
10. Kelvey JL, Adcock LL: Cancer of the vulva. *Obstet Gynecol* 26:455, 1965.
11. Figge DC, Gaudenz R: Invasive carcinoma of the vulva. *Am J Obstet Gynecol* 119:382, 1974.
12. Pratt JH, Watson JR: Carcinoma of the vulva: New incision for one-stage radical vulvectomy and bilateral nodal dissection. *Proc Staff Meet Mayo Clin* 30:23, 1955.
13. Goldberg MI, Belinson JL, Ford JH, et al: Surgical management of invasive carcinoma of the vulva utilizing a lower abdominal midline incision. *Gynecol Oncol* 7:296, 1979.

14. Krupp PJ, Lee FYL, Bohm JW, et al: Therapy of advanced epidermoid carcinoma of vulva: Report of 13 patients, with review of recent literature. *Obstet Gynecol* 46:433, 1975.

15. Daily LJ, Kaplan AL, Kaufman RH: Exenteration for advanced carcinoma of the vulva. *Obstet Gynecol* 36:845, 1970.

16. Thornton WN Jr, Flanagan WC Jr: Pelvic exenteration in the treatment of advanced malignancy of the vulva. *Am J Obstet Gynecol* 117:774, 1973.

17. Green TH Jr, Ulfelder H, Meigs JV: Epidermoid carcinoma of the vulva: An analysis of 238 cases: Pt II. Therapy and end results. *Am J Obstet Gynecol* 75:848, 1958.

18. Twombly GH: The technique of radical vulvectomy for carcinoma of the vulva. *Cancer* 6:516, 1953.

19. Hilliard GD, Massey FM, O'Toole RV Jr: Vulvar neoplasia in the young. *Am J Obstet Gynecol* 135:185, 1979.

20. Massee JS, Welch JS, Pratt JH, et al: Management of urinary-vaginal fistula: Ten-year survey. *JAMA* 190:902, 1964.

21. Symmonds RE: Loss of the urethral floor with total urinary incontinence: A technique for urethral reconstruction. *Am J Obstet Gynecol* 103:665, 1969.

22. Symmonds RE, Hill LM: Loss of the urethra: A report on 50 patients. *Am J Obstet Gynecol* 130:130, 1978.

23. Boronow RC: Management of radiation-induced vaginal fistulas. *Am J Obstet Gynecol* 110:1, 1971.

24. Pride GL, Schultz AE, Chuprevich TW, et al: Primary invasive squamous carcinoma of the vagina. *Obstet Gynecol* 53:218, 1979.

25. Perez CA, Arneson AN, Dehner LP, et al: Radiation therapy in carcinoma of the vagina. *Obstet Gynecol* 44:862, 1974.

26. Pratt JII, Smith GR: Vaginal reconstruction with a sigmoid loop. *Am J Obstet Gynecol* 96:31, 1966.

27. Conway H, Stark RB: Construction and reconstruction of the vagina. *Surg Gynecol Obstet* 97:573, 1953.

28. Cocke WM, Bolasny BL, Sawyers JL: Vaginal reconstruction following extended abdominoperineal resection. *Plast Reconstr Surg* 46:372, 1970.

29. Williams EA: Congenital absence of the vagina: A simple operation for its relief. *J Obstet Gynaecol Br Comm* 71:511, 1964.

30. McCraw JB, Massey FM, Shanklin KD, et al: Vaginal reconstruction with *gracilis* myocutaneous flaps. *Plast Reconstr Surg* 58:176, 1976.

31. Becker DW Jr, Massey FM, McCraw JB: Musculocutaneous flaps in reconstructive pelvic surgery. *Obstet Gynecol* 54:178, 1979.

32. Wheeless CR Jr, McGibbon B, Dorsey JH, et al: Gracilis myocutaneous flap in reconstruction of the vulva and female perineum. *Obstet Gynecol* 54:97, 1979.

33. McCraw JB, Myers B. Shanklin KD: The value of fluorescein in predicting the viability of arterialized flaps. *Plast Reconstr Surg* 60:710, 1977.

Part 3

MEDICAL COMPLICATIONS

11
Venous Thrombosis and Pulmonary Embolism

Herbert L. Kotz

Joseph Giordano

Pulmonary embolism and deep venous thrombosis are serious complications of many medical and surgical disorders. Five hundred thousand new cases of pulmonary embolism occur annually in the United States, and 10%–20% of these patients die (1,2). Autopsy studies have shown pulmonary embolism to be one of the most common causes of death (3,4,5). While mortality from pulmonary embolism on a gynecologic surgical service is low, its unpredictable occurrence in an otherwise routine postoperative course is catastrophic.

ETIOLOGY OF DEEP VENOUS THROMBOSIS

Vessel wall injury, venous stasis, and the hypercoagulable state, Virchow's classic triad (6), have been implicated as responsible for the development of deep venous thrombosis. The veins of the leg and pelvis are subject to trauma during pelvic surgery (7,8). The intima of veins has a negative electric charge that repels negatively charged platelets. Local trauma disrupts the intima and exposes the negatively charged platelets to the more positive potential of the deeper layers of the vessel wall. This process leads to aggregation of platelets and thrombosis (8).

During an operative procedure and in the immediate postoperative period, venous stasis occurs, and many observers feel that this is also a major factor in the development of deep venous thrombosis (9–11). During surgery there is a reduction in venous return to one-half its normal rate (12). This reduction has been attributed to loss of muscle tone secondary to anesthesia. Postoperatively, the blood flow in leg veins undergoes a 75% reduction compared with preoperative levels, and this reduction persists from 4 to 14 days (13).

Surgery has been found to increase the coagulability of blood (14–16). A consistent and significant increase in heparin resistance starting on the first postoperative day and reaching a maximum on the third to fifth postoperative day has been demonstrated (15,17). These changes are greater in older patients and after extensive surgery (18). Factors VIII, IX, and X are increased postoperatively, and platelet count and platelet adhesiveness reach a peak at 10 days after surgery (19,20). Finally, there is an increase in fibrinogen and circulating fibrinolysis inhibitors.

PREVENTION OF DEEP VENOUS THROMBOSIS

Prevention of venous thrombosis must include recognition of high-risk patients. Obesity (21,22), malignant disease (23), heart disease with congestive failure (24), dehydration (23), anemia (23), infection (24), varicose veins (25), and a previous history of thrombophlebitis or embolism (23,26) have been recognized as predisposing factors in venous thrombosis and embolism. Superimposed on all these factors is an age-related risk. Although no age group is exempt, postmortem and clinical studies have shown that the risk of venous thromboembolism increases with age and most of the recorded deaths from this cause occur in patients 50 years of age and over (27).

Preoperatively, the surgeon must assume responsibility for correcting the predisposing factors such as anemia, dehydration, congestive heart failure, and infection. In addition, the patient should be taught breathing and leg exercises that, when employed in the postoperative period, are helpful in reducing venous stasis (8).

During surgery, also, an effort must be made to reduce venous stasis. Localized constriction of the legs, as may occur with electrode straps, should be avoided, since it reduces blood flow and produces turbulence. Postoperatively, leg exercises and deep breathing are encouraged and ambulation is started as soon as possible.

Although compression stockings are in common use, they have not been shown to be effective (28). Only stockings providing graduated limb compression reduce the incidence of isotopically detected thrombosis (29–31).

Attention to the general measures just discussed does not eliminate deep venous thrombosis. It is not surprising, then, that drug therapy has assumed an increasingly important role. Oral anticoagulants were first used in 1959 (32). They may be the most effective method but have not gained wide acceptance because of difficulties in dosage regulation and the hazards of operative and postoperative bleeding (33). Drugs affecting platelet function have been used (34). Both dextran-40 and dextran-70 produce a decrease in platelet adhesiveness and a defect in the release reaction of platelets and platelet aggregation (35). These drugs were effective in some, but not all, series (27). Complications such as occasional renal failure, rare anaphylactic reactions including bronchospasm, and the hazard of pulmonary edema for patients with reduced cardiac reserve have limited their use. Aspirin alone or in combination with dipyridamole (both drugs inhibit platelet aggregation) has been shown to reduce the incidence of isotopically detected venous thrombosis (34,36), but not as effectively as low-dose heparin (37).

Reports of controlled trials with low-dose heparin have revealed new possibilities for the prevention of venous thromboembolism in the postoperative period. Heparin prophylaxis was first used in 1966 for those patients with coagulation times shorter than normal (38). Many studies have subsequently demonstrated the effectiveness of low-dose heparin in reducing the incidence of deep venous thrombosis, scan-detected pulmonary emboli, and fatal pulmonary emboli (39−45).

The formation of significant venous thrombosis depends on the accumulation of activated factor X, the major component of the enzyme complex that converts prothrombin to thrombin. Heparin in low doses accelerates and enhances the action of the major plasma inhibitor of activated factor X. This ability to inhibit the clotting sequence at the activated X stage requires a lower dose of heparin than that necessary to block the clotting process once thrombin is formed (46). Recent studies have suggested that heparin may also work by decreasing blood viscosity, thereby increasing flow (47), and by decreasing the platelet increase seen postoperatively (48).

Low-dose heparin prophylaxis of deep venous thrombosis involves the injection of 5,000 units of heparin subcutaneously in the abdominal wall two or three times daily for 5−7 days or until mobilization is complete. The first dose must be given approximately 2 hours before surgery. With this technique, the circulating blood level of heparin is only a fraction of that achieved by conventional treatment of established thrombosis. However, this low level of heparin is adequate to prevent the initiation of the clotting sequence. Since the patients are not completely heparinized, the risk of bleeding is reduced and the need for laboratory monitoring is eliminated.

In 1974 and 1975 several studies demonstrated, by perfusion scans of the lungs, a decrease in the number and size of postoperative pulmonary emboli in patients treated with prophylactic low-dose heparin (49−51).

Direct evidence of the efficacy of low-dose heparin in the prevention of pulmonary embolism was first presented in 1975 (52) in a controlled prospective trial in patients over the age of 50 having major operations. In this study all patients who died were studied on autopsy. Fatal pulmonary embolism did not occur in any of the 252 treated patients compared with 8 out of 235 patients (3.39%) in the control group.

The best known and largest study on low-dose heparin is the International Multicenter study reported in 1975 (53). This investigation included patients over the age of 40 undergoing a variety of elective surgical procedures. It was a prospective, controlled study with 2,076 patients in the well-matched control group and 2,045 in the heparin group. There were 16 deaths from pulmonary embolus in the control group and 2 in the heparin group, as proven by autopsy.

The most recent report on the prophylactic effect of heparin on postoperative fatal and on clinically apparent but nonfatal thromboembolic complications was a double-blind, prospective, randomized study comprising 1,296 patients (54). Sixteen out of 653 patients in the placebo group had such complications within the treatment period of 1 week compared with 4 out of 643 in the heparin group. Four cases in the placebo group and one in the heparin group were fatal.

Heparin prophylaxis is not without complications. Increased bleeding during surgery and wound hematomas are documented complications (53,55,56). Thrombocytopenia has been reported (57). In general, trials using the highest dose of heparin (15,000 units/day) were associated with more local bleeding than those with the lower dose (10,000 units) (39).

A recent review has documented the efficacy of low-dose heparin in reducing the incidence of deep venous thrombosis, scan-detected pulmonary emboli, and fatal pulmonary emboli (58). The alternatives to the use of low-dose heparin and the dangers in its use were discussed; but, the review concludes that "it is the responsibility of the pelvic surgeon who does not use low-dose heparin to show why not."

Physical measures aimed at reducing venous stasis during and after surgery offer an alternative approach to prophylaxis of deep venous thrombosis. Electrical stimulation of the calf muscles or the use of inflatable boots during the operation and the early postoperative period have been shown to be a highly effective form of prophylaxis (59,60). However, these physical measures of prophylaxis are not entirely free from problems. Patient acceptance is unenthusiastic, and after the first or second postoperative day, the cumbersome and uncomfortable apparatus is often rejected (61). Furthermore, doubt has been cast on the ability of pneumatic compression of the calves to prevent venous thrombosis in surgical patients with malignant disease (62).

DIAGNOSIS OF DEEP VENOUS THROMBOSIS

Clinical Diagnosis

The clinical diagnosis of deep venous thrombosis is difficult and misleading (63−65). The incidence of I125 fibrinogen scan-detected deep venous thrombosis is 15%−29% in general gynecologic surgical patients (66−68) and 14%−42% in general surgical patients (69−71). However, the majority of postoperative patients with deep venous thrombosis do not have localized signs or symptoms (72,73). In addition, if clinical signs are present, they may be secondary to causes other than venous thrombosis. Calf tenderness and Homan's sign are correct in only 50% and 8% of patients, respectively (63,65). Nicolaides (74) reported that of 228 patients with signs and symptoms of deep venous thrombosis, only 57% had this diagnosis confirmed by venography.

Despite its lack of sensitivity, the initial detection of postoperative deep venous thrombosis must be by clinical examination. This principle applies to institutions that do not routinely use postoperative noninvasive screening techniques. Clinical tests using pain responses for diagnosing deep venous thrombosis have been described (8):

1. Pain in the sole of the foot, possibly due to pressure of the thrombosed vein on the plantar nerves
2. Tenderness on the inner side of the foot
3. Tenderness on pressure over the femoral, popliteal, or posterior tibial vessels
4. Tenderness of the calf muscles to deep palpation
5. Homan's sign: pain in the calf muscle with dorsiflexion of the foot
6. Tenderness in the adductor muscles of the thigh
7. Pain in the leg from a blood pressure cuff encircling it and inflated to exert pressure below 150 mm Hg

Lower leg edema may occur, but this depends principally upon the location of the thrombi. The more proximal and therefore the more extensive the thrombi, the more likely that the patient will have lower leg swelling. Iliofemoral vein thrombosis will very frequently cause massive lower leg edema; calf vein thrombosis alone will be more likely to cause just pain and tenderness without lower leg edema.

Venography

Venography is the most reliable and definitive method of diagnosing deep venous thrombosis. The technique has been described as safe, reliable, and simple to perform (75), but it is invasive and does have occasional serious adverse effects.

Contrast material is injected into a superficial vein of the foot; radiographs are then taken at various levels of the lower extremity and pelvis. The major deep venous system is then visualized. Signs of obstruction such as filling defects, abrupt termination of the column of contrast material, nonfilling of a segment of the deep venous system despite proper technique, and the presence of extensive collateralization indicate deep venous thrombosis (76). The test does not routinely visualize the soleal plexus of the calf, the deep femoral vein, and the pelvic veins.

The major complications are the extravasation of contrast material at the injection site, pain during injection, superficial phlebitis, hypersensitivity reactions, and deep venous thrombosis (77,78). The test can be performed as an outpatient service but requires sophisticated x-ray equipment.

While venography is still recognized as the most definitive test for the diagnosis of deep venous thrombosis, noninvasive methods have been developed and play an important role in the diagnosis of this condition. These methods include:

1. Isotope studies
2. Doppler ultrasound
3. Plethysmography

^{125}I Fibrinogen

The radioactive-tagged fibrinogen test came into clinical use in 1968 (70,79) and has added an enormous amount of information to our basic knowledge of deep venous thrombosis. I^{125}-tagged fibrinogen is administered intravenously. Actively forming thrombi pick up the isotope and incorporate it into the clot. Portable scanners then screen the lower extremity and detect areas of increased radioactivity indicating a thrombus. The test can be repeated daily to determine not only new clot formation but also propagation of old clot.

Fibrinogen scanning has become an important tool in the study of the natural history of deep venous thrombosis. By injecting the radioactive-tagged fibrinogen preoperatively and scanning the patient postoperatively, Kakkar (80) and others (67,71) have demonstrated a high incidence of deep venous thrombosis. This technique has made it possible to reliably study the effectiveness of various drug regimens and physical modalities in reducing the incidence of postoperative thrombosis.

The test has a number of disadvantages. Radioactively tagged fibrinogen cannot be reliably used to diagnose established deep venous thrombosis. As mentioned, active formation of a clot is necessary for the incorporation of the tagged isotope. A patient with signs and symptoms of deep venous thrombosis may have large thrombi in major deep venous systems that are not actively forming thrombi; therefore, a false negative test would be obtained. Clots in the iliac veins cannot be diagnosed because of increased background radiation secondary to concentration of radioactive fibrinogen in the urine. The method is expensive because of the equipment, the isotopes, and the technician's time. Each examination takes 15–20 minutes and cannot be performed until 24 hours after the injection of the isotope, making the test useless in an urgent clinical situation (65).

Still, the radioactive-tagged fibrinogen test remains an important tool in the study of the natural history of deep venous thrombosis and, in some institutions, as a screening measure to prospectively study those patients who are at a high risk of developing this disorder.

Doppler Ultrasound

Doppler ultrasound is an effective noninvasive method of diagnosing deep venous thrombosis (81). It evaluates the patency of the deep venous systems by examining the pattern of venous flow. The technique is simple and inexpensive but requires experienced personnel to interpret venous flow patterns. The Doppler technique involves examination of four deep veins of the lower extremity: the posterior tibial, the popliteal, the superficial femoral, and the common femoral. Normally, venous flow is spontaneous and varies with respiration. Variation occurs because during inspiration the descent of the diaphragm increases intra-abdominal pressure, which decreases venous return from the lower extremity. During expiration, the intra-abdominal pressure is reduced and venous flow from the lower extremity is increased. The net result is a phasic pattern in which venous flow is decreased during inspiration and increased during expiration. Venous flow is also tested by proximal and distal compression maneuvers. If the foot is compressed, an augmentation of flow should be appreciated at the posterior tibial vein. If the lower leg proximal to the posterior tibial vein is compressed, venous flow at the posterior tibial vein is disrupted. However, release of the compression should normally elicit an augmented venous flow pattern.

Spontaneous flow, variation with respiration, and response to proximal and distal compression maneuvers are performed on all four deep veins of the lower extremity. Thrombi in any major vein of the lower extremity will alter venous flow pattern and change the normal characteristics just discussed. Appreciation of those abnormal responses by an experienced examiner is the basis for the diagnosis of deep venous thrombosis by the Doppler method.

The major advantage of Doppler ultrasound for the detection of deep venous thrombosis is that it is an inexpensive test that can be used on an outpatient or inpatient basis. It is noninvasive and has no complications associated with it. The accuracy of Doppler ultrasound in the detection of significant deep venous thrombosis when compared with venography has been reported to be as high as 94% (82).

The Doppler ultrasound technique is not capable of detecting small calf thrombi or pelvic vein thrombosis (81). The accuracy of the test decreases considerably if venous collaterals have developed (83). Therefore, the test is most accurate in the immediate period after the development of major deep vein thrombosis. Most important of all, it requires considerable experience to achieve any degree of reliability.

Plethysmography

Plethysmography is a noninvasive technique for the diagnosis of deep venous thrombosis that involves measurement of volume changes produced by temporary venous occlusion. These volume changes can be detected with electrodes measuring resistance across the lower extremity (impedance plethysmography) or by transducers measuring pressure changes in a closed system (volume plethysmography) (84).

The test consists of temporary occlusion of venous outflow in the lower extremity by inflation of a pressure cuff across the upper thigh. The volume of the leg distal to the occluding cuff will slowly increase until the venous pressure in the veins exceeds the pressure of the inflated cuff. The release of the occluding cuff causes a sudden decrease in lower leg volume. Interpretation of these volume changes forms the basis of the plethysmographic technique.

In recent reports, plethysmography has correlated with venography in greater than 95% of the cases (85–87). The test does not require great skill in performance or interpretation; it is noninvasive and can be used at bedside for inpatients or on an outpatent basis.

Plethysmographic testing detects only thrombi that produce obstruction of venous flow. The test will not detect most calf vein thrombi that do not obstruct any outflow tract. There may also be nonocclusive proximal vein thrombi that the test does not detect.

Other Diagnostic Methods

A number of other diagnostic techniques have been evaluated to a limited extent. These have depended on one of three principles: (1) the attachment of isotope-labeled proteins on cells to the thrombus, (2) the use of the gamma camera, and (3) the use of thermography.

Techniques for the preferential attachment of isotope-labeled proteins or cells to the thrombus include injection of isotope-labeled urokinase (88), streptokinase (89), plasmin (90), antifibrin-fibrinogen antibody (91), or leukocytes (92).

The second method is the use of the gamma camera to detect the flow of radioactive particles in the deep veins (93–95). In 1973, a radiopharmaceutical (^{99m}Tc human albumin microspheres or ^{99m}Tc HAM) was described that had the ability to simultaneously define pulmonary emboli and their sites of origin (96). Findings considered definitely positive for venous thrombosis include the loss of visualization of a segment of the venous system, with or without the demonstration of collateral channels, and the appearance of hot spots on delayed imaging of the respective levels. Recent comparative studies showed an 89% and 96% correlation of ^{99m}Tc HAM and venography (94,97).

Polaroid photographs of the gamma-camera scans of the lower limbs are taken 1–2 minutes after the isotope is injected; the conventional lung scan is then performed. While the technique is simple, the apparatus is complex. The labeled particles are readily available, but the apparatus can be used only in the Isotope Department.

The third approach has been the use of thermography as a screening test for thrombosis in high-risk patients (98,99). The principle on which this technique is based is finding raised temperatures and delayed cooling of limbs that contain thrombi. The results of this study were very promising. These more recent techniques require additional clinical evaluation to assess their potential.

Summary of Clinical Diagnostic Procedures

It is now apparent that the physician has a number of options to consider in making a definitive diagnosis of deep venous thrombosis. Clinical examination of the postoperative patient must be the initial step in confirming the presence of signs and symptoms consistent with deep venous thrombosis, if noninvasive screening is not used routinely. However, the inaccuracy of clinical examination for the definitive diagnosis has been well established.

Venography remains the best method of diagnosing deep venous thrombosis. A properly performed positive test constitutes unequivocable evidence of thrombosis. Venography demonstrates not only the presence or absence of thrombi but also their location and whether the clot is loose and therefore likely to embolize (76).

The noninvasive Doppler and plethysmographic tests are a recent and important addition to the clinician's armamentarium. Unequivocal tests can reliably diagnose deep venous thrombosis, and decisions on therapy can be based on these test results. Noninvasive tests that are equivocal should be followed with a venogram for confirmation.

TREATMENT OF DEEP VENOUS THROMBOSIS

Treatment of deep venous thrombosis should begin immediately upon establishment of the diagnosis. The patient should be hospitalized and placed at bed rest with the lower extremity elevated 15 degrees. Heparin therapy is initiated with a bolus of 100 units/kg followed by a continuous intravenous infusion averaging 500–1,500 units/hour. The partial thromboplastin time can be used as a guide to adequate therapy. Coumadin, an oral anticoagulant, is begun at the same time as the heparin therapy, with the goal of establishing a daily dose that will prolong the prothrombin time to approximately twice normal. The patient is maintained at this dose of Coumadin for 3–6 months and her prothrombin time frequently evaluated to ensure adequate anticoagulation.

If anticoagulation is contraindicated or pulmonary emboli develop in the patient despite adequate anticoagulation, inferior vena cava interruption by ligation, plication, or the insertion of a "vena caval umbrella" is indicated.

During hospitalization the patient is fitted with elastic support stockings and instructed on the importance of wearing them when full ambulation begins. She should use these stockings for 6 months. They can be slowly discontinued after that time provided edema does not develop in the affected extremity.

PULMONARY EMBOLISM

Although the main concern of the pelvic surgeon is prevention of pulmonary embolism (PE), no one method or combination of methods has proven infallible. Therefore, a clear understanding of appropriate diagnostic modalities and their limitations is imperative when PE is suspected. The classic picture of PE with infarction manifested by coughing, apprehension, hemoptysis, dyspnea, cyanosis, transient syncope, pleuritic chest pain, sweats, and associated leg phlebitis is easy to recognize.

However, the clinical picture is usually not so clear. The patient may complain of dizziness or dyspnea with fever. There may be an increased pulse rate, temperature elevation, accentuated pulmonary second sound, tachypnea, and S_3 and S_4 gallop sounds. The syndromes that result from PE may lead to such erroneous clinical diagnoses as pleurisy, pneumonia, congestive heart failure, myocardial infarction, stroke, and septicemia (100). Thus, whenever pulmonary embolism is suspected, objective evidence should be obtained to confirm or refute the clinical diagnosis.

What should one do when the diagnosis is suspected? A chest x-ray, an ECG, a complete blood cell count, and arterial bood gases should be ordered. If the diagnosis has not been excluded or remains in doubt, a lung scan should be performed.

Although PE may not cause any change in the roentgenogram, pulmonary infarction usually produces a radiologic abnormality. Areas of decreased vascularity, dilated pulmonary arteries, or pleural fluid may be found. It is felt by some that the diagnosis can be suspected from x-ray films in approximately 50% of patients with PEs (101). The ECG may be useful in some cases in which the diagnosis is in doubt. The classic finding of heart strain on the right side is usually not present. But some significant abnormality concomitant with the acute event may be found in over 60% of the patients (102). The most common findings include QRS changes (65%) and ST-T wave abnormalities (44%) (103).

The most helpful laboratory study is the arterial o_2 (104). In almost all cases the Po_2 is decreased below 80 mm Hg. The Pco_2 is also decreased. The pH is usually greater than 7.4. Although these findings are not specific for PE (they may be seen in cardiac failure), their true value lies in their use as a screening method. A normal Po_2 is very strong evidence against an embolus.

A diagnostic evaluation for PE is incomplete without perfusion lung scanning. The lung scan uses macroaggregates of human serum albumin labeled with technetium, chromium, or iodine. This substance can be completely removed from the blood in a single passage through the lung but is not metabolized during the period of study. Because of their size, the macroaggregates lodge in the pulmonary arterioles and capillaries and their concentration is determined by scanning the lung fields. A diminished concentration in the lung indicates a diminished blood flow to that area of the lung.

A negative lung scan makes the diagnosis of pulmonary embolus highly unlikely. A positive scan in the presence of a normal chest x-ray confirms the diagnosis of pulmonary embolus. A positive scan, in the presence of an abnormal chest x-ray, cannot distinguish between a pulmonary embolus and other pulmonary diseases such as atelectasis, pneumonia, or pneumothorax, which also produce diminished arterial flow. In these cases a ventilation-perfusion scan with ^{133}Xenon is mandatory to reduce the number of false positives.

Pulmonary angiography is the only specific diagnostic test for pulmonary embolism, but it is not without serious complications and should be reserved for those cases in which the diagnosis remains in doubt and the results of angiography are essential to determination of the patient's therapy. The only absolute contraindication to angiography is known allergy to contrast material (105). Two relative contraindications are recent myocardial infarction and ventricular irritability.

To summarize, if the Po_2 and lung scans are normal, the diagnosis of pulmonary embolus may be excluded. If they are abnormal, in the presence of a normal chest x-ray, appropriate therapy can be started.

Although the full treatment of PE is beyond the scope of this chapter, all physicians should recognize the need for prompt administration of intravenous heparin and institution of appropriate supportive measures once the diagnosis is highly suspected.

REFERENCES

1. Dalen JE, Alpert JS: Natural history of pulmonary embolism, in Sasahara AA, Sonnenblick EH, Lesh M (eds): *Pulmonary Emboli.* New York, Grune & Stratton, 1975, pp 77−88.

2. Hume M, Sevitt S, Thomas DP: *Venous Thrombosis and Pulmonary Embolism.* Cambridge, Mass., Howard University, 1970, p 4.

3. Morrell MT, Dunnill MS: The postmortem incidence of pulmonary embolism in a hospital population. *Br J Surg* 55:347, 1968.

4. Smith GT, Dexter L, Dammin GJ: Postmortem quantitative studies in pulmonary thromboembolism, in Sasahara AA, Stein M (eds): *Pulmonary Embolic Disease.* New York, Grune & Stratton, 1965.

5. Freiman DG: Pathologic observation in experimental and human thromboembolism, in Sasahara AA, Stein M (eds): *Pulmonary Embolic Disease.* New York, Grune & Stratton, 1965, p 312.

6. Virchow RLK: Die Pfropfbildugen und Verstopfrangen in den Gefassen *Handb. Spec. Path. w Ther* Band 1, Erlenger, 1954. Cited by Nelson JH Jr: *Atlas of Radical Pelvic Surgery.* New York, Appleton-Century Crofts, 1977, p 54.

7. Gibbs NM: The prophylaxis of pulmonary embolism. *Br J Surg* 47:282, 1959.

8. Marshall R: *Pulmonary Embolism, Mechanism and Management.* Springfield, Ill., Charles C Thomas Publisher, 1965.

9. Strutz WA, Couves CM, Bondar GF, MacKenzie WC: The effects of muscle stimulation on hind limb flow and/or experimentally produced venous thrombosis. *Surg Forum* 10:428, 1960.

10. Marin HM, Stefanini M: Experimental production of phlebothrombosis. *Surg Gynecol Obstet* 100:263, 1960.

11. Wessler S, Freiman DG, Ballon JD, Katz JH, Wolff R, Wolf E: Experimental pulmonary embolism with serum induced thrombi. *Am J Pathol* 38:89, 1961.

12. Doran FSA, Drury M, Swyer A: A simple way to combat venous stasis which occurs in the lower limbs during surgical operations. *Br J Surg* 51:485, 1964.

13. Browse NL: Effect of surgery on resting calf blood flow. *Br Med J* 1:1714, 1962.

14. Fullerton HW, McDonald GA: The recalcified plasma clotting time as a measure of blood coagulability, in Walker W (ed): *Thrombosis and Anticoagulant Therapy*, Dundee, Univ St. Andrews, 1960.

15. Gormsen J, Haxholdt BF: Operative and postoperative changes in blood coagulation. *Acta Chir Scand* 121:377, 1961.

16. Wille P: Der Einfluss von Operation und Narkose auf den Gerinungsablauf. *Folia Haematol* 3:339, 1959. Cited by Nelson JH Jr: *Atlas of Radical Pelvic Surgery*, New York, Appleton-Century-Crofts, 1977, p 55.

17. Holger-Madsen T, Schioler M: Increased heparin resistance after operation measured by the plasma heparin thrombin time. *Acta Chir Scand* 118:257, 1960.

18. Feruglio G, Sandber H, Bellet S: Postoperative changes in blood coagulation in elderly patients. *Am J Cardiol* 5:477, 1960.

19. Dawborne RY, Earlam F, Evans WH: The relation of the blood platelets to thrombosis after operation and parturition. *J Pathol Bact* 31:833, 1928.

20. Wright HP: Changes in adhesiveness of blood platelets following parturition and surgical operations. *J Pathol Bact* 54:461, 1942.

21. Zucker MB: Unexplained bleeding in operations for neoplasia. *Ann NY Acad Sci* 115:225, 1964.

22. Snell AM: The relation of obesity to fatal postoperative pulmonary embolism. *Arch Surg* 15:237, 1927.

23. Barker NW, Priestly JT: Postoperative thrombophlebitis and embolism. *Surgery* 12:411, 1942.

24. DeBakey ME: A critical evaluation of the problem of thromboembolism. *Surg Gynecol Obstet* 98:1, 1954.

25. Coon WW, Coller FA: Some epidemiologic considerations of thromboembolism. *Surg Gynecol Obstet* 109:489, 1959.

26. Kakkar VV, Howe CT, Nicolaides AN, et al: Deep vein thrombosis of the leg: Is there a high risk group? *Am J Surg* 120:529, 1970.

27. Morris GK, Mitchell JRA: Clinical management of venous thromboembolism. *Br Med Bull* 34(2):169−175, 1978.

28. Rosengarten DS, Laird J, Jeyasingh K, et al: The failure of compression stockings to prevent deep vein thrombosis after operation. *Br J Surg* 57:296, 1970.

29. Holford LP: The effect of graduated static compression on isotopically diagnosed deep venous thrombosis of the leg. *Br J Surg* 63:157, 1976.

30. Scurr JH, Ibrahim SZ, Faber RG, LeQuesne LP: The efficacy of graduated compression stockings in the prevention of deep vein thrombosis. *Br J Surg* 64:371, 1977.

31. Sigel B, Edelstein AL, Savitch L, et al: Type of compression for reducing venous stasis. *Arch Surg* 110:171, 1975.

32. Sevitt S, Gallagher NG: Prevention of venous thrombosis and pulmonary emblism in injured patients. *Lancet* (2):981−989, 1959.

33. Morris GK, Mitchell JRA: Prevention and diagnosis of venous thrombosis in patients with hip fractures. *Lancet* (2):867−869, 1976b.

34. Salzman EW, Harris WH, DeSanctis RW: Reduction in venous thromboembolism by agents affecting platelet function. *N Engl J Med* 284:1287, 1971.

35. Kline A, Hughes LE, Campbell H, et al: Dextran 70 in prophylaxis of thromboembolic disease after surgery. *Br Med J* 2:109, 1975.

36. Renney JTG, O'Sullivan EF, Burke PF: Prevention of postoperative deep vein thrombosis with dipyridamole and aspirin. *Br Med J* 1:992, 1976.

37. Cotton LT, Roberts VC: TThe prevention of postoperative deep venous thrombosis by intermittent compression of the legs, in Bergan JJ and Yao JST (eds): *Venous Problems*. Chicago, Year Book Medical Publishers Inc, 1978, p 554.

38. Sharnoff JG: Results in the prophylaxis of postoperative thromboembolism. *Surg Gynecol Obstet* 123:303, 1966.

39. Verstreete M: The prevention of postoperative deep vein thrombosis and pulmonary embolism with low dose subcutaneous heparin and dextran. *Surg Gynecol Obstet* 143:981, 1976.

40. Gallus AS, Hirsh J, O'Brien SE, et al: Prevention of venous thrombosis with small subcutaneous doses of heparin. *JAMA* 235:1980, 1976.

41. VanGeloven F, Wittebol P, Sixma JJ: Comparison of postoperative Coumadin, dextran 40 and subcutaneous heparin in the prevention of postoperative deep vein thrombosis. *Acta Med Scand* 202:367, 1977.

42. Kutnowski, Vendendris M, Steinberger R, Kraytman M: Prevention of postoperative deep vein thrombosis by low-dose heparin in urological surgery. *Urol Res* 5:123, 1977.

43. Kakker VV, Corrigan TP, Fossard DP, Sutherland I, Thirwell J: Prevention of fatal postoperative pulmonary embolism by low doses of heparin: Reappraisal of results of International Multicentre Trial. *Lancet* 1 (8011):567, 1977.

44. Jackaman JR, Perry BJ, Siddons H: Deep vein thrombosis after thoracology. *Thorax* 33:761, 1978.

45. Sherry S: Preventing pulmonary embolism with heparin in low doses. *Postgrad Med* 59:80, 1976.

46. Wessler S, Yin ET: Theory and practice of minidose heparin in surgical patients: A status report. *Circulation* 47:671, 1973.

47. Erde A, Kakkar VV, Thomas DP, et al: Effect of low dose subcutaneous heparin on whole blood viscosity. *Lancet* 2:342, 1976.

48. Verda D: Discussion in *Venous Disorders.* Chicago, Year Book Medical Publishers Inc, 1978, p 305.

49. Ribaudo JM, Hoellrick RG, McKinnon WMP, et al: Evaluation of minidose heparin administration as a prophylaxis against postoperative pulmonary embolism: A prospective double blind study. *Am J Surg* 5:289, 1975.

50. Lahnborg G, Bergstrom K, Friman L, Lagerglen H: Effect of low dose heparin on incidence of postoperative pulmonary embolism detected by photoscanning. *Lancet* 1:329, 1974.

51. Abernethy EA, Hartsuck JM: Postoperative pulmonary embolism: A prospective study. *Am J Surg* 128:739, 1974.

52. Sagar S, Massey J, Sanderson JM: Low dose heparin prophylaxis against fatal postoperative pulmonary embolism. *Br Med J* 4:257, 1975.

53. Kakkar VV, Corrigan TP, Fossard DP: Prevention of fatal postoperative pulmonary embolism by low doses of heparin: An International Multicentre Trial. *Lancet* 2:45, 1975.

54. Kiil J, Axelsen F, Anderson D: Prophylaxis against postoperative pulmonary embolism and deep vein thrombosis by low dose heparin. *Lancet* 1(8074):1115, 1978.

55. Gruber UF, Duckert F, Fridrich R, Tonhorst J, Rem J: Prevention of postoperative thromboembolism by dextran 40, low doses of heparin or xantinol nicotinate. *Lancet* 1(8005):207, 1977.

56. Pachter HL, Riles TS: Low dose heparin: Bleeding and wound complications in the surgical patient. *Ann Surg* 186:669, 1977.

57. Galle PC, Moss HB, McGrath KM, et al: Thrombocytopenia in two patients treated with low dose heparin. *Obstet Gynecol* 52(1 suppl), 1978, pp 95−115.

58. Kotz HL, Geelhoed GW: Why not low-dose heparin? Lethal thromboembolism and its prevention in pelvic surgery. *Gynec Oncol* 12:271, 1981.

59. Cotton LT, Roberts VC: The prevention of deep vein thrombosis with particular reference to mechnical methods of prevention. *Surgery* 81:228, 1977.

60. Browse NL, Negus D: Prevention of postoperative leg vein thrombosis by electrical muscle stimulation: An evaluation with 125I-labelled fibrinogen. *Br Med J* 3:615−618, 1970.

61. Salzman EW: Physical methods for prevention of venous thromboembolism. *Surgery* 81(2):123, 1977.

62. Hill NH, Pflug JJ, Jeyasingh K, et al: Prevention of deep vein thrombosis by intermittent pneumatic compression of the calf. *Br Med J* 1:131−135, 1972.

63. Kakkar VV: The problems of thrombosis in the deep veins of the leg. *Ann Roy Coll Surg Eng* 45:257, 1969.

64. Nicolaides AN: Diagnosis of venous thrombosis by phlebography, in Bergan JJ and Yao JST (eds): *Venous Problems.* Chicago, Year Book Medical Publishers Inc, 1978, p 123.

65. Browse N: Diagnosis of deep vein thrombosis. *Br Med Bull* 34:163, 1978.

66. Friend J: Personal communication to Nicolaides AN, Hobbs JT, in *Venous Disorders.* Chicago, Year Book Medical Publishers Inc, 1978.

67. Ballard RM, Bradley-Watson PJ, Johnstone FD, et al: Low doses of subcutaneous heparin in the prevention of deep vein thrombosis after gynecologic surgery. *J Obstet Gynecol* 80:469, 1973.

68. Bonnar J, Walsh J: Prevention of thrombosis after pelvic surgery by British dextran 70. *Lancet* 1:614, 1972.

69. Gallus AS, Hirsh J, Tuttle RJ, et al: Small subcutaneous doses of heparin in prevention of venous thrombosis. *N Engl J Med* 288:545, 1973.

70. Flanc C, Kakkar VV, Clarke MB: The detection of venous thrombosis of the legs using 125I-labelled fibrinogen. *Br J Surg* 55:742, 1968.

71. Gordon-Smith IC, Grundy DJ, LeQuesne LP, et al: Controlled trial of two regimes of subcutaneous heparin in prevention of postoperative deep vein thrombosis. *Lancet* 1:1133, 1972.

72. Browse N: Deep vein thrombosis. *Br Med J* 4:676, 1969.

73. Sevitt S, Gallagher N: Venous thrombosis and pulmonary embolism. *Br J Surg* 48:475, 1961.

74. Nicolaides AN: The current status of small-dose subcutaneous heparin in the prevention of venous thromboembolism, in *Venous Disorders*. Chicago, Year Book Medical Publishers Inc, 1978, p 517.

75. DeWeese JA: Venous and lymphatic disease, in Schwartz, (ed): *Principles of Surgery* 2. McGraw-Hill Book Co Inc, 1974, p 916.

76. Neiman HL: Philosophy in the diagnosis of venous thrombosis, in Bergan JJ and Yao JST (eds): *Venous Problems*. Chicago, Year Book Medical Publishers Inc, 1978, p 111.

77. Albrechtsson V, Olsson CG: Thrombotic side-effects of lower limb phlebography. *Lancet* 1:723, 1976.

78. Beltmann MA, Paulin S: Leg phlebography: The incidence, nature and modification of undesirable side effects. *Radiology* 122:101, 1977.

79. Negus D, Pinto DJ, LeQuesne LP, Brown N, Chapman M: 125I-labelled fibrinogen in the diagnosis of deep vein thrombosis and its correlation with phlebography. *Br J Surg* 55:835, 1968.

80. Kakkar V: The diagnosis of deep vein thrombosis using the 125I fibrinogen test. *Arch Surg* 104:152, 1972.

81. Sumner DS: Diagnosis of venous thrombosis by ultrasound, in Bergan JJ and Yao JST (eds): *Venous Problems*. Year Book Medical Publishers Inc, 1978, p 159.

82. Barnes RW: Doppler ultrasonic diganosis, in *Noninvasive Diagnostic Techniques in Vascular Disease*. St. Louis, The CV Mosby Co, 1978, pp 344–350.

83. Sigel B, Felix R, Pophy GL, Ipsen J: Diagnosis of lower limb venous thrombosis by Doppler ultrasound techniques. *Arch Surg* 104:174, 1972.

84. Wheeler HB, Pearson D, O'Connell D, Mullich SG: Impedance phlebography: Technique, interpretation and results. *Arch Surg* 104:164, 1977.

85. Kay SM, Peura RA, Wheeler HB, Anderson FA Jr: Quantitation of the venous outflow portion of an impedance phlebogram. *Proc 3rd Ann Bioengineering Conf* 159, Elmsford, N.Y., Pergamon Press, 1975.

86. Wheeler HB, O'Donnell JA, Anderson FA, et al: Bedside screening for venous thrombosis using occlusive impedance phlebography. *Angiology* 26:199, 1975.

87. Wheeler HB: Impedance phlebography: The diagnosis of venous thrombosis by occlusive plethysmography, in *Noninvasive Diagnostic Techniques in Vascular Disease*. St. Louis, The CV Mosby Co, 1978, pp 259–373.

88. Millar WT, Smith JFB: Localization of deep venous thrombosis using technetium 99^m labeled urokinase. *Lancet* 2:695, 1974.

89. Kempe V, VanDerlinden W, VonScheele C: Diagnosis of deep vein thrombosis with 99^m Tc-streptokinase: A clinical comparison with phlebography. *Br Med J* 4:748, 1974.

90. Ouchi H, Warren R: Detection of intravascular thrombi by means of 131I-labelled plasma. *Surgery* 51:142, 1962.

91. Reich T, Reynolds BM, Healy M, et al: Detection of venous thrombosis in the human by means of radio-iodination antifibrin-fibrinogen antibody. *Surgery* 6:1211, 1966.

92. Charkas ND, Dugan MA, Malmud LS, et al: Labelled leukocytes in thrombi. *Lancet* 2:600, 1974.

93. Highman JH, O'Sullivan E, Thomas E: Isotope venography. *Br J Surg* 60:52, 1973.

94. Henken RE, Yao JST, Quinn JL III, Bergen JJ: Radionuclide venography in lower extremity venous disease. *J Nucl Med* 15:171, 1974.

95. Rosenthall L: Combined inferior vena cavography: Iliac venography and lung imaging with 99ᵐTc albumin macroaggregates. *Radiology* 98:623, 1971.

96. Yao JST, Henkin RE, Conn J Jr, et al: Combined isotope venography and lung scanning. *Arch Surg* 107:146, 1973.

97. Dean RH: Radionuclide venography and simultaneous lung scanning: Evaluation of clin applications of noninvasive diagnostic technique, in *Vascular Disease*. St. Louis, The CV Mosby Co, 1978.

98. Cooke ED, Pilcher MF: Deep vein thrombosis: A preclinical diagnosis by thermography. *Br J Surg* 61:971, 1974.

99. Bergovist D, Hallböök T: Thermography in screening postoperative deep vein thrombosis: A comparison with the 125I fibrinogen test. *Br J Surg* 65:443, 1978.

100. Horowitz RE, Tatter D, in Sherry S, Brinkhaus KM, Genton E, Stingle JM (eds): *Thrombosis*, Washington, D.C., National Academy of Sciences, 1969, pp 19–28.

101. Stein GN, Chen ST, Goldstein F, Israel HL, Finkelstein A: The importance of chest roentgenography in the diagnosis of pulmonary embolism. *Am J Roentgenol Radium Ther Nucl Med* 81:255, 1959.

102. Henderson RR: Pulmonary embolism and infarction. *Med Clin North Am* 48:1425, 1964.

103. Sasahara AA, Sharma GVRL, Tow DE, et al: Methodology in diagnosis of pulmonary embolization, in *Venous Disorders*. Chicago, Year Book Medical Publishers Inc, 1978, p 309.

104. Szucs MM, Brooks HL, Grossman W, et al: Diagnostic sensitivity of laboratory findings in acute pulmonary embolism. *Ann Int Med* 74:161, 1971.

105. Dalen JE, Brooks HL, Johnson LW, et al: Pulmonary angiography in acute pulmonary embolism: Indications, techniques and results in 367 patients. *Am Heart J* 81:175, 1971.

12
Chemotherapy Complications

Jeane P. Hester

The threat of bone marrow myelosuppression and fatal complications from neutropenia and thrombocytopenia to patients receiving multiagent chemotherapeutic regimens has been diminished, but not erased, by the effective use of platelet replacement therapy and granulocytes in conjunction with antibiotics. Although clinical observations since the mid-1960s have documented the impact on survival of replacement with these components, their use has lagged somewhat behind that of red cell replacement.

This lag relates in part to several factors: (*1*) the technology required to collect platelets and granulocytes is more complex than that for red cells; (*2*) standard units of these components cannot be uniformly collected; (*3*) the cell dose that constitutes appropriate physiologic replacement is not totally understood; (*4*) the short half-life of granulocytes and platelets prevents long-term storage; (*5*) alloimmunization remains a major barrier to replacement, and a clinically useful typing system for identification of compatible donor-recipient pairs does not yet exist outside the histocompatibility and ABO typing systems; (*6*) criteria for therapeutic replacement remain somewhat controversial. Prophylactic replacement remains conjectural and currently investigational; (*7*) patient response to replacement is too complex to characterize quantitatively, and clinical observations of improvement used to date do not lend themselves to easy statistical analysis.

These major factors and some of the variables that have an impact on them will be discussed. The data presented here reflect experience with component collection by continuous-flow centrifugation technology and transfusion observations in adult leukemia patients with pancytopenias secondary to bone marrow hypoplasia or leukemic infiltrate, but the physiologic principles of replacement

Supported in part by grants No. CA-19806 and CA-28153 from the Department of Health, Education, and Welfare, Public Health Service, National Cancer Institute, National Institutes of Health, Bethesda, Maryland, and the IBM Corporation, Dayton, New Jersey.

should apply to patients with solid tumors, if therapeutic modalities are used that result in severe myelosuppression.

COLLECTION TECHNOLOGY

The simple centrifugation of a single unit of anticoagulated normal whole blood provided the first blood components: packed red cells and platelet-rich plasma. This technology was available in the 1950s and was described by Adams et al. (1). The quantitative differences in peripheral blood concentration of red cells (10^{12}/l), platelets (10^{11}/l), and leukocytes (10^9/l) demonstrated that the total yield of platelets and leukocytes contained in a single unit of whole blood would be inadequate for replacement. This fact provided the impetus for the development of technology directed toward collection of these two cellular components.

Leukocyte Collection

The development in the 1960s of the NCI-IBM blood cell separator provided the first clinically useful closed, sterile system for collection of leukocytes from the blood of hematologically normal donors (2). By means of extracorporeal anticoagulation with citrate and donor attachment to the instrument by venipuncture, large volumes of normal donor blood could be continually extracted and separated in a centrifugal field and returned to the donor after a small fraction of leukocytes (approximately 30%) to be used for replacement were extracted. An average of 10 liters of donor blood was processed in 180 minutes. Granulocyte collection was greatly enhanced by adding a macromolecular red cell sedimenting agent, usually 6% hydroxyethyl starch, and by inducing granulocytosis in the donor by using oral or intravenous steroids or other agents such as intramuscular etiocholanolone (3,4). Without these modifications, leukocyte yields were usually well below 10 billion (10×10^9) and were predominantly mononuclear leukocytes.

Variables relating to granulocytes harvested from normal donors by continuous-flow centrifugation techniques developed in the 1970s using the single-stage disposable channel were described by Hester et al. (5). They define the statistically important contribution of the donor leukocyte/granulocyte count preprocedure to the granulocyte yield. This is a biologic variable that can be only partially manipulated through the use of leukocytosis-inducing agents and that will always result in a variable dose of cells collected for transfusion. However, it was possible to construct a mathematical model relating donor precount, blood volume, and collect volume variables by which the granulocyte yield can be predicted, and when the cell dose (minimum and maximum) is defined that correlates with infection prevention or infection control, it should be possible to modify the donor-procedure variables so that an optimal cell dose can be collected. Average leukocyte yields through the late 1970s from conventional technology were $15-20 \times 10^9$ leukocytes, of which 50%–80% were granulocytes. The mean leukocyte yield in the disposable single-stage channel after 8.8 liters of blood was processed in 165 minutes was 33×10^9 cells, a significant increment.

The relationship of donor precount to total leukocyte yield for the IBM 2997 single-stage channel is shown in Figure 1. The relevance of premedicating the donor to produce a shift in the differential to granulocytosis and of producing a leukocytosis is also shown. This figure demonstrates that in unstimulated donors, the percent of granulocytes in the collect generally parallels the donor peripheral blood differential and is considerably lower than that achieved in premedicated donors, in whom 80%−90% of circulating leukocytes are granulocytes.

Donor Selection for Granulocyte Replacement

Primary family members (siblings, parents, offspring) are screened and selected on the basis of ABO and HLA compatibility. Donors who are both HLA− and ABO− compatible are selected as first donors followed by HLA− incompatible/ABO-compatible donors, then HLA- and ABO-incompatible donors. The genetic distribution of HLA antigens indicates that a sibling has a 25% chance of sharing both HLA haplotypes and of being HLA-compatible, a 50% chance of sharing one HLA haplotype, and a 25% chance of sharing no HLA haplotypes. Parents and offspring always share one haplotype. If HLA typing is not available, selection of ABO-compatible primary family members is considered appropriate. If ABO-incompatible donors must be used, limitation of crosscellular red blood cell contamination in the granulocyte pack to hematocrits <5% reduces the risk of unacceptable toxicity to the recipient, which might be manifested as anaphylaxis and/or intravascular hemolysis. In the absence of sufficient donors from the primary family unit, second-degree relatives (aunts, uncles, grandchildren) are screened as potential donors because they may share one HLA haplotype with the patient.

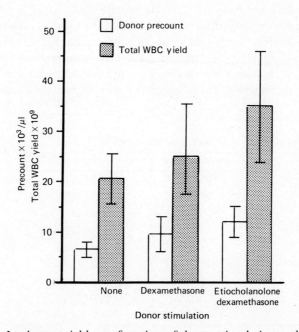

Figure 1. Leukocyte yield as a function of donor stimulation and precount.

Guidelines for frequency of donation are arbitrary, but male donors are allowed to donate on four consecutive days and females on three consecutive days. An average interval of ≥ 30 days is then required before redonation. This interval has also been chosen arbitrarily, and final donation-frequency guidelines will depend on studies in progress that fully define long-term risks of exposure to leukocytosis-inducing agents, anticoagulants, and red cell sedimenting agents used in the procedure. Donor risks from such procedures include (1) citrate-induced hypocalcemia with circumoral and/or peripheral parasthesias, nausea, vomiting, carpopedal spasm, QT interval changes; (2) plasma expansion from macromolecular sedimenting agents with resultant weight gain, peripheral edema, and headaches from fluid shifts; (3) technology-related risks such as red cell hemolysis, infusion of air emboli, macroscopic and/or microscopic platelet aggregates and/or inappropriate cellular depletion (usually platelets). Granulocyte donors responding to a survey questionnaire indicated that hypocalcemic symptoms were the most commonly experienced ones encountered during collection procedures. Other symptoms and their frequency are listed in Table 1.

Recipient Response

Clinical experience has indicated for some time that granulocyte replacement is beneficial in the therapeutic setting of progressive infection unresponsive to antibiotic therapy. These benefits were clearly shown by Graw et al. in 1972 (6) for neutropenic patients with bacteremia. Antibiotic management is, without a doubt, sufficient for infection control in some patients, but prognostic variables that would predict a favorable response to antibiotics alone do not currently exist. Complete protective environment isolation has significantly reduced, but not eliminated, bacterial/fungal flora and infection (7). Scientific data were lacking that would quantitatively characterize the many variables influencing the course of neutropenic infections to substantiate the clinical observations. Neutropenic animal models that would yield conclusive data through systematic study and correlation of each of the variables have now been reported and provide us with some of the clearest data relative to neutropenia, infection, and survival. They delineate the relationship between the dose of bacterial inoculum and the

Table 1. Granulocyte Donor Survey: Intrapheresis Symptoms

Variable	+ Symptoms	− Symptoms	Unknown[a]
1. Hypocalcemia	135 (58%)	80 (35%)	16 (7%)
2. Headache	56 (24%)	137 (59%)	38 (17%)
3. Weight gain	50 (22%)	145 (63%)	30 (15%)
4. Muscular cramps	22 (10%)	163 (71%)	46 (19%)
5. Nausea	21 (9%)	168 (73%)	42 (18%)
6. Visual disturbances	15 (7%)	176 (76%)	40 (17%)
7. Chest pain	13 (6%)	171 (74%)	47 (20%)
8. Indigestion	9 (4%)	175 (76%)	47 (20%)
9. Menses	6 (6%)	96 (94%)	

[a]Questionnaire not answered.

onset of infection, the subsequent response to antibiotics and/or granulocyte replacement by reduction in intravascular bacterial growth, and the alloim-munizing influence of prior granulocyte transfusions (8,9). Such studies cannot be duplicated in human trials, but this animal work may provide us data from which we can derive guidelines for determining criteria for replacement.

Protocols commonly used for adult leukemia patients with a circulating neutrophil concentration $<1 \times 10^3/\mu l$ call for initiation of antibiotic therapy for temperature elevations $\geq 38°C$, when pyrexia is unrelated to blood component transfusions, immunotherapy, or chemotherapy. Granulocyte replacement therapy may be initiated after 48–72 hours of antibiotic trials if a reduction in temperature below 38°C has not been achieved, if blood cultures remain positive, or if there is evidence of progressive infection (pneumonia, cellulitis, etc.). Granulocyte replacement is usually carried out until control of infection is achieved or bone marrow recovery occurs. McCredie et al. (10) reported that control of infection correlated with the number of granulocyte transfusions given during neutropenic sepsis. Patients who received four to eight transfusions had a better clinical response than those who received one or two replacement transfusions. Patients who received nine or more transfusions had a lower response rate. This result was interpreted as a failure to control the underlying neoplastic disease or prolonged marrow aplasia, rather than a failure per se of granulocytes. The appearance of antibody-mediated immune destruction of the transfused granulocytes could not be ruled out. The organisms responsible for the majority of infections (pneumonia and/or septicemia) in this study were *Klebsiella, Candida,* and *Pseudomonas.*

Randomized trials of therapeutic granulocyte replacement showing survival advantage to patients receiving such replacement are reported by Higby et al. (11). Vogler et al. (12) have reported a correlation between cell dose $\geq 20 \times 10^9$ and survival. Prophylactic granulocyte replacement (13) resulted in a decrease in serious infection and a reduction in the percentage of neutropenic days febrile >38° but did not prevent infection. Prophylactic replacement is promising but still investigational until problems of cell dose, alloimmunization, and procedure-induced donor toxicity are solved.

The duration of neutropenia is a biologic variable in patients that cannot be predicted, that varies with each course of chemotherapy, and that has an impact on infection and the need for granulocyte replacement. An analysis of patients receiving prophylactic or therapeutic granulocyte replacement (Table 2) revealed that a significant number of them experienced no infection if the duration of neutropenia was ≤ 10 days (13). Patients having fever of unknown origin or local infection averaged <15 days of neutropenia, compared with a median of 17 days of neutropenia in patients with pneumonia and bacteremia. No course of chemotherapy that produced neutropenia for ≥ 16 days was associated with an absence of infection.

The most common infections associated with death in adult leukemia patients during induction chemotherapy are pneumonia and/or bacteremia and/or disseminated fungal infection. In a recently completed analysis of the cause of death in patients failing to enter remission (14), 59% died of infection alone, suggesting that optimal supportive care regimens of antibiotics and granulocyte replacement have still not been achieved. Deaths occurring during the first 2

Table 2. Comparisons of Infection Between Prophylactic and Therapeutic P.M.N. Replacement

	Patients Experiencing Infection(%)							
	Duration of Myelosuppression (Days)							
	0	10	11	15	16	20	>21	
Type of Infection	PP[b]	TP[c]	PP	TP	PP	TP	PP	TP
None	23%	47%	8%	0	0	0	0	0
FUO-local[a]	54%	15%	69%	53%	17%	27%	50%	9%
Pneumonia-bacteremia	23%	37%	23%	47%	83%	63%	50%	91%

[a]Fever of unknown origin.
[b]Prophylactic P.M.N.
[c]Therapeutic P.M.N.

weeks tended to be bacterial. Fungal-related deaths tended to predominate late in the course of treatment (J.P. Hester, unpublished data). Survival advantage could be seen for patients receiving granulocyte replacement in addition to antibiotics, compared with those who did not, although death ultimately occurred when recovery of normal bone marrow did not take place.

A median survival time of 50 days (range 19–95) was observed in leukemia patients receiving granulocyte replacement who subsequently failed to enter complete remission. This period of time permitted at least two courses of chemotherapy to be administered in an effort to achieve remission.

The effectiveness of granulocyte replacement has been clinically evaluated in terms of lysis of fever, clearing of infection, and survival. The quantitative response to granulocyte replacement is usually evaluated in terms of the posttransfusion granulocyte count. The observed posttransfusion increment is directly related to the number of cells transfused and inversely related to the recipient blood volume. The absolute granulocyte increment and its relationship to the number of granulocytes transfused is shown in Figure 2 and suggests that transfusion cell doses of 30×10^9 cells will be needed to give a mean posttransfusion peripheral count of $1 \times 10^3/\mu l$, the level described by Bodey et al. (15) to correlate with risk of spontaneous infection. The standard deviation is as great as the mean, indicating that numerous other variables are also affecting the transfusion response. Two of these variables relate to ABO and HLA typing of donor-recipient pairs.

The influence of ABO and HLA compatibility on the immediate (t=0) and 1-hour (t=1) posttransfusion corrected increments is shown in Table 3 for approximately 1,000 therapeutic replacement transfusions. A forward stepwise regression analysis relating the increment to (1) pretransfusion granulocyte level, (2) height of temperature, (3) ABO compatibility, (4) HLA compatibility, and (5) dose of cells transfused indicated ABO and HLA compatibility between donor-recipient pairs were statistically the most significant determinants of the posttransfusion corrected increment.

Granulocyte recovery after transfusion is complicated by the kinetic properties of granulocytes as well as by patient variables. Kinetic studies indicate that

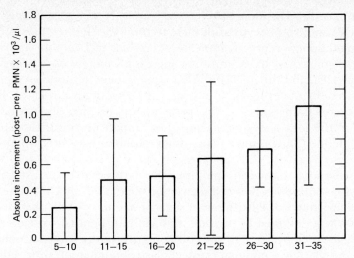

Figure 2. The relationship of absolute granulocyte increment to total granulocytes transfused.

Table 3. Posttransfusion Corrected Increments[a] Related to HLA and ABO

| HLA | | ABO | |
		Compatible	Incompatible
	t=0	.624	.288
Compatible			
	t=1	.652	.408
	t=0	.476	.150
Incompatible			
	t=1	.464	.212

[a]P.M.N. $\times$ $10^3/\mu l/10^{10}$ P.M.N./M² body surface area.

a large portion of granulocytes are not in the circulating pool but in the marginating pool and cannot be measured. Additionally, the rate of egress into infected tissues is variable and cannot be measured. The posttransfusion granulocyte count reflects only that fraction of cells in the circulating pool. The short half-life predicts the impossibility of maintaining an adequate peripheral blood granulocyte level for 24 hours based on the number of cells it is possible to collect and transfuse by current technology.

PLATELET COLLECTION AND REPLACEMENT

Collection

For many years the primary sources of platelet concentrates have been pooled units of platelets harvested from single units of whole blood drawn for RBC replacement, multiple-bag plateletpheresis from single donors, and the semicontinuous-flow Haemonetics blood cell separator. Crosscellular contamination with RBC and lymphocytes with these technologies is often macroscopic and requires an additional centrifugation step to reduce it. Lymphocyte contamination was recognized to have immunologic disadvantages to the recipient by Herzig et al. (16), and the need for ABO compatibility of donor-recipient pairs was suggested by Aster (17). However, the quantitative role of RBC and lymphocyte contamination and the presence or absence of lymphocytotoxic antibodies in the sera of recipients and their impact on transfusion have been difficult to define (18,19), since many other variables may alter the transfusion response.

Platelet collection has been simplified by a disposable dual-stage channel developed for continuous-flow cell separation technology by IBM. This channel, which combines the two centrifugation steps of manual plateletpheresis into one process (20), was designed to provide uniformly suspended platelets ready for transfusion at the completion of the collection procedure (no resuspension time required) and that have minimal crosscellular contamination with red cells and lymphocytes. Like granulocyte collection in the single-stage continuous-flow channel, platelet collection in this system correlates with the height of the donor platelet count, the amount of blood processed, and the volume of concentrate collected. Platelet yield will be sufficiently predictable to allow collection of a cell dose appropriate for physiologic replacement.

Replacement

Effective platelet replacement results in either prevention of hemorrhage (prophylactic replacement) or restoration of hemostasis in a thrombocytopenic patient with active hemorrhage. There is a quantitative relationship between the degree of platelet depletion in the peripheral blood and the risk of hemorrhage. While this relationship is not absolute, spontaneous life-threatening hemorrhage is more likely to occur at platelet counts below $20,000/\mu l$ (22). In acute leukemia patients, cerebrovascular and massive gastrointestinal hemorrhage are the most common causes of fatal hemorrhage. In a recent study, 11% of leukemia patients failing to enter remission died of hemorrhage alone, and 16% died of hemorrhage and infection (14).

Djerassi and Farber observed in 1965 (22) that hemostasis was more consistently apparent in patients whose posttransfusion platelet counts were increased by $\geq 40,000/\mu l$ than in those whose counts were increased by $<20,000/\mu l$.

The value of prophylactic replacement was demonstrated by Higby et al. (23) in a randomized study in which patients received three units of platelet concentrates/M^2 or equal volumes of platelet-poor plasma twice weekly. Deaths attributed to hemorrhage alone occurred in 15% of patients receiving platelet concentrates and in 63% of controls.

Short-term replacement therapy has been effective with platelets collected and transfused from random donors. It has been appreciated for many years that successful long-term replacement depends in large part on whether alloimmunization occurs. Immunologic destruction of platelets is difficult to evaluate. Antibody production in patients exposed to blood products is nonuniform in terms of the type of antibody produced, the time to onset of antibodies, the dose of incompatible cells required to induce an antibody response, and the ability of the patient to mount an immune response (24,25,26).

Yankee (27) recognized the relevance of the HLA typing system in identifying related compatible donor-recipient pairs and demonstrated that aplastic anemia patients could be supported for prolonged periods. The HLA system was subsequently used for unrelated donors as well. Improved increments could be identified in patients receiving platelets from unrelated donors who shared at least two of the HLA antigens. For patients with splenomegaly, the posttransfusion increment was poor and appeared to be independent of HLA antigen sharing with the donor (28).

Because of the difficulty in finding HLA-compatible unrelated donors, Duquesnoy et al. (29) investigated and reported the feasibility of identifying donors with lesser degrees of histocompatibility. Many HLA antigens show serologic cross-reactivity, and there is some experimental evidence that they may have low immunogenicity to transplant or transfusion recipients (30). Platelet recovery in alloimmunized refractory patients averaged 35%−40% using this identification system. Schiffer (31) reported that lymphocytotoxic antibodies were commonly present in 50%−60% of adult leukemia patients within 3− weeks after platelet replacement transfusions were initiated. The patients on whom he reported received an average of 11 replacement transfusions during 3−4 weeks of induction chemotherapy, suggesting that alloimmunization may have a significant impact on most patients. Schiffer (32) also directed attention to the fact that potential transmission of hepatitis, cytomegalovirus, toxoplasmosis, and secondary bacterially contaminated concentrates is a small but real risk to patients receiving blood component replacement.

Recipient clinical variables that also reduce the effectiveness of platelet replacement include (1) splenomegaly with sequestration, (2) disseminated intravascular coagulopathies, (3) active hemorrhage, and (4) pyrexia/infection. Other variables such as platelet viability and chemoimmunotherapy that may alter transfusion effectiveness are under investigation.

Patient response has been commonly reported in terms of the number of units transfused and the posttransfusion platelet increment/unit transfused/M^2 of body surface area. Most investigators correct the calculations for an assumed 30% sequestration by the spleen. The number of platelets in each unit is quite variable and ranges from $\leq 0.4 \times 10^{11}$ to $\geq 1.0 \times 10^{11}$, so that the evaluation of the response to transfusion in terms of units is imprecise and impedes the understanding of dose-response relationships. Table 4, derived from data obtained from five patients and eight transfusions, illustrates the relationship between cell dose ($\times 10^{11}$ cells) and blood volume estimates (2.5L/M^2) and illustrates that a low posttransfusion count may merely reflect transfusion of an inadequate number of cells. Additionally, recovery of 95% of the transfused platelets in one patient suggests that splenic sequestration may or may not be present in patients without clinical splenomegaly.

The posttransfusion increment is related to the number of platelets transfused, the blood volume of the recipient, and the presence or absence of single or multiple variables known to diminish platelet recovery.

The expected posttransfusion count, if 100% of transfused platelets could be recovered, is shown in Figure 3 for a range of cell doses and recipient blood

Table 4. Relationship of Recipient Body Surface Area, Cell Dose Transfused, and Posttransfusion Increment, Dual-Stage Channel

Blood Volume (Liters)	Number of Cells Transfused ($\times 10^{11}$)	Posttransfusion Increment $\times 10^3/\mu l$ Observed	Expected[a]	% Recovery
1.25	4.4	215	270	80
3.7	6.6	99	162	62
3.75	7.0	174	184	95
4.25	1.6	25	35	72
4.25	3.6	69	80	87
4.25	5.0	101	115	88
5.0	1.05	14	20	70
5.0	7.2	109	140	78

[a] 100% recovery.

volume estimates and serves as a baseline for our current evaluation of response to platelet replacement. Calculating the absolute increment observed (I_0 = pre-post count $\times 10^3/\mu l$) gives clinically useful information because it establishes whether or not a concentration of platelets was achieved that could be expected to restore hemostasis. A level $\geq 40,000/\mu l$ was observed to correlate with a corrected bleeding time (30) if the patient was not receiving drugs known to inhibit platelet function. Calculation of the expected increment (I_E = number of cells transfused/blood volume) and percent recovery after transfusion ($I_0/I_E \times$ 100%) allows some evaluation of recipient clinical variables that may be influencing recovery.

Platelet recovery in adult leukemia patients receiving single-donor platelets collected in the dual-stage channel ranged from 0%–100%, but the mean was 40% for all studies, testifying to the many variables contributing to the transfusion response. Based on this mean recovery, a cell dose of $\geq 1.0 \times 10^{11}$ cells/1.0 l blood volume ($I_E = 1 \times 10^5/\mu l$) would in general provide a posttransfusion increment sufficient to provide hemostasis ($I_0 = 0.4 \times I_E$). Efforts should then be directed toward ensuring adequate cell doses from all collecting technologies.

Single-donor platelets for patients requiring long-term support are preferred over pooled units from multiple donors, because they reduce the number of donor antigens (HLA, B-cell, non-B-cell) to which the patient is exposed. Like granulocyte donors, primary family members (siblings, parents, offspring) who share HLA antigens can be selected as donors. Secondary family members (grandchildren, aunts, uncles, cousins) can be screened for family haplotypes. If patients will subsequently require granulocyte replacement from such family donors, prior exposure to platelets may sensitize patients to granulocyte replacement. Data do not yet exist to support this statement, but granulocyte concentrates have crosscellular contamination with lymphocytes and platelets. Unrelated/random single donors may be used for nonimmunized patients until evidence of alloimmunization appears.

The use of autologous frozen platelets collected from patients during remission has been reported by Schiffer (31) as an alternative in management of alloimmunized patients. Investigation of platelet-freezing technology is un-

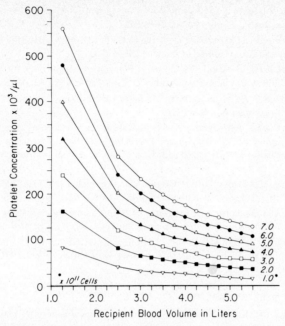

Figure 3. Absolute platelet increment ($\times 10^3/\mu$l) relative to recipient blood volume and number of cells transfused.

derway so that freeze-thaw losses that significantly reduce the number of cells available for transfusion can be minimized. Refinement in techniques would allow more widespread use of frozen platelets.

REFERENCES

1. Adams WS, Blahd WH, Basseth SH: A method of human plasmapheresis. *Proc Soc Exp Biol Med* 80:377, 1952.

2. Freireich EJ, Judson G, Levin RH: Separation and collection of leukocytes. *Cancer Res* 25:1516, 1965.

3. McCredie KB, Freireich EJ, Hester JP, Vallejos C: Increased granulocyte collection with the blood cell separator and the addition of etiocholanolone and hydroxyethyl starch. *Transfusion* 14:357, 1974.

4. Mischler JM, Higby DJ, Rhomberg W, Cohen E, Nicora RW, Holland JF: Hydroxyethyl starch and dexamethasone as an adjunct to leukocyte separation with the IBM blood cell separator. *Transfusion* 14:352, 1974.

5. Hester JP, Kellogg RM, Mulzet AP, Kruger VR, McCredie KB, Freireich EJ: Principles of blood separation and component extraction in a disposable continuous-flow single-stage channel. *Blood* 54:254, 1979.

6. Graw RG, Herzig G, Perry S, Henderson G: Normal granulocyte transfusion therapy: Treatment of septicemia due to gram negative sepsis. *N Engl J Med* 287:367, 1972.

7. Rodriguez V, Bodey GP, Freireich EJ, McCredie KB, Gutterman JU, Keating MJ, Smith TL, Gehan EA: Randomized trial of protected environment: Prophylactic antibiotics in 145 adults with acute leukemia. *Medicine* 3:253, 1978.

8. Epstein RB, Waxman FJ, Bennett BT, Andersen BR: Pseudomonas septicemia in neutropenic dogs: I. Treatment with granulocyte transfusions. *Transfusion* 14:51, 1974.

9. Applebaum FR, Trapani RJ, Graw RG Jr: Consequences of prior alloimmunization during granulocyte transfusion. *Transfusion* 17:460, 1977.

10. McCredie KB, Freireich EJ, Hester JP, Vallejos C: Leukocyte transfusion therapy for patients with host-defense failure. *Transplant Proc* 3:1285, 1973.

11. Higby DJ, Yates J, Henderson E, Holland JF: Filtration leukapheresis for granulocyte transfusion therapy: Clinical and laboratory studies. *N Engl J Med* 292:761, 1975.

12. Vogler WR, Winton EF, Larson DH: Methods of collection and results of transfusion of granulocytes. *Exp Hematol* 6(3):93, 1978.

13. Hester JP, McCredie KB, Freireich EJ: Advances in supportive care: Blood component transfusion, in *Care of the Child with Cancer,* Proceedings of the American Cancer Society National Conference on the Care of the Child with Cancer, Philadelphia, George F Stickley Co, 1979, pp 93–N100.

14. Estey E, Keating MJ, Bodey GP, McCredie KB, Freireich EJ: Causes of failure of remission induction in acute myelogenous leukemia (AML). *Am Soc Clin Oncol* 21:436, 1980.

15. Bodey GP, Buckley M, Sathe YS, Freireich EJ: Quantitative relationships between circulating leukocytes and infection in patients with acute leukemia. *Ann Intern Med* 64:328, 1966.

16. Herzig RH, Herzig GP, Bull MI, Decter JA, Lohrmann HP, Stout RG, Yankee RA, Graw RG Jr: Correction of poor platelet transfusion responses with leukocyte-poor HLA matched platelet concentrates. *Blood* 46:743, 1975.

17. Aster R: Effect of anticoagulant and ABO incompatibility on recovery of transfused human platelets. *Blood* 26(6):732, 1965.

18. Mannoni P, Bracq C, Rodet M, Duedari N: Immunological aspects of platelet transfusions, in *Proceedings of the XVII Congress of the International Society of Hematology,* 1978, p. 317.

19. Herzig RH, Terasaki PI, Trapani RJ, Herzig GP, Graw RG Jr: The relationship between donor-recipient lymphocytotoxicity and the transfusion response using HLA matched platelet concentrates. *Transfusion* 17:657, 1977.

20. Hester JP, Kellogg RM, McCreide KB, Freireich EJ: Platelet (Plt) collection and transfusion (Tx) with IBM 2997 two stage disposable channel. *Am Soc Clin Oncol* 19:416, 1978.

21. Gaydos LA, Freireich EJ: The quantitative relation between platelet count and hemorrhage in patients with acute leukemia. *N Engl J Med* 266:905, 1962.

22. Djerassi I, Farber S: Control and prevention of hemorrhage: Platelet transfusion. *Cancer Res* 25:1499, 1965.

23. Higby DJ, Cohen E, Holland JF, Sinks L: The prophylactic treatment of thrombocytopenic leukemic patients with platelets: A double blind study. *Transfusion* 5:440, 1974.

24. Shulman NR: Immunological considerations attending platelet transfusion. *Transfusion* 6:39, 1966.

25. Thorsby E, Astri H, Gjmedal E: Repeated platelet transfusion from HLA compatible unrelated and sibling donors. *Tissue Antigens* 2:397, 1972.

26. Bondevik H: Antibody response after single dose human alloimmunization. *Transplantation* 21:57, 1976.

27. Yankee RA: Importance of histocompatibility in platelet therapy. *Vox Sang* 20:419, 1971.

28. Hester JP, McCredie KB, Freireich EJ: Platelet replacement *Progress in Clinical and Biological Research—The Blood Platelet in Transfusion Therapy.* New York, Alan R Liss Inc, 1978, pp 281–293.

29. Duquesnoy RJ, Filip DJ, Aster RH: Influence of HLA-A2 on the effectiveness of platelet transfusions in alloimmunized thrombocytopenic patients. *Blood* 50(3):407, 1977.

30. Columbani J, Colombani M, Degos J, Terrier E, Gandy Y, Dastot H: Effect of cross reactions on HLA antigen immunogenicity. *Tissue Antigens* 4:135, 1974.

31. Schiffer CA, Lichtenfeld JL, Wiernik PH: Antibody response in patients with acute nonlymphocytic leukemia. *Cancer* 37(5):2177, 1976.

32. Schiffer CA, Aisner J, Wiernik PH: Platelet transfusion therapy for patients with leukemia, in Greenwalt TJ, Jamieson GA (eds): *Progress in Clinical and Biological Research—The Blood Platelet in Transfusion Therapy.* New York, Alan R Liss Inc, 1978, pp 267–279.

13

Complications of Parenteral and Oral Alimentation, Subclavian Catheter Insertion, Thoracentesis, and Paracentesis

C. Robert Stanhope

Complications of parenteral and oral alimentation, subclavian catheter insertion, thoracentesis, or paracentesis are apt to occur on any gynecologic oncology service. Early recognition of complications lessens their potential adversity and is accomplished by close attention to details and frequent, careful examination of the patient.

COMPLICATIONS OF TOTAL PARENTERAL NUTRITION

Total parenteral nutrition (TPN), a modern technique of intravenous feeding, is indicated for patients not able to maintain adequate nutrition by oral alimentation. In gynecologic oncology, TPN is commonly used after intestinal bypass for radiation injury or obstruction; while indolent wounds or bowel fistulas heal; and when the gastrointestinal tract is shortened, nonfunctional, or being rested in a patient with severe enteritis or colitis.

TPN solutions combine essential amino acids, electrolytes, and hypertonic dextrose and are highly hyperosmolar (1,800–2,400 mOsm/l). If infused through a peripheral vein, such a hypertonic solution would cause severe phlebitis and thrombosis; therefore, a central venous catheter is commonly used for TPN administration.

Complications of TPN use may be metabolic (resulting from the effects of

255

hyperosmolar electrolyte solutions), infective, or traumatic (resulting from the insertion of a central venous catheter).

Metabolic Complications Associated with TPN

Metabolic complications result from the use of hypertonic glucose or amino acid solutions, or from deficiencies that develop in fatty acids, trace elements, or vitamins. Because TPN solutions contain hypertonic dextrose, infusion must begin slowly, to allow the body to increase endogenous insulin in response to the large amount of glucose. If the production of endogenous insulin is inadequate or if the rate of TPN infusion is too rapid, glucose will not be metabolized adequately and hyperglycemia will result. Therefore, the patient's blood and urine sugar levels should be carefully monitored. Ideally, the blood sugar should not exceed 200 mg% and the urine sugar should be 2+ or less. Values in excess of these indicate hyperglycemia and are treated by adding insulin or by decreasing the rate of TPN infusion.

Hyperglycemia

Persistent severe hyperglycemia can lead to hyperosmolar hyperglycemic non-ketotic coma (1). This condition is the result of an intense osmotic diuresis that can cause profound dehydration, progressive lethargy, mental confusion, coma, or even death. Hyperosmolar hyperglycemic nonketotic coma is further characterized by the absence of acetone in the serum or urine, serum blood sugar in the range of 700–1,200 mg%, and serum osmolality in the range of 270–500 mOsm/l.

Treatment involves infusion of 5–9 liters of hypotonic saline (0.45 NS) and injection of insulin. Insulin requirements vary; markedly sensitive patients may experience unexpected lowering of blood sugar after as little as 10 units of regular insulin has been administered, whereas other patients seem resistant to insulin and require a total of 300–700 units of regular insulin for their blood sugar to be lowered. During fluid replacement, hypokalemia sometimes develops and potassium replacement may be necessary. Outcome is poor when there are delays in diagnosis or inadequate fluid or insulin therapy.

Hypoglycemia

Hypoglycemia can occur after any significant decreases in the rate of infusion of TPN. The pancreatic islet cells are stimulated to produce insulin during infusion of TPN, and this elevated level of insulin may decrease slowly after cessation of TPN. Therefore, TPN should be discontinued gradually over a 12- to 36-hour period. If a patient is suspected of being hypoglycemic, her blood sugar level should immediately be determined and additional intravenous glucose given. After TPN administration is completed, the patient should be given isotonic glucose for at least 6 hours, to make certain hypoglycemia will not occur.

Hyperammonemia

Hyperammonemia occurs in neonates or in patients with hepatic dysfunction who receive either protein hydrolysates or crystalline amino acid solutions.

Tension pneumothorax must be recognized immediately and treated. Patients experience pleural pain, hypoxia, and acute air hunger; systolic blood pressure may drop suddenly and cardiopulmonary arrest may occur.

Physical findings in patients experiencing tension pneumothorax include a shift in the location of the cardiac apical pulse, a contralateral tracheal shift, hyperresonance on percussion, and an absence of breath sounds over the affected lung. The immediate steps to relieve tension pneumothorax are aspiration of the involved pleural space using a large-bore needle inserted into the second anterior interspace, followed by thoracostomy and insertion of a chest tube connected to closed waterseal drainage.

Embolic Phenomena

Air embolism is a fatal but avoidable complication of central venous catheterization. The catheter tip, when positioned within a large vessel such as the superior vena cava, is subject to the negative pressure of the thorax and a considerable amount of air may suddenly enter the circulatoy system during deep inspiration, particularly if the needle is open and the patient is not supine or is not in Trendelenburg's position. The sign of an air embolus is a sudden rise in venous pressure concomitant with hypotension. A rapid thready pulse, syncope, and cyanosis occur. A loud "milk wheel" murmur, a result of air in the right atrium and pulmonary artery, may be heard directly over the precordium. This air partially blocks the flow of blood into the right side of the heart and out of the heart to the lungs. The immediate treatment is to place the patient in the left lateral position to allow the air in the right ventricle to rise into the right atrium and superior vena cava. The patient's head should be lowered to prevent air from entering the cerebral circulation in case arterial air embolization has occurred. Aspiration of the air may be accomplished if there is a catheter present in the right atrium or superior vena cava. Immediate thoracotomy and needle aspiration of the right ventricle are possible life-saving measures (6,7,8).

Thrombosis of the subclavian vein causes pain and swelling of the affected upper extremity and can be confirmed by venogram. Continuous intravenous heparin therapy is suggested for 7–10 days, at which time the thrombus should be organized and propagation is unlikely. Upper extremity swelling may persist for an extended period of time.

Pulmonary Embolism

Pulmonary embolism can occur in association with the use of the intravenous polyethylene subclavian catheter. Supportive care after pulmonary embolism is discussed elsewhere in this book.

Catheter Embolism

Catheter embolism has also been reported. The most common cause of this condition is breaking or shearing of the catheter by the sharp beveled needle used for insertion. Extreme caution must be taken never to withdraw the catheter through the sharp beveled needle. In the event that a piece of polyethylene catheter is missing and embolization is suspected, a chest x-ray film should be taken to determine the exact position of the catheter. If the patient's condition allows it, cardiac catheterization or thoracotomy for removal of the segment is recommended (9). Leaving the catheter in situ can result in sepsis, endocarditis, or perforation of the heart.

COMPLICATIONS OF THORACENTESIS

Pneumothorax

The most common complication of thoracentesis is pneumothorax, in which an air leak is caused either by puncture or laceration of the lung or by the improper use of a three-way stopcock. Patients are frequently asymptomatic; however, some experience shoulder pain or a heavy feeling in the chest. Occasionally, a chest x-ray film taken immediately after thoracentesis shows no evidence of pneumothorax, but a subsequent film 12–24 hours later, after symptoms have developed, reveals a large pneumothorax. The treatment for pneumothorax has been considered earlier in this chapter. The risk of lung puncture or laceration by a needle during thoracentesis is reduced if coughing can be suppressed. This can usually be accomplished by pretreating the patient with meperidine or codeine.

Empyema

Contamination of the pleural space or puncture of an infected lung may lead to the development of an empyema. Treatment consists of surgical drainage and appropriate antibiotics. Antibiotics have greatly reduced the frequency of this complication.

Hemorrhage

Hemorrhage into the pleural cavity may occur after injury of a pulmonary or intercostal blood vessel. In addition, hemorrhage into the peritoneal cavity can occur after thoracentesis if the diaphragm is markedly elevated or if the tap has been performed too low and the spleen, liver, or other abdominal viscera have been injured.

COMPLICATIONS OF PARACENTESIS

Perforation of a Viscus

In most situations, the introduction of a needle into the abdominal cavity carries little risk, even if the needle punctures the bowel. If the bowel is greatly distended, however, or if the perforating instrument is not a needle but a large-bore trochar, leakage and widespread peritonitis are likely. After leakage of intestinal contents into the abdominal cavity, patients experience abdominal pain and progressive signs of peritonitis. Abdominal x-ray films frequently show free air. A patient in whom there is a suspicion of leakage should be observed carefully and broad-spectrum antibiotic coverage should be initiated early. If signs and symptoms of peritonitis progress, the patient should undergo surgical exploration and repair or resection of the injured intestine.

Hemorrhage

Large-bore needles or trochars may perforate the inferior epigastric vessels, causing extensive bleeding within the abdominal wall. Another hazard during insertion of the trochar is laceration of a vessel located in the mesentery of the bowel or in a large tumor, or laceration of an enlarged liver or spleen. After paracentesis, patients must be observed closely for evidence of severe internal bleeding.

REFERENCES

1. Ashworth CJ, Sacks Y, Williams LF, et al: Hyperosmolar hyperglycemic non-ketotic coma: Its importance in surgical problems. *Ann Surg* 167:556−560, 1968.
2. Dudrick SJ, MacFadyen BV, Van Buren CT, et al: Parenteral hyperalimentation—metabolic problems and solutions. *Ann Surg* 176:259−264, 1972.
3. Ryan JA, Able RM, Abbott WM, et al: Catheter complications in total parenteral nutrition. *N Engl J Med* 290:757−761, 1974.
4. French G, Shenoi V: Disseminated moniliasis with demonstration of organisms in blood. *Can Med Assoc J* 71:238−241, 1954.
5. Taschdjian CL, Kozinn PS, Okas A, et al: Serodiagnosis of systemic candidiasis. *J Infect Dis* 117:180−187, 1967.
6. Levinsky WJ: Fatal air embolism during insertion of CVP monitoring apparatus. *JAMA* 209:1721−1722, 1969.
7. Durant TM, Long J, Oppenheimer MJ: Pulmonary (venous) air embolism. *Am Heart J* 33:269−281, 1947.
8. Shires T, O'Banion J: Successful treatment of massive air embolism producing cardiac arrest. *JAMA* 167:1483−1484, 1958.
9. Doering RB, Stemmer EA, Connolly JE: Complication of indwelling venous catheters. *Am J Surg* 114:259−266, 1967.

14
Infection

Peter E. Schwartz

Infection is a frequent cause of death in patients with solid tumors. A review of fatal infections in cancer patients revealed that 70% of the patients with acute leukemia, 51% of the patients with lymphoma, and 47% of the patients with solid tumors died as a direct result of infection (1). Pneumonia was the most common infection in solid-tumor patients, followed by disseminated infections and peritonitis. Unlike acute leukemia patients, in whom fungi represent approximately one-third of the etiologic agents causing fatal infections, 94% of solid-tumor patients die as a result of bacterial infection. The source of infection in most gynecologic cancer patients is the pelvis and the gastrointestinal tract. Therefore, the gynecologic oncologist must be prepared to prevent or treat infections arising from the pelvic reproductive organs and the gastrointestinal tract.

This chapter will discuss host defenses, infectious complications of surgery, radiation, chemotherapy, and combined-modality treatment, the bacteriologic flora of the gastrointestinal and female reproductive tracts, and antibiotic therapy for control of infection in patients with gynecologic malignancies.

HOST DEFENSES

Host defenses may be divided into mechanical barriers, phagocytic defenses, cell-mediated immunity, and humoral immunity (2). Each of these defenses can be altered by the tumor itself, by therapy for the management of the tumor, and by nonspecific factors.

Mechanical Barriers

The skin and mucous membranes represent the first line of defense against bacterial and fungal infection (2). These barriers are often interrupted by the growth of the tumor or its metastases into the gastrointestinal tract or vagina in patients with pelvic malignancies. Surgical therapy for the management of these tumors also results in violation of the mucous membranes and may further potentiate the source of seeding of bacteria. Changes occur in the vaginal

265

bacterial flora after hysterectomy for benign disease, and a significant increase in positive cultures for potential pathogens, including *Escherichia coli* and *Bacteroides fragilis,* has been demonstrated (3–5).

Endotracheal tubes, urinary catheters, and intravenous lines, including hyperalimentation lines, may result in violation of the skin and irritation of the mucous membranes, resulting in bacteremia. Fungicemia has been reported in association with hyperalimentation lines (6). Radiation therapy for managing gynecologic malignancies may lead to significant irritation of the mucous membranes of the small and large bowel, creating sites for bacterial invasion. Similarly, chemotherapy for controlling gynecologic malignancies may produce ulcerations of the mucous membrane that may then serve as the source for bacterial seeding (7). Certain chemotherapeutic agents may potentiate radiation effects, resulting in greater desquamation of the skin and mucous membranes than is attained with either mode of therapy alone (7). Decubitus ulcers may also serve as a source of infection, particularly in the compromised host (8).

Phagocytic Defenses

Polymorphonuclear neutrophils are able to ingest and kill a large variety of microorganisms. However, a decline in the neutrophil count to a level below 1,500 is associated with an increasing incidence of infection (1). The incidence of infection may be quantified with the absolute number of neutrophils present. A drop in the neutrophil count to 100 or less is associated with a significant incidence of infection, which in patients with acute leukemia frequently results in fatal infections. Neutropenia in gynecologic cancer patients is usually secondary to chemotherapy and is a self-limited phenomenon. Usually it will spontaneously reverse itself provided the patient is given supportive care. Radiation therapy, as well as chemotherapy, will at times produce significant depression of bone marrow function. When whole-abdomen irradiation is employed in the management of ovarian cancer, or when pelvic irradiation in which the radiation fields are extended to cover the paraaortic lymph nodes is employed in the management of cervical cancer, one is frequently irradiating approximately one-half of the active adult bone marrow. Metastases to the bone marrow are extremely infrequent in gynecologic malignancies, but in other malignancies, they can be a significant cause of bone marrow suppression (8). The sequential use of chemotherapy and radiation may result in severe bone marrow suppression and was found in one large series of ovarian cancer patients to be a common cause of interruption in or failure to complete radiation therapy in patients in whom primary chemotherapy had failed (9).

Mature neutrophil bactericidal and candidacidal function may be impaired by radiation, steroids, and chemotherapy (10–13). Steroids may impair leukocyte migration to the infection site, and hyperalimentation may cause hypophosphatemia, resulting in restriction of neutrophil locomotion and bactericidal activity by reducing the energy available to the neutrophil from phosphate metabolism (14).

Cell-Mediated Immunity

Successful control of infection due to viruses, protozoa, intracellular bacteria (such as *Listeria, Salmonella, Mycobacterium tuberculosis*), and most fungi requires an intact lymphocyte-macrophage defense system (15,16). Fortunately, these infections are not common in gynecologic cancer patients. Cell-mediated immunity may be studied in cancer patients by correlating skin test anergy to in vitro lymphocyte dysfunction (17). T-lymphocyte function is impaired by malnutrition, advanced age, and surgery, all of which may be associated with gynecologic cancer patients (2,16). Steroids, not frequently used in the care of gynecologic malignancies, may have a significant effect on cell-mediated immunity (18).

Humoral Immunity

The humoral immunity system defends primarily against bacterial infections by direct serum microbicidal activity or by opsonizing bacteria for phagocytosis and subsequent killing (16,19,20). This system is also important in preventing viral reinfection. Hypogammaglobulinemia usually parallels impaired antibody response to antigenic stimuli, but it is not directly linked to it (2). Abnormalities in humoral immunity are particularly pronounced to chronic lymphocytic leukemia and multiple myeloma and may be seen in Hodgkin's disease and other lymphomas (21). Chemotherapy will markedly diminish primary antibody responses and may contribute to hypogammaglobulinemia. Malnutrition and advanced age may further impair primary and secondary antibody responses in cancer patients (16,22,23).

Although multiple defects in host defense may exist in any individual cancer patient, usually one is dealing with disruption of mechanical barriers or impairment of the phagocytic defense in the gynecologic oncology patient. A rational approach to the diagnosis and management of infection in these patients is based upon an understanding of the possible exogenous and endogenous factors resulting in infections and the microbial agents causing the infection.

INFECTIOUS COMPLICATIONS

Infectious complications of surgery, radiation, chemotherapy, and combined-modality therapy in patients with malignancies in the reproductive organs may often be prevented. Infections, when recognized early, may be controlled, but the most severe complications of infections, abscess formation and septicemia, must be aggressively managed.

The next section of this chapter will briefly discuss prophylaxis, control of infection, and management of abscesses and septicemia from the point of view of surgery, radiation therapy, chemotherapy, and combined-modality treatment.

SURGERY

Surgery frequently results in interference with mechanical barriers, increasing the risk of bacterial infection (24). Simple measures to prevent infection include preoperative bowel preparation of patients undergoing gastrointestinal surgery. This preparation, which may be either the mechanical or antibiotic type (25), is indicated for patients who are about to undergo pelvic exenterations, resections for advanced ovarian cancer, second-look surgery in which bowel resection may be anticipated to be part of the procedure, bowel bypasses for radiation enteritis, or surgery for recurrent partial small bowel obstruction secondary to ovarian cancer and colostomies. Surgery should be carefully planned, and incisions should not be made in heavily irradiated areas. Patients who have radiation enteritis often do better with bowel bypasses than with resections because the sites of radiation enteritis are often chronically infected and resection exposes these patients to an increased chance of bacterial infection (26). Complications in patients undergoing simple hysterectomies after completion of radiation therapy for barrel-shaped cervical cancers may be decreased by reducing the intracavitary radiation component of the planned program of therapy (27). Radical hysterectomies for recurrent cancer of the cervix in heavily irradiated pelves often result in infectious complications. The selection of a surgical procedure must always be carefully weighed in an irradiated pelvis because the need to do extensive resections in areas with a poor blood supply may result in vascular compromise of the ureters and bladder and an increased risk of necrosis and fistula formation (26).

Proper preoperative evaluation is extremely important. For example, patients undergoing small bowel bypass for either radiation enteritis or partial small bowel obstruction secondary to recurrent ovarian cancer should routinely receive a large bowel radiologic evaluation to be certain that occult obstruction in the large bowel is not present. If one bypasses the small bowel into the obstructed distal large bowel, increased pressure will develop at the anastomosis site, resulting in compromise of the anastomosis, fever, abscess formation, and eventually an enterocutaneous fistula. Patients should be evaluated for routine prophylactic anticoagulation, particularly those patients with a prior history of thrombophlebitis or significant lower-extremity varicose veins. All patients about to undergo prolonged surgery for gynecologic cancer are at high risk for thrombophlebitis. Impaired healing in malnourished cancer patients may be reversed by preoperative hyperalimentation (28).

Prophylactic antibiotics to reduce the size of the bacterial inoculum have been studied extensively in benign pelvic surgery for gynecologic problems (29). The routine use of prophylactic antibiotics in gynecologic procedures employing a vaginal approach is well established, but the value of prophylactic antibiotics for patients undergoing transabdominal surgery has yet to be established. Nevertheless, patients with gynecologic malignancies frequently are older, have compromised host defense mechanisms, and are suitable candidates for prophylactic antibiotic therapy. No objective studies have appeared in the literature comparing the effects of prophylactic antibiotic therapy on patients with gynecologic malignancies undergoing surgery versus a control group of patients. Clearly there is a need for such studies.

Ledger et al. have established the following guidelines for prophylactic antibiotics (30): The operations should carry a significant risk of postoperative site infection and significant bacterial contamination. The antibiotic used for prophylaxis should have laboratory evidence of effectiveness against some of the contaminating microorgansims and demonstrable clinical effectiveness. Antibiotics should be present in the wound in effective concentrations at the time of the incision, and only short-term, low-toxicity antibiotics should be used. Antibiotics needed to combat resistant infections should be reserved and not used for prophylaxis. The benefits of prophylactic antibiotics must outweigh the dangers of their use. These principles are appropriate for gynecologic cancer patients.

Newer antibiotics, particularly of the cephalosporin type, may be quite appropriate as single agents in prophylaxis for patients undergoing gynecologic cancer surgery, but studies have not been reported. Prophylactic antibiotics are never a substitute for meticulously performed surgery.

Percutaneous suction drainage of the retroperitoneal space, to reduce the volume of fluid present, is routinely employed at Yale–New Haven Hospital in the patient undergoing pelvic lymphadenectomy in association with a radical hysterectomy. T-tube suction drainage of the retroperitoneal space may reduce the nutritive source of bacterial growth after a routine hysterectomy for benign disease and may be a suitable alternative to prophylactic antibiotics in benign gynecologic procedures (31).

Control of Infection

Control of infection in surgical patients is extremely important. Simple procedures will often control infection, and avoidance of them on a routine basis may lead to the formation of abscesses and subsequent septicemia. Patients operated on and found to have unsuspected infections such as pelvic inflammatory disease should undergo vigorous irrigation of the pelvic cavity after the infected tubes and ovaries are removed (25). Antibiotic solutions containing kanamycin sulfate may be used for this purpose, but their value has been questioned (16,25). The routine use of drains brought out from the pelvis retroperitoneally to the skin may also reduce the chance of abscess formation, but again their value except in closed systems has been questioned (16). Diverticular abscesses may be confused with pelvic masses suggestive of gynecologic malignancies and may not always be detectable by a barium enema. If diverticular abscesses are found at the time of an exploratory laparotomy, it may be appropriate to elect to perform a two- or three-stage procedure with a diverting colostomy as part of the initial surgery, in order to reduce the likelihood of anastomosis leaks (32). The occurrence of an accidental enterostomy may be readily treated by primary closure and vigorous irrigation of the peritoneal cavity to reduce the effect of fecal spillage (16). However, it is appropriate in the management of accidental enterostomies, if the length of the enterostomy is greater than one-half of the diameter of the small bowel, to resect the enterostomy site and perform a primary end-to-end anastomosis. Wound infections often occur in patients who have been operated on in prior radiation sites, who have undergone bowel surgery, or who have had infections in the incision site after surgical procedures (24). Recognition of the infection is extremely important, and once the wound has become fluctuant, it should be opened the entire length of the infected site. Control of wound infections requires adequate drainage that a small opening in the skin may not provide.

Management of Abscess and Septicemia

When an abscess is identified, prompt surgical drainage and vigorous debridement, if at all possible, are required (16,24). Patients with abscesses in heavily irradiated areas may experience impaired wound healing after adequate drainage and debridement. Recent developments in the management of nonhealing wounds in heavily irradiated sites using myocutaneous grafts have resulted in an opportunity to bring well-vascularized tissue to heavily irradiated areas, allowing rapid healing that, in the past, may not have been possible or may have required extremely long recuperative periods (33).

Septicemia in the surgical patient usually occurs as the result of a preceding infection such as a urinary tract infection, pneumonia, peritonitis, septic thrombophlebitis, an infected intravenous catheter line, or a wound infection (16). A careful search for the site of infection is mandatory. The site may be very difficult to localize in patients with pelvic infections. Patients who have undergone recent gastrointestinal surgery may require colostomies or ileostomies to control infections secondary to anastomosis leaks and abscess formation. The identification of *Bacteroides* spp. in the bloodstream demands a vigorous search for a pelvic abscess. Effective management of *Bacteroides* septicemia is dependent on the identification and drainage of the pelvic abscess (34).

Broad-spectrum antibiotic therapy must be initiated after thorough culturing (blood, urine, sputum, drain sites, discharges) and evaluation of the patient with septicemia. Broad-spectrum antibiotics may then be adjusted, depending on the patient's response and the antibiotic sensitivities determined by microbiologic assays. Inadequate control of severe infection will lead to poor or inadequate tissue perfusion, resulting in septic shock (16).

RADIATION THERAPY

Radiation therapy may interrupt mechanical barriers such as the mucous membranes of the gastrointestinal tract and the skin, leading to secondary bacterial infection, and may also reduce the phagocytic response when an excessive amount of the active adult bone marrow is included in the radiation field. Nevertheless, certain precautions can be taken to prevent radiation resulting in infectious complications. The use of modern megavoltage radiation units has reduced the incidence of moist desquamation and skin necrosis because the maximum radiation depth dose is well below the skin surface. Avoiding excessive radiation dosages will also result in avoiding severe radiation-associated injuries to the gastrointestinal and genitourinary tract. A dormant infection may flare up when the patient is exposed to radiation (35). Removing the fallopian tubes and ovaries in a patient with a history of active pelvic inflammatory disease is appropriate before initiating radiation therapy for carcinoma of the cervix (35).

Once an infection has been established, control is based on interrupting or discontinuing radiation therapy, providing supportive care to the patient, and draining or resecting pelvic abscesses and pyometra. Septicemia from radiation-induced injuries should be treated vigorously with broad-spectrum antibiotics, and long-term gastrointestinal or gentiourinary complications may require bowel or urinary diversions (26).

CHEMOTHERAPY

Chemotherapy may result in impaired phagocytic defenses and interruption of mechanical barriers (2). Prophylaxes against such complications include careful monitoring of bone marrow function and subsequent dose reduction if the patient exhibits significant bone marrow depression after initiation of chemotherapy. Chemotherapy may result in local complications secondary to extravasation, causing localized necrosis (36). The simple expedient of injecting chemotherapeutic agents into the intravenous tubing of a fast-running intravenous catheter may prevent this complication.

The routine use of trimethoprim-sulfamethoxazole when the neutrophil count appears to be decreasing after the administration of a course of chemotherapy has been thought to be useful in ameliorating the effects of neutropenia by reducing the endogenous flora of the gastrointestinal tract (37). Lithium carbonate has been advocated as a means of stimulating neutrophil release into the peripheral circulation and potentially minimizing the effects of neutropenia in patients receiving chemotherapy (38). The prompt initiation of broad-spectrum antibiotic therapy has been demonstrated to be advantageous in nongynecologic cancer patients who are granulocytopenic as a result of chemotherapy administration (39). In gynecologic cancer patients who are receiving combination chemotherapy, it would appear appropriate to initiate broad-spectrum antibiotic therapy when they become febrile and have demonstrated a decrease in total white count to less than 1,000. A regimen consisting of clindamycin and gentamicin has been successfully employed at Yale–New Haven Hospital in gynecologic cancer patients who become febrile and neutropenic while being treated with a variety of combination chemotherapies for nonepithelial cancers of the ovary and high-risk trophoblast disease.

Preliminary data suggest that intravenous hyperalimentation (I.V.H.) may reverse immunologic nonreactivity in cancer patients secondary to malnutrition and reduce the degree of chemotherapy-induced bone marrow suppression while patients are receiving it (28,40). Studies have also suggested that I.V.H. therapy may increase patients' tolerance for higher doses of chemotherapy or more frequent administration and potentially increase response rates (40).

The development of septicemia and abscess formation in patients on chemotherapy requires the prompt introduction of broad-spectrum antibiotics. Granulocyte transfusions are usually unnecessary in the management of these patients because the bone marrow suppression is self-limited (1). Nevertheless, an occasional patient does require granulocyte transfusions. The role of protected environments has not been adequately evaluated in patients with gynecologic malignancies, but it is unlikely that such environments will add substantially to the management of these patients, and costs may be prohibitive (1,37).

ETIOLOGIC AGENTS

The overwhelming number of infections associated with gynecologic cancers are caused by the endogenous flora of the cervical-vaginal and gastrointestinal tracts (41,42). The same organisms, for the most part, are present in each of these sites (43). Pathogens include Gram-negative aerobic bacteria such as *E. coli,* the predominant organism in this group, as well as *Proteus mirabolis, Klebsiella* spp., and *Enterobacteriacea* spp. *Pseudomonas* spp. and indole-positive strains of *Proteus* are less frequent causes of infection. The other major group of endogenous organisms is anaerobes, which are frequently associated with infections arising from the pelvis or gastrointestinal tract. These include *Peptococcus* spp., *Peptos-treptococcus* spp., and *Bacteroides* spp., with *B. fragilis* predominating (44). Most infections in patients with gynecologic malignancies are associated with mixed bacterial flora consisting of anaerobic and facultative or aerobic bacteria (42). So-called nonpathogenic organisms (*Streptococcus viridans,* coagulase-negative staphylococci, *Veillonella,* and several anaerobic Gram-positive non-spore-forming bacilli—*Bifidobacterium, Eubacterium, Lactobacillus* spp., and *Propionibac-terium*) may act synergistically in pelvic infections by lowering tissue oxidation production potential sufficiently to allow anaerobic bacteria to grow (42).

Selection of Antimicrobial Agents

The selection of antimicrobial agents should be based upon the known suscep-tibilities of the infectious agents to the available antimicrobial preparations. Some antibiotics are of limited efficacy in patients with impaired host defenses, especially neutropenic patients. In general, it is preferable to use a bactericidal rather than a bacteriostatic antibiotic.

Penicillin-Cephalosporins

Penicillins are bactericidal and have been reported to be the most effective antibiotics in patients with impaired host defenses (1). Penicillin G is the choice drug for all anaerobic infections except those due to *B. fragilis* and isolates of fusobacteria that are resistant to it. Toxicity to penicillin G other than allergies is uncommon and is usually manifest in about 3% of the population. Allergic reactions are usually of the delayed type and include fever, erythema, urticaria, and arthritis. Immediate reactions, i.e., anaphylaxis, is rare. Penicillin G is usually supplied as a potassium salt, resulting in the patient receiving 1.7 mEq of potassium for every 1 million units of penicillin administered. Sodium salt is available for patients with renal failure. Patients with serious infections should receive 20–50 million units of penicillin daily (42). High-dose prolonged therapy may produce neurotoxicity (myoclonic contractions, depressed sen-sorium, grand mal seizures), electrolyte disturbances, and metabolic alkalosis (45).

Ampicillin

Ampicillin is more active against *E. coli* and *P. mirabolis* than penicillin G, but it is less active for anaerobes and some *Streptococcus* spp. (44). However, the spectrum of activity for ampicillin and penicillin G is the same when doses of penicillin approximating 30–50 million units a day are used (42). Adverse effects of ampicillin include rashes, which occur more frequently than with penicillin G. The usual dosage of ampicillin for serious infections is 1–2 g I.V. every 4 hours.

Oxacillin

Oxacillin is a semisynthetic penicillin and the drug of choice for treatment of *Staphylococcus* soft-tissue infections, an infrequent complication for patients with gynecologic malignancies (42). It is preferred over methicillin because of the lower incidence of associated interstitial nephritis (45). Adverse effects are similar to those of penicillin G. The usual dose of oxacillin is 1–2 g I.V. every 4 hours.

Carbenicillin

Carbenicillin has been extensively studied in cancer patients because of its activity against *Pseudomonas aeruginosa,* both indole-positive and negative *Proteus* spp., and some Enterobacteriaceae spp. and *E. coli.* A daily dosage of at least 30 g (5 g every 4 hours I.V.) is necessary for treatment to be effective. Skin rashes, sodium and fluid overload, hypertension, pulmonary edema, and platelet dysfunction have been reported with carbenicillin administration (45).

Ticarcillin

Ticarcillin is a newly introduced semisynthetic penicillin with a spectrum of antibacterial activity similar to that of carbenicillin (46). It is somewhat more active against *P. aeruginosa* in vitro and is more active than carbenicillin on a weight basis. It is active in the presence of neutropenia and has been administered at a dose of 3.5 g I.V. every 4 hours. The spectrum includes *E. coli, Serratia* and some enterobacteria, *Proteus* spp., *Streptococcus* spp., pneumococci, Gram-positive bacilli, and anaerobes, including *B. fragilis.* Toxic reactions include allergic reactions, hypokalemia, and platelet dysfunction.

Cephalosporins

The cephalosporins are similar to the penicillins structurally and in spectrum of activity and are active against Gram-negative bacteria including *E. coli, Klebsiella* spp., and *P. mirabolis* (42). However, they are generally considered not to be active in the management of *B. fragilis* infections. Recently, a group of new cephalosporin-type agents were introduced, including cephapirin sodium, cefamandole nafate, and cefoxitin. All cephalosporins are excreted by the kidneys (45).

Cephapirin Sodium

Cephapirin sodium has a spectrum of activity similar to that of cefalothin, the first cephalosporin to become available for clinical use (47). It is highly resistant to the staphylococcus beta-lactamases. The bactericidal spectrum includes *E. coli, Klebsiella, P. mirabolis, Salmonella, Shigella, Staphylococcus aureus, Staphylococcus epidermidis, Streptococcus* spp. (except for enterococci), pneumococci, and anaerobes, excluding *B. fragilis.* It is available only as a parenteral drug and is used primarily for *Klebsiella* spp. and *S. epidermidis.* The usual dose is 1–2 g I.V. every 4 hours. Toxic reactions include phlebitis in approximately 5%–10% of patients, allergy, and rare bone marrow suppression, hemolysis, and neutropenia.

Cefamandole Nafate

Cefamandole nafate, a cephalosporin derivative, has a greater resistance to Gram-negative beta-lactamases than cefalothin, cefazolin, or cephapirin sodium

(48). It has enhanced activity against *E. coli, Klebsiella, Proteus* spp., and *Enterobacteriaceae* spp., as well as *Haemophilus influenza*. It is somewhat less active against Gram-positive cocci than cephalothin. It is indicated for *Klebsiella, E. coli, H. influenza,* and Enterobacteriaceae spp., and is possibly active in mixed intra-abdominal infections. It is not yet approved by the Federal Drug Administration for use in *B. fragilis* infections. Signs of toxicity are similar to those of cephapirin except that phlebitis is less frequently observed. It has a nephrotoxicity similar to that seen with other cephalosporins. Its usual dose range is 0.5–2 g I.V. every 4–6 hours.

Cefoxitin

Cefoxitin is a bactericidal agent that is highly resistant to degradation by beta-lactamases (41,49). It appears to have a better spectrum than cephalothin for all Gram-negative rods, has better coverage of indole-positive *Proteus* infections than cefamandole, and is very active against *Serratia* and *B. fragilis* (44). It is less active against Gram-positive cocci than all other cephalosporins. Cefoxitin indications are the same as those of cefamandole nafate. Toxic reactions include a significant incidence of phlebitis, pain when the drug is injected intramuscularly, and reactions similar to those caused by the other cephalosporins. Its dosage range is 0.5–2 g I.V. every 4–6 hours.

Chloramphenicol

Chloramphenicol is an extremely important bacteriostatic agent in the management of patients with gynecologic malignancies (42). It is active in approximately 75% of most hospital strains of Gram-negative bacilli except for *Pseudomonas* and is very active in controlling anaerobes, including *B. fragilis*. It is given in an intravenous form, usually at a dosage of 50 mg/kg/day in four equally divided doses. Its toxicity is associated with a rare occurrence of aplastic anemia. There are two forms of bone marrow toxicity associated with chloramphenicol. The first is inhibition of red cell synthesis resulting in an increased serum iron concentration, a decrease in reticulocyte counts, anemia, and vacuolization of red cell precursors in the bone marrow. This is a dose-dependent reaction and is reversible. A second form of toxicity, an idiosyncratic, non-dose-related aplastic anemia, is extremely infrequent, is usually not associated with intravenous administration, and is generally not reversible (42).

Tetracyclines

Tetracyclines are no longer commonly used in the management of gynecologic infections because resistant strains of anaerobic bacteria, including *Bacteroides*, have evolved (42). Newer tetracyclines, including doxycycline and minocycline, are more active against anaerobic bacteria than other tetracyclines. Minocycline is substantially more active against *B. fragilis* than doxycycline. However, a number of side effects have been associated with minocycline, including nausea, vertigo, dizziness, and light-headedness, making it infrequently the agent of first choice in the management of pelvic infections. Tetracycline is usually given in an oral dosage of 250–500 mg every 6 hours. When given parenterally, it is infused at a rate of 500 mg every 12 hours. Doxycycline is administered orally: 100 mg every 12 hours for two doses and then 100 mg every 24 hours. Minocycline is given orally: 200 mg initially followed by 100 mg every 12 hours. Doxycycline is the only tetracycline that may be used in the presence of renal failure (45).

Aminoglycoside Antibiotics

Aminoglycoside antibiotics have very broad spectra of activity. Gentamicin has been used extensively for infections in cancer patients because of its activity against most Gram-negative bacilli including *P. aerugenosa* (1). Gentamicin is very effective in patients with adequate neutrophils but has been reported to have suboptimal effects when neutropenia is present (1). All members of the aminoglycoside group can cause renal and ototoxicity (45). Streptomycin and gentamicin primarily affect balance; kanamycin may cause deafness. Gentamicin nephrotoxicity is similar to kanamycin nephrotoxicity. The frequency may be enhanced with multiple courses, and an occasional patient will develop acute renal failure after only a few days of therapy. Nephrotoxicity is usually reversible, but the patient may require dialysis until recovery occurs. Gentamicin dosage should be based on serum creatinine levels, and maintenance dosage should be based on the peak and trough levels of the drugs (45). Gentamicin is usually given at a dosage of 3−5 mg/kg/day in three equally divided doses in patients with normal renal function.

Two aminoglycoside antibiotics, tobramycin and amikacin, have recently become available for clinical use. Tobramycin is closely related to kanamycin and gentamicin and is active against *Staphylococcus*. It appears to be more active against *Pseudomonas* than gentamicin (46,50). It has no activity against anaerobes or pneumococci. It is indicated primarily for systemic *Pseudomonas* infections and is often used in combination with carbenicillin or ticarcillin. Its toxicity is similar to that of gentamicin (ototoxicity, nephrotoxicity, allergic reactions), and monitoring the blood levels of patients while they are receiving tobramycin treatment is mandatory. Patients with severe infections should receive a loading dose of 1.5−2.0 mg/kg of lean body weight (LBW) × 40% "fat weight" I.V. and maintenance doses of 1.0−1.5 mg/kg of LBW every 8 hours.

Amikacin is structurally similar to kanamycin but has a spectrum of activities similar to tobramycin and gentamicin, including many aerobic Gram-negative rods that may be inactivated by the latter agents (*Serratia* spp., *P. aeruginosa*) (44,51). Its indications are the same as those for gentamicin or tobramycin, but in hospitals where gentamicin resistance is not a major problem, it should be reserved for proven or suspected gentamicin-tobramycin−resistant bacteria. Its toxicity is identical with that of gentamicin and tobramycin, and therefore it is mandatory to monitor I.V. levels of the drug. An I.V. loading dose of 5.0−7.5 mg/kg is recommended, followed by 5.0 mg/kg I.V. every 8 hours (44).

Clindamycin

Clindamycin is a synthetic antibiotic that is extremely active against most anaerobes, including *B. fragilis* (42). It is not active against aerobic Gram-negative bacilli or enterococci although it is active against most Gram-positive cocci including penicillinase-producing staphylococci. It is extremely useful in managing patients with gynecologic malignancies in whom infectious complications develop and is usually given at a dose of 600 mg I.V. every 6 hours. A major serious adverse effect of clindamycin therapy has been the development of a pseudomembranous enterocolitis. Pseudomembranous entercolitis has been associated with other antibiotics (52). Enterocolitis associated with clindamycin is usually preceded by diarrhea, crampy abdominal pain, fever, abdominal distention, leukocytosis, and blood or mucus in the stool. It can be diagnosed by sigmoidoscopy, which reveals a characteristic edema and erythema of the rectal mucosa with raised whitish-yellow plaques. Ulceration is unusual. If pseudomembranes are present, clindamycin should be promptly stopped. The pseudomembranous enterocolitis may be self-limited. Severe cases require more aggressive therapy because it appears to be caused by toxin-producing *Clostridia* spp. (52).

Trimethoprim-Sulfamethoxazole

Trimethoprim-sulfamethoxazole is a fixed combination of two drugs that act sequentially in the pathway of tetrahydrofolate synthesis (44). This combination is often bactericidal and is active against Gram-positive cocci (except for enterococci), Gram-positive bacilli, aerobic Gram-negative rods (except for *Pseudomonas*), *Nocardia*, and *Pneumocystis* (53,54). It is well absorbed orally and is indicated in recurrent urinary tract infections, typhoid fever, otitis media, and *Pneumocystis carinii*. Also, it is possibly prophylactic against sepsis in neutropenic patients (40). Toxic reactions include gastrointestinal irritation, bone marrow suppression (in high doses), hypersensitivity, and cross-reactivity with other sulfonamides.

Combination Antimicrobial Therapy

The choice of antimicrobial therapy is based on known etiologic agents from the cervical-vaginal and gastrointestinal flora and should cover both aerobic and anaerobic bacteria. Laboratory animal studies have demonstrated that septic complications of colonic perforation involve mixed bacterial flora that are best treated with coverage for Gram-negative rods as well as for anaerobes (55). A variety of broad-spectrum antibiotic combinations are effective in managing septic complications in patients with gynecologic malignancies (43). Gentamicin and clindamycin have been extremely active in controlling infections at Yale—New Haven Hospital, but the combination does not cover enterococci. The role of enterococci in pelvic sepsis has been questioned (41). The addition of ampicillin to gentamicin and clindamycin provides adequate coverage for enterococci. Carbenicillin and gentamicin have been strongly advocated in bone marrow—suppressed patients, because carbenicillin is active against aerobes and anaerobes, including *B. fragilis* (1). This combination must be used cautiously in patients with compromised renal function. Chloramphenicol in combination with gentamicin provides excellent anaerobic as well as aerobic coverage. The use of the newer cephalothins such as cefoxitin or cephamandole nafate with gentamicin may provide adequate coverage of the anaerobes as well as aerobes; however, insufficient information is available at this time to recommend the latter combination (56). Cephalothin in combination with gentamicin has been reported to increase renal toxicity (57).

Resistent *Pseudomonas* infections may respond to ticarcillin and tobramycin, resistant *Klebsiella* and *E. coli* may respond to cephalosporin in combination with gentamicin, and resistant enterococci and *Staphylococcus* may respond to vancomycin in combination with gentamicin (46).

DURATION OF TREATMENT

Patients with soft-tissue infections in the pelvis or abdomen should be treated for 3−5 days after they are clinically stable, that is, have no clinical evidence of persistent infection, including an absence of fever and abdominal tenderness. Patients with group A beta-hemolytic *Streptococcus* should be treated for a minimum of 10 days, and patients with *Staphylococcus* bacteremia are usually treated for a minimum of 4 weeks (42). Patients with bacteremia due to other organisms are treated for 1 week after apparent clinical cure.

Patients treated with combination chemotherapy in whom fever develops while they are neutropenic should be started promptly on combination antibiotic therapy. The preference at Yale−New Haven Hospital is to employ gentamicin and clindamycin, thereby providing adequate anaerobic and aerobic coverage. These patients should be maintained on antibiotics until the neutrophil count starts rising, which is usually a matter of 4 or 5 days. Antibiotics may be discontinued when the temperature returns to normal in the presence of a rising neutrophil count.

TREATMENT FAILURE

The choice of antibiotic therapy in managing infections associated with gynecologic malignancies is extremely important. Inappropriate selection of an antibiotic or an antibiotic combination and inappropriate administration of the antibiotic may lead to failure to respond to initial therapy. Serious infections usually require 48−72 hours before a clear response manifests itself. Inappropriate early discontinuation of antibiotic therapy may only confuse the clinical management. Antibiotic failure is most often due to inadequate surgical drainage, the presence of obstructed ureters, atelectasis, drug allergies, and thromboembolic phenomena, all of which will fail to respond to a change in the antibiotic regimen. However, the selection of ineffective antibiotics may be corrected for in patients with persistent fever when culture reports are available, allowing the clinician to change therapy to effective agents.

FUNGAL INFECTION

The incidence of fungal infections is increasing, particularly in cancer patients (1,38). Fungal infections are infrequent in gynecologic cancer patients. They tend to occur most often in patients with acute leukemia (1). The most common fungal infections are associated with *Candida* spp.; however, other fungal infections have been reported including *Aspergillus* spp., *Phycomycetes* spp., *Torulopsis glabratta*, and *Geotrichum candidum*. These organisms seldom cause infection unless one is dealing with patients with severely impaired host defense mechanisms. A second group of fungal infections includes *Cryptococcus neofor-*

mans, Histoplasma capsulatum, Coccidioides immitus, and *Nocardia asteroides.* Superficial *Candida* infections may arise in the groin and perianal areas, particularly in patients receiving antibiotics, and will respond to topical antifungal agents (1). Oropharyngeal candidiasis may be treated with nystatin, but the value of this therapy in cancer patients has been questioned (1). *Candida* fungicemia associated with I.V. hyperalimentation lines may be treated by removing the lines. Disseminated candidiasis infrequently occurs in patients with solid tumors and responds poorly to amphotericin-B therapy (1). Fungicemia has been managed with 5-fluorocytosine, but disseminated disease usually responds poorly regardless of the specific fungal organism present.

Viral Infections

Viral infections are infrequent in patients with gynecologic malignancies but may be a major problem in the management of patients with lymphoma because lymphoma patients tend to have deficiencies in cell-mediated immunity (1,2). Interferon and macrophages appear to be the most important host defenses against viral infection (58). Antibodies may play a role in preventing dissemination and recurrence (59). The most serious infections are caused by the herpes virus group. Hepatitis occurs relatively frequently in cancer patients but may be either drug-or virus-induced. The distinction may be difficult to determine. Mortality secondary to hepatitis may be increased in cancer patients with impaired host defenses (1).

Protozoan Infections

Protozoan infections are rare in patients with gynecologic malignancies. *Pneumocystis carinii* has been reported to cause an interstitial pneumonitis, particularly in young patients with leukemia or lymphoma (60). It has been reported to respond to pentamidine isethionate and the combination of trimethoprim-sulfamethoxazole (1,53). *Toxoplasma gondii* may infrequently cause pneumonia, chorioretinitis, and a disease similar to infectious mononucleosis, particularly in patients with Hodgkin's disease (1). Treatment entails the use of pyrimethamine and sulfonamides, but the prognosis when there is central nervous system involvement is extremely poor (1).

REFERENCES

1. Bodey GP: Infections in cancer patients. *Ca Treat Rev* 2:89–127, 1975.
2. Dilworth JA, Mandell GL: Infections in patients with cancer. *Semin Oncol* 2:349–359, 1975.
3. Ohm MU, Galask RP: The effect of antibiotic prophylaxis on patients undergoing vaginal operations: I. Alterations of the microbial flora. *Am J Obstet Gynecol* 123:597–603, 1975.
4. Ohm MJ, Galask RP: The effect of antibiotic prophylaxis on patients undergoing total abdominal hysterectomy: II. Alterations of microbial flora. *Am J Obstet Gynecol* 125:448–454, 1976.
5. Grossman JH III, Adams RL: Vaginal flora in women undergoing hysterectomy with antibiotic prophylaxis. *Obstet Gynecol* 53:23–26, 1979.
6. Ryan JA Jr, Abel RM, Abbott WM, et al: Catheter complications in total parenteral nutrition: A prospective study of 200 consecutive patients. *N Engl J Med* 290:757–761, 1974.

7. Adrian RM, Hood AF, Skarin AT: Mucocutaneous reactions to antineoplastic agents. *CA J Clinicians* 30:143–157, 1980.

8. Bodey GP: Infections in patients with cancer, in Holland JF, Frei E III (eds): *Cancer Medicine.* Philadelphia, Lea & Febiger, 1973, pp 1135–1165.

9. Schwartz PE, Smith JP: Second look surgery in the management of ovarian cancer. *Am J Obstet Gynecol* 138: 1124–1130, 1980.

10. Lehrer RI, Cline MJ: Leukocyte candidacidal activity and resistance to systemic candidiasis in patients with cancer. *Cancer* 27:1211–1217, 1971.

11. Dale DC, Petersdorf RG: Corticosteroids and infectious diseases. *Med Clin North Am* 57:1277–1287, 1973.

12.. Bachner RL, Neiburger RG, Johnson DE, et al: Transient bactericidal defect of peripheral blood phagocytes from children with acute lymphoblastic leukemia receiving craniospinal irradiation. *N Engl J Med* 289:1209–1213, 1973.

13. Webel ML, Ritts RD Jr, Taswell HF, et al: Cellular immunity after intravenous administration of methylprednisolone. *J Lab Clin Med* 289:1209–1213, 1973.

14. Craddock PR, Yawata Y, VanSanten L, et al: Acquired phagocyte dysfunction: A complication of the hypophosphatemia of parenteral hyperalimentation. *N Engl J Med* 290:1403–1407, 1974.

15. World Health Organization Scientific Group: Cell-mediated immunity and resistance to infection. WHO technical Report Series No. 159, 1973.

16. Alexander JW: Life-threatening sepsis, in Condon, RE, DeCosse JJ (eds): *Surgical Care: A Physiologic Approach to Clinical Management.* Philadelphia, Lea & Febiger, 1980, pp 302–313.

17. Hersh EM, Mavligit GM, Gutterman JU: Immunologic evaluation of malignant disease. *JAMA* 236:1739–1742, 1976.

18. Rinehart JJ, Sagone AL, Balcerzak SP, et al: Effects of corticosteroid therapy on human monocyte function. *N Engl J Med* 292:236–241, 1975.

19. Stossel TP: Phagocytosis. *N Engl J Med* 290:717–723, 774–780, 833–839, 1974.

20. Maddison SE: Structure and function of human immunoglobulins. *Health Lab Sci* 9:167–177, 1972.

21. Harris J, Copeland D: Impaired immunoresponsiveness in tumor patients. *Ann NY Acad Sci* 230:56–85, 1974.

22. Law DK, Dudrick SJ, Abdou NI: Immunocompetence of patients with protein-calorie malnutrition: The effects of nutritional repletion. *Ann Intern Med* 79:545–550, 1973.

23. Ram JS: Aging and immunological phenomena—a review. *J Gerontol* 22:92–107, 1967.

24. Dineen P: Infections following surgical operations, in Hoeprich PD (ed): *Infectious Diseases,* ed 2. Hagerstown, Md., Harper & Row Publishers Inc, 1977, pp 1159–1161.

25. Hoeprich PD: Chemoprophylaxis of infectious diseases, in Hoeprich PD (ed): *Infectious Diseases,* ed 2. Hagerstown, Md., Harper & Row Publishers Inc, 1977, pp 190–206.

26. Smith JP: Management of bowel and bladder complications from irradiation to pelvis and abdomen, in Fletcher GH (ed): *Textbook of Radiotherapy,* ed 2. Philadephia, Lea & Febiger, 1973, pp 702–705.

27. O'Quinn AG, Fletcher GH, Wharton JT: Guidelines for conservative hysterectomy after irradiation. *Gynecol Oncol* 9:68–79, 1980.

28. Silberman H: Hyperalimentation in patients with cancer. *Surg Gynecol Obstet* 150:755–757, 1980.

29. Duff P, Park RC: Antibiotic prophylaxis in vaginal hysterectomy: A review. *Obstet Gynecol* 55:1935–2025, 1980.

30. Ledger WJ, Gee C, Lewis WP: Guidelines for antibiotic prophylaxis in gynecology. *Am J Obstet Gynecol* 121:1038–1045, 1975.

31. Swartz WH, Tanaree P: T-tube suction drainage and/or prophylactic antibiotics. *Obstet Gynecol* 47:665–670, 1976.

32. Storer EH, Lockwood RA: Colon, rectum and anus, in Schwartz SI (ed): *Principles of Surgery.* New York, McGraw-Hill Book Co, 1969, pp 958–1019.

33. Morrow CP, Lacey CG, Lucas WE: Reconstructive surgery in gynecologic cancer employing the gracilis myocutaneous pedicle graft. *Gynecol Oncol* 7:176–187, 1979.

34. Fry DE, Garrison RN, Polk HC: Clinical implications in Bacteroides bacteremia. *Surg Gynecol Obstet* 149:189–192, 1979.

35. Rutledge FN, Wharton JT: Surgical procedures associated with radiation therapy for cervical cancer, in Fletcher GH (ed): *Textbook of Radiotherapy,* ed 2. Philadelphia, Lea & Febiger, 1973, pp 705–719.

36. Ignoffo RJ, Friedman MA: Therapy of local toxicities caused by extravasation of cancer chemotheraputic drugs. *Ca Treat Rev* 7:17–28, 1980.

37. Wiernik PH: The management of infection in the cancer patient. *JAMA* 244:185–187, 1980.

38. Greco FA, Brereton HD: Effect of lithium carbonate on the neutropenia caused by chemotherapy: A preliminary clinical trial. *Oncology* 34:153–155, 1977.

39. Schimpff SC: Therapy of infection in patients with granulocytopenia. *Med Clin North Am* 61:1101–1118, 1977.

40. Issell BF, Valdivieso M, Zaren HA, et al: Protection against chemotherapy toxicity by IV hyperalimentation. *Ca Treat Rep* 62:1139–1143, 1978.

41. Sweet RL, Ledger WJ: Cefoxitin: Single-agent treatment of mixed aerobic-anaerobic pelvic infections. *Obstet Gynecol* 54:193–198, 1979.

42. Mead PB, Gump DN: Antibiotic therapy in obstetrics and gynecology. *Clin Obstet Gynecol* 19:109–129, 1976.

43. Bartlett JG: Choosing and using antibiotics, in Condon RE, DeCosse JJ (eds): *Surgical Care: A Physiologic Approach to Clinical Management.* Philadelphia, Lea & Febiger, 1980, pp 273–301.

44. Hoeprich PD: Current principles of antimicrobial therapy. *Obstet Gynecol* 55 (suppl):121s–127s, 1980.

45. Whelton A: Theraputic considerations in the use of antibiotics in renal insufficiency. *Obstet Gynecol* 55 (suppl):128s–138s, 1980.

46. Parry MF, Neu HC: A comparative study of ticarcillin plus tobramycin versus carbenicillin plus gentamycin for the treatment of serious infections due to gram-negative bacilli. *Am J Med* 64:961–966, 1978.

47. Mandell GL: Cephalosporins, in Mandell GL, Douglas RG Jr, Bennett JE (eds): *Principles and Practice of Infectious Disease.* New York, John Wiley & Sons, 1979, pp 238–248.

48. Moellering RC Jr(ed): Symposium on cefamandole. *J Infect Dis* 137:s1–s194, 1978.

49. Future prospects and past problems in antimicrobial therapy: The role of cefoxitin. *Rev Infect Dis* 1:1–244, 1979.

50. Tobramycin. *J Infect Dis* 134:s1–s234, 1976.

51. Symposium on Amikacin. *Am J Med* 62:863–966, 1977.

52. Bartlett JG, Chang TW, Gurwith M, et al: Antibiotic-associated pseudomembranous colitis due to toxin producing Clostridia. *N Engl J Med* 298:531–534, 1978.

53. Trimethoprim-sulfamethoxazole. *J Infect Dis* 128:s433–s792, 1973.

54. Lau WK, Young LS: Cotrimoxazole treatment of Pneumocystis carinii pneumonia. *N Engl J Med* 295:716–718, 1976.

55. Weinstein WM, Onderdonk AB, Bartlett JG, et al: Antimicrobial therapy of experimental intraabdominal sepsis. *J Infect Dis* 132:282–286, 1975.

56. Gentry LO: Efficacy and safety of cefamandole plus either gentamicin or tobramycin in therapy of severe gram-negative bacterial infections. *J Infect Dis* 137 (suppl):s144–s149, 1978.

57. Wade JC, Smith CR, Petty BG, et al: Cephalothin plus an aminoglycoside is more nephrotoxic than methicillin plus an aminoglycoside. *Lancet* 2:604–606, 1978.

58. Merigan TC: Host defense against viral disease. *N Engl J Med* 290:323–329, 1974.

59. Heath RB: Virus infections in patients with malignant disease. *Postgrad Med* 45:36–39, 1969.

60. Goodell B, Jacobs JB, Powell RD, et al: Pneumocystis carinii: The spectrum of diffuse interstitial pneumonia in patients with neoplastic diseases. *Ann Intern Med* 72:337–340, 1970.

Index